Temporomandibular Joint Diseases:
Diagnosis and Management

Temporomandibular Joint Diseases: Diagnosis and Management

Editor

Luis Eduardo Almeida

MDPI • Basel • Beijing • Wuhan • Barcelona • Belgrade • Manchester • Tokyo • Cluj • Tianjin

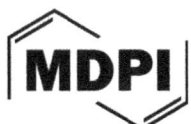

Editor
Luis Eduardo Almeida
Surgical Sciences
Marquette University
Milwaukee
United States

Editorial Office
MDPI
St. Alban-Anlage 66
4052 Basel, Switzerland

This is a reprint of articles from the Special Issue published online in the open access journal *Diagnostics* (ISSN 2075-4418) (available at: www.mdpi.com/journal/diagnostics/special_issues/Temporomandibular_Joint_Diagnosis).

For citation purposes, cite each article independently as indicated on the article page online and as indicated below:

LastName, A.A.; LastName, B.B.; LastName, C.C. Article Title. *Journal Name* **Year**, *Volume Number*, Page Range.

ISBN 978-3-0365-4290-4 (Hbk)
ISBN 978-3-0365-4289-8 (PDF)

© 2022 by the authors. Articles in this book are Open Access and distributed under the Creative Commons Attribution (CC BY) license, which allows users to download, copy and build upon published articles, as long as the author and publisher are properly credited, which ensures maximum dissemination and a wider impact of our publications.

The book as a whole is distributed by MDPI under the terms and conditions of the Creative Commons license CC BY-NC-ND.

Contents

About the Editor vii

Preface to "Temporomandibular Joint Diseases: Diagnosis and Management" ix

Benedikt Sagl, Ferida Besirevic-Bulic, Martina Schmid-Schwap, Brenda Laky, Klara Janjić and Eva Piehslinger et al.
A Novel Quantitative Method for Tooth Grinding Surface Assessment Using 3D Scanning
Reprinted from: *Diagnostics* 2021, *11*, 1483, doi:10.3390/diagnostics11081483 1

Roger Alonso-Royo, Carmen María Sánchez-Torrelo, Alfonso Javier Ibáñez-Vera, Noelia Zagalaz-Anula, Yolanda Castellote-Caballero and Esteban Obrero-Gaitán et al.
Validity and Reliability of the Helkimo Clinical Dysfunction Index for the Diagnosis of Temporomandibular Disorders
Reprinted from: *Diagnostics* 2021, *11*, 472, doi:10.3390/diagnostics11030472 11

Soo-Hwan Byun, Chanyang Min, Dae-Myoung Yoo, Byoung-Eun Yang and Hyo-Geun Choi
Increased Risk of Migraine in Patients with Temporomandibular Disorder: A Longitudinal Follow-Up Study Using a National Health Screening Cohort
Reprinted from: *Diagnostics* 2020, *10*, 724, doi:10.3390/diagnostics10090724 21

Simona Tecco, Vincenzo Quinzi, Alessandro Nota, Alessandro Giovannozzi, Maria Rosaria Abed and Giuseppe Marzo
Electromyography-Guided Adjustment of an Occlusal Appliance: Effect on Pain Perceptions Related with Temporomandibular Disorders. A Controlled Clinical Study
Reprinted from: *Diagnostics* 2021, *11*, 667, doi:10.3390/diagnostics11040667 33

Grzegorz Zieliński, Aleksandra Byś, Jacek Szkutnik, Piotr Majcher and Michał Ginszt
Electromyographic Patterns of Masticatory Muscles in Relation to Active Myofascial Trigger Points of the Upper Trapezius and Temporomandibular Disorders
Reprinted from: *Diagnostics* 2021, *11*, 580, doi:10.3390/diagnostics11040580 45

Xiao-Chuan Fan, Lin-Sha Ma, Li Chen, Diwakar Singh, Xiaohui Rausch-Fan and Xiao-Feng Huang
Temporomandibular Joint Osseous Morphology of Class I and Class II Malocclusions in the Normal Skeletal Pattern: A Cone-Beam Computed Tomography Study
Reprinted from: *Diagnostics* 2021, *11*, 541, doi:10.3390/diagnostics11030541 57

Diego Fernando López, Valentina Ríos Borrás, Juan Manuel Muñoz, Rodrigo Cardenas-Perilla and Luis Eduardo Almeida
SPECT/CT Correlation in the Diagnosis of Unilateral Condilar Hyperplasia
Reprinted from: *Diagnostics* 2021, *11*, 477, doi:10.3390/diagnostics11030477 71

Masahiko Terauchi, Motohiro Uo, Yuki Fukawa, Hiroyuki Yoshitake, Rina Tajima and Tohru Ikeda et al.
Chemical Diagnosis of Calcium Pyrophosphate Deposition Disease of the Temporomandibular Joint: A Case Report
Reprinted from: *Diagnostics* 2022, *12*, 651, doi:10.3390/diagnostics12030651 83

Mattias Ulmner, Rachael Sugars, Aron Naimi-Akbar, Nikolce Tudzarovski, Carina Kruger-Weiner and Bodil Lund
Synovial Tissue Proteins and Patient-Specific Variables as Predictive Factors for Temporomandibular Joint Surgery
Reprinted from: *Diagnostics* 2020, *11*, 46, doi:10.3390/diagnostics11010046 93

Andrea Duarte Doetzer, Roberto Hirochi Herai, Marília Afonso Rabelo Buzalaf and Paula Cristina Trevilatto
Proteomic Expression Profile in Human Temporomandibular Joint Dysfunction
Reprinted from: *Diagnostics* **2021**, *11*, 601, doi:10.3390/diagnostics11040601 . . . . **107**

Xiao-Chuan Fan, Diwakar Singh, Lin-Sha Ma, Eva Piehslinger, Xiao-Feng Huang and Xiaohui Rausch-Fan
Is There an Association between Temporomandibular Disorders and Articular Eminence Inclination? A Systematic Review
Reprinted from: *Diagnostics* **2020**, *11*, 29, doi:10.3390/diagnostics11010029 . . . . **145**

Dion Tik Shun Li and Yiu Yan Leung
Temporomandibular Disorders: Current Concepts and Controversies in Diagnosis and Management
Reprinted from: *Diagnostics* **2021**, *11*, 459, doi:10.3390/diagnostics11030459 . . . . **165**

Lauren Covert, Heather Van Mater and Benjamin L. Hechler
Comprehensive Management of Rheumatic Diseases Affecting the Temporomandibular Joint
Reprinted from: *Diagnostics* **2021**, *11*, 409, doi:10.3390/diagnostics11030409 . . . . **181**

About the Editor

Luis Eduardo Almeida

Dr. Luis Eduardo Almeida is Clinical Associate Professor and program director of Oral and Maxillofacial Surgery at Marquette University School of Dentistry, Milwaukee, Wisconsin, USA. He received his DDS degree from Federal University of Parana State, Curitiba, Parana, Brazil. After that, Dr. Almeida did his residency in Oral and Maxillofacial Surgery at Northwestern University, Chicago, Illinois, USA. Going back to Brazil, Dr. Almeida continued his path in education, culminating with a Master of Sciences and a PhD from Pontific Catholic University, Parana, Brazil. Dr. Almeida has an extent surgical experience, with more than 300 TMJ Surgical cases and more than 2500 orthognathic surgeries. His research field is Temporomandibular Joint and inflammation. He has more than 50 peer-reviewed papers published in research journals and participation as co-investigator in NIH grants. His passion for teaching is demonstrated by having more than 50 residents graduated through his life.

Preface to "Temporomandibular Joint Diseases: Diagnosis and Management"

The temporomandibular joint (TMJ) is capable of remodeling even after growth has stopped, allowing it to make structural changes and adapt to different physiological demands. Temporomandibular disorders (TMD) are a group of degenerative disorders involving the components of the TMJ, which can lead to displacement of the disc, joint remodeling, and eventually osteoarthritis. Different methods of diagnosis and treatments of TMD have been described in the literature in the past years. This reprint was created to provide updated information regarding all methods of diagnosis of TMD, from clinical exams to immunohistologic and molecular diagnosis and novel treatments for this disease, ranging from non-invasive techniques, such as physical therapy, ultrasound, low-level laser therapy, and splints, to surgical treatments of TMJ.

Luis Eduardo Almeida
Editor

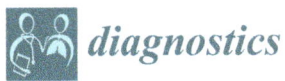

Article

A Novel Quantitative Method for Tooth Grinding Surface Assessment Using 3D Scanning

Benedikt Sagl [1,*], Ferida Besirevic-Bulic [2], Martina Schmid-Schwap [2], Brenda Laky [1], Klara Janjić [1], Eva Piehslinger [2] and Xiaohui Rausch-Fan [1]

[1] Center of Clinical Research, University Clinic of Dentistry, Medical University of Vienna, 1090 Vienna, Austria; brenda.laky@meduniwien.ac.at (B.L.); klara.janjic@meduniwien.ac.at (K.J.); xiaohui.rausch-fan@meduniwien.ac.at (X.R.-F.)
[2] Division of Prosthodontics, University Clinic of Dentistry, Medical University of Vienna, 1090 Vienna, Austria; ferida.besirevic-bulic@meduniwien.ac.at (F.B.-B.); martina.schmid-schwap@meduniwien.ac.at (M.S.-S.); eva.piehslinger@meduniwien.ac.at (E.P.)
* Correspondence: benedikt.sagl@meduniwien.ac.at

Abstract: Sleep bruxism is an oral parafunction that involves involuntary tooth grinding and clenching. Splints with a colored layer that gets removed during tooth grinding are a common tool for the initial diagnosis of sleep bruxism. Currently, such splints are either assessed qualitatively or using 2D photographs, leading to a non-neglectable error due to the 3D nature of the dentition. In this study we propose a new and fast method for the quantitative assessment of tooth grinding surfaces using 3D scanning and mesh processing. We assessed our diagnostic method by producing 18 standardized splints with 8 grinding surfaces each, giving us a total of 144 surfaces. Moreover, each splint was scanned and analyzed five times. The accuracy and repeatability of our method was assessed by computing the intraclass correlation coefficient (ICC) as well reporting means and standard deviations of surface measurements for intra- and intersplint measurements. An ICC of 0.998 was computed as well as a maximum standard deviation of 0.63 mm^2 for repeated measures, suggesting an appropriate accuracy of our proposed method. Overall, this study proposes an innovative, fast and cost effective method to support the initial diagnosis of sleep bruxism.

Keywords: sleep bruxism; digital dentistry; diagnostic bruxism splint

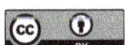

1. Introduction

Traditionally, bruxism is defined as an oral parafunction involving involuntary tooth grinding and clenching [1]. Moreover, a distinction is made between awake and sleep bruxism, which potentially have different origins and pathophysiology [2]. Bruxism is a possible risk factor for different pathologies and can lead to severe abrasion of teeth, tooth hypermobility, masticatory muscle pain, headache, periodontal tissue damage as well as temporomandibular joint (TMJ) pain. Most people will go through phases of tooth grinding or clenching during the course of their lifetime [3] with studies reporting approximately 5–13% of adults as frequent tooth grinders [4–6].

Diagnosis of bruxism is a challenging task due to its involuntary nature. Initial assessment often relies on reports of tooth grinding sounds and symptoms such as flattened teeth, which already imply a rather late time of diagnosis. The American Academy of Sleep Medicine defined diagnostic criteria for sleep bruxism, which involve the occurrence of abnormal tooth wear, associated sounds and jaw discomfort [5]. A polysomnographic (PSG) investigation, including video, audio as well as a multitude of different respiratory, muscular and other parameters, is generally seen as the gold standard for a definitive diagnosis of sleep bruxism [7]. Since PSG is very expensive and time consuming for the patient, many studies have used electromyography (EMG) [8] devices to measure masticatory muscle activity during sleep, investigating rhythmic masticatory muscle activity

(RMMA), which is a diagnostic sign of sleep bruxism [9,10]. Another approach using an instrumented splint to measure peaks in bite force has been proposed previously [11].

While EMG gives reliable information on RMMA occurrence and, as a consequence, helps with detecting bruxism [10], portable EMG devices are still rather expensive and most clinics do not own enough devices to easily use them for every potential patient. A previously proposed simple and cost-effective tool for bruxism diagnosis is a colored splint to monitor tooth contact during sleep. The first reports of this method go back to the 1970s [12,13]. The proposed splint consists of four colored layers comprising an overall thickness of 0.51 mm. During grinding of the teeth, one or multiple, depending on the amount of grinding force, colored layers are ground off, revealing information on occlusal contact areas. More recently a semi-automatic method to analyze such splints has been published [14,15]. The method uses standardized pictures to measure the abraded area in a 2D projection but neglects the 3D nature of the tooth shape. Another comparable product was developed by a group at the Kanagawa Dental College [16]. While their splint only has a single colored layer, reducing the diagnostic information on bruxing force, it is very thin (0.1 mm thickness), which potentially limits the alteration of muscular activity during sleep caused by the splint [17]. To the best of our knowledge, analysis of this tool has also solely focused on quantitative assessments of occlusal grinding patterns in 2D projections (photographs) [18–21]. All analysis methods that rely on 2D projections infer an error, which increases with the angle between the projection plane and the tooth facet. With the advance of digital dentistry and improvements in the quality as well as the accessibility of 3D scanning devices, a logical next step would be the digitalization of occlusal splints and the detailed diagnostic analysis of the occlusal contacts using 3D mesh analysis approaches.

Consequently, the presented study proposes a novel method for the semi-automated 3D analysis of colored occlusal splints for the diagnostic investigation of tooth contacts in the context of bruxism. This method has the potential to gather more accurate information on nocturnal occlusal contacts in an easy and reliable fashion, helping clinicians to collect the information necessary for bruxism diagnosis, while only using equipment accessible in a dental practice.

2. Materials and Methods

To test and validate our diagnostic method a model consisting of an idealized gingiva arch with a total of 8 embedded icosahedrons was designed using the Autodesk® Meshmixer toolkit (Autodesk, San Rafael, CA, USA) (Figure 1).

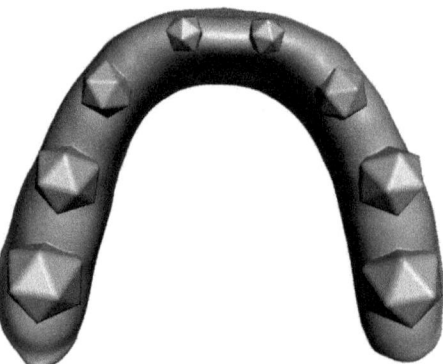

Figure 1. Top view of the 3D model created in the Meshmixer toolkit.

To later test the performance of the presented method for different sizes of grinding surfaces, the geometrical bodies varied in size. The triangular surfaces of the icosahedrons' faces decreased from posterior to anterior, with respective triangle heights of 5 mm, 4 mm, 3 mm and 2 mm. The base model was produced with an additive manufacturing approach using a Formlabs® Form 2 printer (Formlabs, Somerville, MA, USA) and the Formlabs® Dental LT Clear V1 resin (Formlabs, Somerville, MA, USA). The model was used in combination with a pressure molding device (Biostar®, Scheu Dental, Iserlohn, Germany) to produce the splints themselves from a dedicated pressure molding foil with one red-colored side and a thickness of 0.1 mm (Bruxchecker®, Scheu Dental, Iserlohn, Germany). After production the splints are relatively translucent and normally turn opaque in the patient's mouth. To get the same effect in vitro, we submerged the finished splints in water with some added toothpaste for 6 h. After this step the splints showed surface opaqueness comparable to clinical splints.

To simulate tooth grinding, one triangle per icosahedron was prepared using a KaVo K4 handpiece (KaVo Dental, Biberach an der Riß, Germany) and the red layer was ground off to leave the respective surface transparent. Processed triangles varied between splints and were used to test the performance of our method for different surface angles. Scanning of the transparent surfaces lead to rather severe 3D reconstruction artifacts—consequently, we spray-painted the inside of the splint using a colored (green) powder spray (Occlu®Spray Plus, Hager & Werken, Duisburg, Germany) (Figure 2).

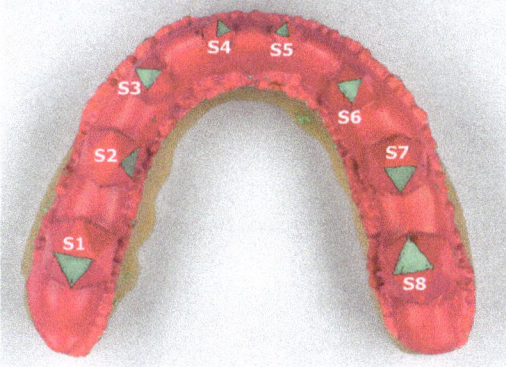

Figure 2. Example splint after "grinding surface" preparation and powder spraying. S1 to S8 depict the respective grinding surfaces.

After preparation, splints were scanned using an optical 3D scanner (Primescan™ AC, Dentsply Sirona, Bensheim, Germany) and mesh files were exported as .ply files including vertex position as well as vertex color information. To check for intrascan accuracy of the method, each splint was scanned 5 times. Meshes were imported into the Meshmixer software toolkit (version 3.4) and the "grinding surfaces" were segmented using a semi-automatic method. For this purpose, an initial vertex inside the grinding surface was selected and the selection was expanded using a similarity measure of vertex color for the abraded areas. The abraded areas were green and the rest of the splint remained red. The surface area of each grinding facet was recorded for 18 splints for 5 repeated measurements, giving 90 scans and 720 grinding surfaces. A detailed description of our software workflow can be found in Appendix A.

Intraclass correlation coefficient (ICC) over the 5 repeated measures was evaluated and an analysis of variance (ANOVA) of repeated scans of the same physical splint was performed. To better describe the grinding surfaces we moreover reported the maximum, minimum, mean and relative standard deviations over the repeated measures for each grinding surface. Additionally, to showcase the differences in results computed using a 2D projection approach with respect to the proposed 3D method, all 18 splints were photographed using a standardized set-up and grinding areas were segmented in 2D using ImageJ (https://imagej.nih.gov/ij, [22]). We report mean surface areas and standard deviations for each grinding surface for both measurement methods and compared 2D photographs to 3D scans using an independent-samples *t*-test. Statistical assessment was performed using IBM SPSS Statistics 26® (IBM, Armonk, NY, USA).

3. Results

The proposed workflow allowed for the successful completion of all necessary substeps. Using the colored powder spray enabled easy and fast scanning, without any artifacts caused by the transparent grinding areas on the splint (Figure 3). Moreover, the clear difference in color between the red splint and the green grinding surfaces allowed for easy segmentation of the grinding surfaces (Figure 4). To assess this statement, the repeatability and accuracy of the scanning procedure were tested as follows.

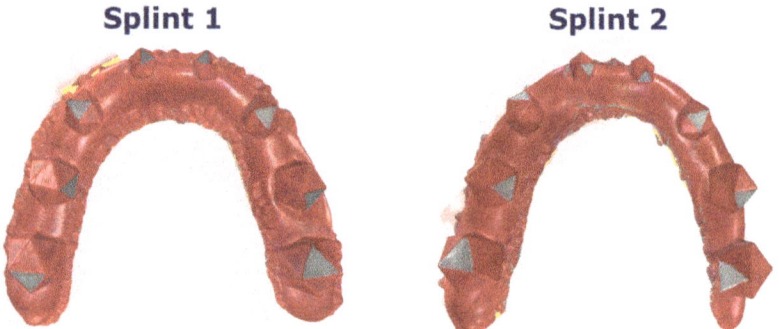

Figure 3. Example scans of two out of the 18 different splints; different combinations of triangles were prepared for each splint to investigate different surface angles.

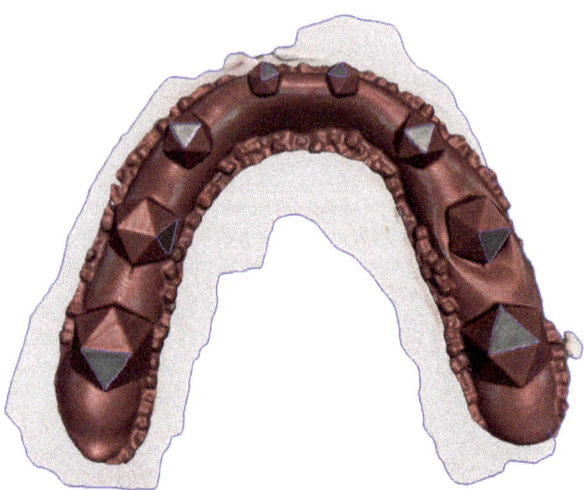

Figure 4. Example of a scanned splint after successful segmentation.

The ICC score of 0.998 (95% confidence interval, CI 0.997–0.998; $p < 0.001$), for single measures using a two-way mixed effects model assessing absolute agreement, suggests a high repeatability and reliability of our proposed method. No significant differences between repeated scans and segmentations were detected, suggesting an appropriate repeatability of our approach (F = 1.112; $p = 0.350$).

Table 1 reports the mean surface area and standard deviation for each grinding surface for all 18 scans using the 2D and 3D methods. For 2D measurements only a single measurement was completed, while we report the mean over the five repetitions for our new method. Generally speaking, higher standard deviations can be seen for the 2D measurements. Moreover, the independent-samples t-test showed statistically significant differences for all grinding surfaces between surface areas measured in 2D and 3D. Figure 5 shows the results of the 2D measurements for an example splint (Splint 2) and depicts clear differences in grinding size for similarly sized icosahedrons.

Table 1. Mean surface area and standard deviation for all 8 grinding surfaces over the 18 prepared splints measured from 2D photographs and 3D scans. *p*-values are reported for independent-samples *t*-test for differences between the measurement methods.

	Surface Area in 2D [mm^2]	Surface Area in 3D [mm^2]	*p*-Value
Surface 1	13.2 ± 2.85	17.41 ± 1.2	<0.001
Surface 2	7.61 ± 2.27	11.20 ± 0.61	<0.001
Surface 3	4.90 ± 1.47	6.46 ± 0.61	<0.001
Surface 4	1.98 ± 0.37	2.78 ± 0.29	<0.001
Surface 5	2.01 ± 0.57	2.97 ± 0.32	<0.001
Surface 6	4.80 ± 1.66	6.45 ± 0.71	<0.001
Surface 7	8.80 ± 1.12	10.65 ± 0.44	<0.001
Surface 8	13.56 ± 3.16	16.93 ± 0.86	<0.001

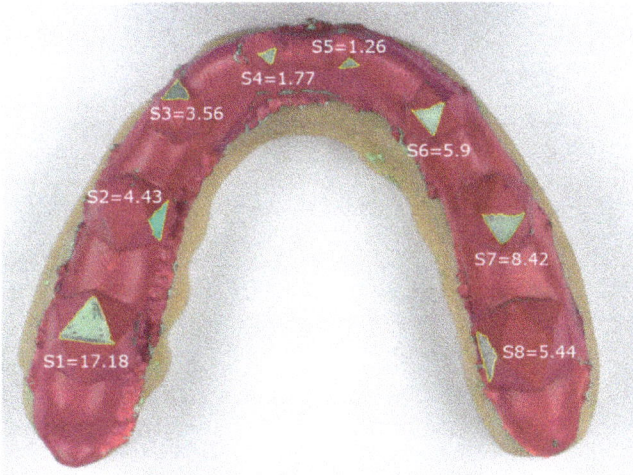

Figure 5. Example of a 2D measurement (Splint 2 shown). Surface area for each grinding surface is reported in mm^2. While measurements on the same size icosahedrons should be relatively close, stark differences can be seen, e.g., between S1 and S8.

The accuracy of the presented method was assessed by reporting the maximum, minimum and mean standard deviations between the five repeated scans of the same splint reported in absolute mm^2 and relative to the mean size of the grinding area (%; Table 2). The highest maximum standard deviation was 0.63 mm^2. Generally, a trend for larger absolute variation was found for the measurements of larger grinding surfaces. Taking the size of the grinding surface into account, the largest relative variation was found to be 10.36%. Generally, the relative standard deviation was larger for the smaller grinding surfaces.

Table 2. Standard deviation of repeated measures for each surface over 18 prepared splints.

	Maximum [mm^2]	Minimum [mm^2]	Mean [mm^2]	Percentage of Mean Surface
Surface 1	0.41	0.11	0.25	2.35
Surface 2	0.59	0.14	0.28	5.28
Surface 3	0.48	0.09	0.19	7.43
Surface 4	0.29	0.03	0.12	10.36
Surface 5	0.26	0.08	0.15	8.91
Surface 6	0.35	0.04	0.17	5.38
Surface 7	0.59	0.15	0.28	5.5
Surface 8	0.63	0.15	0.32	3.73

4. Discussion

The presented study established and reports a novel method for the semi-automatic, quantitative, 3D assessment of grinding surfaces on a colored occlusal splint; a task that, to the best of the authors' knowledge, has not been accomplished in the previous literature so far. Our measurements suggest a high repeatability and accuracy of the presented method. Overall, the proposed workflow could be a valuable tool for future investigations regarding occlusal variables and has the potential to increase the understanding of various functional, parafunctional and dysfunctional tasks of the masticatory system.

Generally speaking, occlusal splints are a cheap, non-invasive and easy-to-use method to assess the grinding pattern of a patient [14,17]. Consequently, they are a great tool for the initial assessment in bruxism diagnosis [20]. Currently these splints are mostly qualitatively assessed by defining the involved regions of the occlusal grinding patterns (e.g., "canine guided", "premolar and/ or molar involved") [16], which limits their diagnostic value. Some quantitative methods have been proposed, but they all use 2D photographs of the splints [14,15]. Those methods so far cannot calculate the grinding area precisely, since the 3D nature of human teeth induces a non-negligible error caused by the 2D projection of a photograph. This error increases with the angle between the 2D projection plane and the grinding facet plane. When models are photographed from above, the largest error can be seen on steep tooth surfaces, e.g., on the canines. By using an optical 3D scanner, we solved this problem and computed accurate 3D shapes.

One major problem during initial testing of the presented method was the detection of the grinding areas during 3D scanning. The patient (or, in our case, the polishing device) grinds off the colored layer on the splint, leaving translucent grinding areas. While these areas are easy to register visually, the translucency of the foil makes them very hard for an optical scanner to detect, which leads to non-repeatable and noisy results, where the scanner sometimes detects the splint and sometimes scans the dental model below the splint. This problem often induces sharp edges and switching of the surface between the level of the cast and the splint, which leads to an overestimation of the grinding surfaces and a generally cumbersome scanning process. We solved this problem by using a colored powder spray with a different color with respect to the splint color. We chose a green spray because it gave good contrast to the red color of the splint and since red and green are well separated in RGB (red, green, blue) color space, we expected this color decision to further improve the segmentation process. This simple and cost-effective solution enabled us to drastically increase the scan quality, while simultaneously reducing scanning time.

To assess the repeatability of our results we scanned each splint five times, segmented the grinding surfaces and compared the differences between the repeated scans. The high ICC of 0.998 detected with the presented method suggests an excellent repeatability. Moreover, this finding was confirmed by detecting no significant differences between the repeated measurements, giving us confidence in the results computed with the proposed method.

In general, the same grinding surface on different splints should be relatively comparable in surface area (e.g., Splint1 S1 and Splint2 S1) with only minor differences caused by the manual grinding process. Moreover, since the triangles on the left and right sides have the same size in our model, differences between the respective surfaces (e.g., S1 and S8) should be minimal. This was indeed true and we could only detect statistically significant differences between the grinding areas of surfaces on differently sized icosahedrons.

To further evaluate accuracy of the measurement method, we investigated the standard deviation of the grinding surfaces between the repeated measurements and compared them to the standard deviation between the grinding surfaces on different splints. Standard deviations were larger between models, compared to repeated measures of the same splint. The largest standard deviation for the repeated measures was 0.63 mm^2 for surface 8. Relative to the mean grinding area of the surface, the computed standard deviation for surface 8 is equal to 3.73%. As expected, the largest relative difference was found for the smallest grinding surfaces, with 10.36% for Surface 4, which represents an absolute surface of 0.29 mm^2. These maximum values represent the worst case and when looking at the mean standard deviations for each surface we see values of approximately half the value of these maximums. We think that these relatively small differences suggest an appropriate accuracy for clinically relevant differences in grinding areas.

Additionally, we showcased our novel measurement method by comparing it to the currently used method of assessing surface areas on 2D photographs. Larger standard deviations for the surfaces were found when using the 2D method. As described above, this is due to the fact that, in addition to the standard deviation caused by the actual differences from manual preparation of the grinding areas, an additional variability is included by using grinding facets with different angles with respect to the imaging plane. This can clearly be seen in Figure 5 when comparing S1 and S8. These surfaces are roughly the same size, apart from small variances caused by the manual grinding, but due to the projection error S8 is substantially smaller than S1 when using photographs. By using the presented method this error is drastically reduced. On the other hand, the projection error for S1 is relatively small since the surface is well aligned with the projection plane of the photograph. Consequently, our data show that if a grinding surface with a large angle to the imaging plane is chosen, the surface area was underestimated drastically. As expected, significant differences in grinding area were detected between the two measurement methods (photographs vs. 3D scanning) for all grinding surfaces.

While our study computed convincing results, some limitations remain. Firstly, the occlusal splint used in our study can only assess the direction of the grinding movement, the area and number of occlusal grinding surfaces, but it cannot define the magnitude, frequency and duration of the applied grinding force, which are relevant parameters related to the pathogenesis of TMD [23]. Other splint designs have been proposed that use multiple layers of colored material, inferring some information on grinding force magnitude [14], but some authors have reservations regarding the thickness of these multilayer splints [24]. It was suggested that the thicker splints act in the same way as an actual therapeutic splint and reduce muscle activity, which would make them infeasible as a diagnostic tool. Nevertheless, colored splints have proven to be a valuable first diagnostic tool in bruxism diagnosis [16,17,19,20] and we are confident that our method is transferable to other splint designs. Secondly, we did not compare our optical scans to a different physical measurement of the grinding surface. Optical scanning has been shown to be a valuable and accurate tool in digital dentistry [25–27] and is used for various dental applications [28,29]. More specifically, the trueness and precision of the 3D scanner used in this study has been assessed for complete arch scans by multiple previous studies [30–32]. Schmidt et al. found a mean deviation of 33.8 ± 31.5 μm. Moreover, Dutton et al. assessed the performance of the Primescan over multiple materials and found a trueness of 17 μm and a precision of 25 μm. Lastly, Ender et al. report a trueness of 33.9 ± 7.8 μm and a precision of 31.3 ± 10.3 μm. Consequently, we do not think that the initial validation of the correctness of the overall geometry has to be proven for our specific study.

Future studies could, for example, focus on the assessment of a potential correlation between occlusal grinding areas in 3D and muscle activity EMG, in order to include additional information on the frequency and magnitude of the grinding events. This could provide important clues to predict diseases of traumatic occlusion and TMJ disorders.

5. Conclusions

In conclusion, this study proposes an innovative, fast and cost effective method to support the initial diagnosis of sleep bruxism. Moreover, due to the 3D nature of the presented method, it facilitates the fast and easy quantitative assessment of the surface area of the respective grinding facets. The study results suggest a high accuracy as well repeatability of the proposed method, which will allow for better quantitative assessment and comparison of the grinding areas in future clinical studies. This will potentially help in gathering knowledge and developing better screening and treatment methods for patients in the early stages of sleep bruxism.

Author Contributions: Conceptualization, B.S., F.B.-B., M.S.-S., E.P. and X.R.-F.; methodology, B.S., F.B.-B., M.S.-S., K.J. and B.L.; software, B.S., B.L.; validation, B.S. and B.L.; formal analysis, B.S and B.L.; investigation, B.S. and K.J.; resources, M.S.-S., E.P. and X.R.-F.; data curation, B.S.; writing—original draft preparation, B.S.; writing—review and editing, F.B.-B., M.S.-S., B.L., K.J., E.P. and X.R.-F.; visualization, B.S. All authors have read and agreed to the published version of the manuscript.

Funding: This research received no external funding.

Institutional Review Board Statement: Not applicable.

Data Availability Statement: The data presented in this study are available on request from the corresponding author.

Acknowledgments: The authors want to thank Dominique Flechl for her support during splint creation and Denisa Hani for her support during 3D scanning of the splints.

Conflicts of Interest: The authors declare no conflict of interest. The Bruxchecker® foils were sponsored by Scheu Dental. The company had no role in the design of the study; in the collection, analyses, or interpretation of data; in the writing of the manuscript, or in the decision to publish the results.

Appendix A. —Software Workflow

This appendix will briefly describe the software settings and procedures used during the various digital processing and production steps.

Model design: The model is based on the idealized morphology of a gingival arch. We idealized the arch using manual smoothing in the Autodesk® Meshmixer toolkit. Afterwards we selected icosahedrons under Meshmix → Primitives and pulled them onto the appropriate positions on the arch. The offset was kept at 0 and the dimension was used to change the size as described in the Methods section. The icosahedrons were added using the Boolean Union composition mode.

Model 3D Printing: The model was printed in a layer density of 0.05 mm with a total of 413 layers. It was printed within approximately 3 h, consuming 18.48 mL of resin. The object was printed on full rafts, including a raft label and internal supports. Rafts had a touchpoint size of 0.60 mm and a density value of 1. Automated advanced settings included a flat spacing of 5 mm, a slope multiplier value of 1, 5 mm height above raft, 2 mm raft thickness, a Z-compression correction of 0.75 mm and an early layer merge of 0.30 mm. After printing, the object was washed in isopropanol (IPA) for 15 min. Washing was repeated in fresh IPA for another 5 min, followed by drying overnight. The next day, the printed model was cured in a Formlabs® Form Cure for 20 min at 80 °C, following the recommendations of the manufacturer. After curing, all support structures were removed manually.

Splint 3D Scanning: The colored splints were scanned using the dedicated scanning software using the standard parameters. Afterwards the saved .ply files were collected and exported for post-processing.

Splint 3D assessment: .ply files of the scanned splints were opened using the Autodesk® Meshmixer toolkit and the function under Select → Filters → Vertex Color Similarity was used. Back face selection was not enabled and no crease angle threshold was used. Each grinding facet was segmented and separated into its own component (Edit → Separate). Afterwards, each grinding facet was selected and the surface area was computed using Analysis →Stability. Values were computed and collected for all grinding areas of all splints and used for statistical analysis.

References

1. Ferro, K.J.; Morgano, S.M.; Driscoll, C.F.; Freilich, M.A.; Guckes, A.D.; Knoernschild, K.L.; Mc Garry, T.J. The Glossary of Prosthodontic Terms: Ninth Edition. *J. Prosthet. Dent.* **2017**, *117*, e1–e105. [CrossRef]
2. Carra, M.C.; Huynh, N.; Lavigne, G. Sleep Bruxism: A Comprehensive Overview for the Dental Clinician Interested in Sleep Medicine. *Dent. Clin. N. Am.* **2012**, *56*, 387–413. [CrossRef] [PubMed]
3. Bader, G.; Lavigne, G. Sleep bruxism; an overview of an oromandibular sleep movement disorder: Review Article. *Sleep Med. Rev.* **2000**, *4*, 27–43. [CrossRef]
4. Lavigne, G.J.; Montplaisir, J.Y. Restless Legs Syndrome and Sleep Bruxism: Prevalence and Association Among Canadians. *Sleep* **1994**, *17*. [CrossRef]
5. Sateia, M.J. International Classification of Sleep Disorders-Third Edition. *Chest* **2014**, *146*, 1387–1394. [CrossRef] [PubMed]
6. Manfredini, D.; Winocur, E.; Guarda-Nardini, L.; Paesani, D.; Lobbezoo, F. Epidemiology of Bruxism in Adults: A Systematic Review of the Literature. *J. Orofac. Pain* **2013**, *27*, 99–110. [CrossRef] [PubMed]
7. Lavigne, G.; Rompre, P.; Montplaisir, J. Sleep Bruxism: Validity of Clinical Research Diagnostic Criteria in a Controlled Polysomnographic Study. *J. Dent. Res.* **1996**, *75*, 546–552. [CrossRef]
8. Thymi, M.; Lobbezoo, F.; Aarab, G.; Ahlberg, J.; Baba, K.; Carra, M.C.; Gallo, L.M.; de Laat, A.; Manfredini, D.; Lavigne, G.; et al. Signal acquisition and analysis of ambulatory electromyographic recordings for the assessment of sleep bruxism: A scoping review. *J. Oral Rehabilitation* **2021**, *48*, 846–871. [CrossRef]
9. Lavigne, G.; Rompré, P.; Poirier, G.; Huard, H.; Kato, T.; Montplaisir, J. Rhythmic Masticatory Muscle Activity during Sleep in Humans. *J. Dent. Res.* **2001**, *80*, 443–448. [CrossRef]
10. Mayer, P.; Heinzer, R.; Lavigne, G. Sleep Bruxism in Respiratory Medicine Practice. *Chest* **2016**, *149*, 262–271. [CrossRef] [PubMed]
11. Robin, O.; Claude, A.; Gehin, C.; Massot, B.; McAdams, E. Recording of bruxism events in sleeping humans at home with a smart instrumented splint. *Cranio* **2020**, 1–9. [CrossRef] [PubMed]
12. Forgione, A.G. A Simple but Effective Method of Quantifying Bruxing Behavior. *J. Dent. Res.* **1974**, *53*, 127.
13. Heller, R.F.; Forgione, A.G. An Evaluation of Bruxism Control: Massed Negative Practice and Automated Relaxation Training. *J. Dent. Res.* **1975**, *54*, 1120–1123. [CrossRef]
14. Ommerborn, M.; Giraki, M.; Schneider, C.; Schaefer, R.; Gotter, A.; Franz, M.; Raab, W.H.M. A new analyzing method for quantification of abrasion on the Bruxcore device for sleep bruxism diagnosis. *J. Orofac. Pain* **2005**, *19*, 232–238.
15. Isacsson, G.; Bodin, L.; Selden, A.; Barregård, L. Variability in the quantification of abrasion on the Bruxcore device. *J. Orofac. Pain* **1996**, *10*, 362–368.
16. Onodera, K.; Kawagoe, T.; Sasaguri, K.; Protacio-Quismundo, C.; Sato, S. The Use of a BruxChecker in the Evaluation of Different Grinding Patterns During Sleep Bruxism. *Cranio* **2006**, *24*, 292–299. [CrossRef]
17. Tao, J.; Liu, W.; Wu, J.; Zhang, X.; Zhang, Y. The study of grinding patterns and factors influencing the grinding areas during sleep bruxism. *Arch. Oral Biol.* **2015**, *60*, 1595–1600. [CrossRef]
18. Padmaja Satheeswarakumar, L.; Elenjickal, T.J.; Ram, S.K.M.; Thangasamy, K. Assessment of Mandibular Surface Area Changes in Bruxers Versus Controls on Panoramic Radiographic Images: A Case Control Study. *Open Dent J.* **2018**, *12*, 753–761. [CrossRef] [PubMed]
19. Sugimoto, K.; Yoshimi, H.; Sasaguri, K.; Sato, S. Occlusion Factors Influencing the Magnitude of Sleep Bruxism Activity. *Cranio* **2011**, *29*, 127–137. [CrossRef] [PubMed]
20. Hokama, H.; Masaki, C.; Mukaibo, T.; Tsuka, S.; Kondo, Y.; Hosokawa, R. The effectiveness of an occlusal disclosure sheet to diagnose sleep bruxism: A pilot study. *Cranio* **2017**, *37*, 5–11. [CrossRef]
21. Tokiwa, O.; Park, B.-K.; Takezawa, Y.; Takahashi, Y.; Sasaguri, K.; Sato, S. Relationship of Tooth Grinding Pattern During Sleep Bruxism and Dental Status. *Cranio* **2008**, *26*, 287–293. [CrossRef] [PubMed]
22. Schneider, C.A.; Rasband, W.S.; Eliceiri, K.W. NIH Image to ImageJ: 25 years of image analysis. *Nat. Methods* **2012**, *9*, 671–675. [CrossRef] [PubMed]
23. Sagl, B.; Schmid-Schwap, M.; Piehslinger, E.; Kundi, M.; Stavness, I. Effect of facet inclination and location on TMJ loading during bruxism: An in-silico study. *J. Adv. Res.* **2021**. [CrossRef]
24. Pierce, C.; Gale, E. Methodological Considerations Concerning the Use of Bruxcore Plates to Evaluate Nocturnal Bruxism. *J. Dent. Res.* **1989**, *68*, 1110–1114. [CrossRef] [PubMed]
25. Persson, A.S.; Odén, A.; Andersson, M.; Englund, G.S. Digitization of simulated clinical dental impressions: Virtual three-dimensional analysis of exactness. *Dent. Mater.* **2009**, *25*, 929–936. [CrossRef]
26. Medina-Sotomayor, P.; Pascual-Moscardo, A.; Camps, I. Accuracy of 4 digital scanning systems on prepared teeth digitally isolated from a complete dental arch. *J. Prosthet. Dent.* **2019**, *121*, 811–820. [CrossRef]

27. Bosniac, P.; Rehmann, P.; Wöstmann, B. Comparison of an indirect impression scanning system and two direct intraoral scanning systems in vivo. *Clin. Oral Investig.* **2018**, *23*, 2421–2427. [CrossRef]
28. Akhlaghian, M.; Khaledi, A.-A.; Farzin, M.; Pardis, S. Vertical marginal fit of zirconia copings fabricated with one direct and three indirect digital scanning techniques. *J. Prosthet. Dent.* **2020**. [CrossRef]
29. Mizumoto, R.M.; Yilmaz, B. Intraoral scan bodies in implant dentistry: A systematic review. *J. Prosthet. Dent.* **2018**, *120*, 343–352. [CrossRef]
30. Schmidt, A.; Klussmann, L.; Wöstmann, B.; Schlenz, M.A. Accuracy of Digital and Conventional Full-Arch Impressions in Patients: An Update. *J. Clin. Med.* **2020**, *9*, 688. [CrossRef]
31. Dutton, E.; Ludlow, M.; Mennito, A.; Kelly, A.; Evans, Z.; Culp, A.; Kessler, R.; Renne, W. The effect different substrates have on the trueness and precision of eight different intraoral scanners. *J. Esthet. Restor. Dent.* **2020**, *32*, 204–218. [CrossRef] [PubMed]
32. Ender, A.; Zimmermann, M.; Mehl, A. Accuracy of complete- and partial-arch impressions of actual intraoral scanning systems in vitro. *Int. J. Comput. Dent.* **2019**, *22*, 11–19. [PubMed]

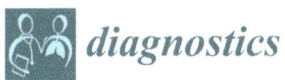

Article

Validity and Reliability of the Helkimo Clinical Dysfunction Index for the Diagnosis of Temporomandibular Disorders

Roger Alonso-Royo [1], Carmen María Sánchez-Torrelo [1], Alfonso Javier Ibáñez-Vera [2,*], Noelia Zagalaz-Anula [2], Yolanda Castellote-Caballero [2], Esteban Obrero-Gaitán [2], Daniel Rodríguez-Almagro [2] and Rafael Lomas-Vega [2]

[1] FisioMedic Clinic, Dos Hermanas, 41701 Sevilla, Spain; rar00032@red.ujaen.es (R.A.-R.); fisiomedic.dh@gmail.com (C.M.S.-T.)
[2] Department of Health Sciences, Campus las Lagunillas, University of Jaen, 23071 Jaén, Spain; nzagalaz@ujaen.es (N.Z.-A.); mycastel@ujaen.es (Y.C.-C.); eobrero@ujaen.es (E.O.-G.); dalmagro@ujaen.es (D.R.-A.); rlomas@ujaen.es (R.L.-V.)
* Correspondence: ajibanez@ujaen.es; Tel.: +34-953-211935

Abstract: The Helkimo Clinical Dysfunction Index (HCDI) is a simple and quick test used to evaluate subjects affected by temporomandibular disorders (TMDs), and its psychometric properties have not been tested. The test evaluates movement, joint function, pain and musculature, providing a quick general overview that could be very useful at different levels of care. For this reason, the aim of this study was to validate the use of the HCDI in a sample of patients with TMD. Methods: The sample consisted of 107 subjects, 60 TMD patients and 47 healthy controls. The study evaluated concurrent validity, inter-rater concordance and predictive values. Results: The HCDI showed moderate to substantial inter-rater concordance among the items and excellent concordance for the total scores. The correlation with other TMD assessment tests was high, the correlation with dizziness was moderate and the correlation with neck pain, headache and overall quality of life was poor. The prediction of TMD showed a sensitivity of 86.67%, a specificity of 68.09% and an area under the curve (AUC) of 0.841. Conclusions: The HCDI is a valid and reliable assessment instrument; its clinimetric properties are adequate, and it has a good ability to discriminate between TMD-affected and TMD-unaffected subjects.

Keywords: temporomandibular disorder; validity and reliability; questionnaires and survey validity study

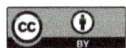

1. Introduction

Temporomandibular joint disorders (TMDs) are a very prevalent condition that, according to some authors, are present in 27.4% of adolescents [1] and 25% of adults [2]. Costs in European public hospitals due to erroneous diagnosis of TMD exceed a minimum of €52 and a maximum of €425, with a mean of €146, according to the amounts received from mutual insurance companies and insurers [3]. The analysis of the aetiology of TMDs has focused on several factors such as inflammatory diseases [4], fractures and trauma [5,6], as well as biomedical models related to temporomandibular joints, muscles of mastication and occlusal factors [7]. The management of TMDs includes clinical examination [8] and the use of imaging techniques both for diagnosis and for monitoring the efficacy of treatments [9,10], which classically included the use of botulinum toxin [11], occlusal splint therapy [12] and polyphenols as potential therapeutic agents [13]. TMDs are related to headache, neck pain, shoulder pain, insomnia, vertigo, ocular pain and hearing loss [14], and 91% of TMD patients reported pain, 61.2% joint clicks or crepitation and 53.3% temporomandibular joint limited range of movement [15].

Due to the wide list of related symptoms, diagnostic criteria for temporomandibular disorders (DC/TMDs) were designed for the performance of an exhaustive assessment of each patient [16]; for this reason, an important requirement of time is needed for adequate evaluation with these internationally accepted criteria, which are considered the gold-standard reference test for the diagnosis of temporomandibular disorders. The test examines 12 dimensions that evaluate mandibular movement, type of bite, pain on movement, pain on touch of the musculature, alterations in mandibular movement and headache [16].

According to the cost of misdiagnosis and the time necessary to perform the reference test for TMD diagnosis, it would be beneficial to find a simpler and quicker tool to use as a diagnostic method for TMD in primary care. The Helkimo Clinical Dysfunction Index (HCDI) has been widely used for the clinical diagnosis of TMDs [17–19]. It is a simple and quick test that assesses limitations of mandibular movement, pain and joint function. However, the studies that analysed the reliability [20,21] and validity of this tool are old, used a very small sample, applied incorrect statistical techniques and were limited to the analysis of a single clinimetric property [22,23].

Therefore, a thorough analysis of the main properties of the HCDI is necessary, using the DC/TMD protocol as a reference. For this reason, the aim of the study was to assess and test the psychometric properties of the HCDI in patients with TMD.

2. Materials and Methods

2.1. Participants

To meet the objectives of this work, a cross-sectional validation study was designed. The protocol of this study received the approval of the Research Ethics Committee of Jaén, Spain (date of approval: 27 April 2020; internal code ABR.20/2.TFM). This study was conducted in accordance with the Declaration of Helsinki, good clinical practice guidelines and all applicable laws and regulations, and written informed consent was obtained from all subjects to participate in the study.

The sample size calculation was carried out using the recruitment of at least 10 subjects per item of the scale as a criterion, with a minimum of 80 subjects for validity studies and 20 for reliability [24]. This study was developed between May and August 2020. The sample was selected from the patients of the Dental Medical Center Doctores López Collantes, which provides stomatology services (Dos Hermanas, Sevilla, Spain). and from those at the FisioMedic Clinic (Dos Hermanas, Sevilla, Spain), which provides physiotherapy, general medicine and traumatology services. Recruitment was performed by telephone contact and personal interviews.

2.2. Measurements

Once the patients were selected, demographic data were recorded: age, sex, height, weight, body mass index (BMI), educational level, work situation, smoking status, alcoholic habits and physical activity [25].

The diagnostic validity of the HCDI was measured according to the DC/TMD protocol, which is the gold-standard diagnostic test for TMD. The DC/TMD protocol is composed of 12 items that assess muscle and joint pain, pain during jaw movement, headache, bites, noise, obstacles or blockages during jaw movement and discomfort in the palpation of the muscles of the temporomandibular joint. Finally, a diagnostic tree is used to specify a diagnostic result. The DC/TMD protocol has a sensitivity of 86%, a specificity of 98% and an inter-examination reliability of 85% [16].

The main measure was the HCDI. The instrument is comprised of five items, with each assessment having three possible answers, scored as 0, 1 or 5. The first item (A) is related to the limitation in the range of jaw movement and is subdivided into four sections: the maximum opening of the mouth and the protrusion and lateral shift to both sides. In the opening of the mouth, a value of more than 40 mm scores 0 points, a value between 30 and 39 mm scores 1 point and opening less than 30 mm scores 5 points; protrusion and lateral mouth shifts score 0 if the measurement is 7 mm or more, 1 point if the range of motion is between 4 and 6 mm and 5 points if the range is less than 4 mm. These subsections of item A are added together to obtain a subtotal that scores 0 if the sum of the four sections is 0, 1 point if the subtotal is between 1 and 4 points and 5 points if the subtotal is greater than 4 points. The second item (B) evaluates the alterations of joint function that produce deviations, sounds and/or joint locks or blockages; the third item (C) evaluates the presence of pain when performing some movements; the fourth item (D) evaluates muscular pain in the masticatory muscles; and the fifth item (E) evaluates the presence of discomfort or pain in the prearticular area of the temporomandibular joint (TMJ) through palpation. From the sum of the 5 items, we identify no TMJ involvement if the score is 0, mild TMJ involvement when the score ranges from 1 to 9, moderate TMJ involvement if the score ranges between 10 and 19 and severe TMJ involvement for a score between 20 and 25. Previous studies have shown that the HCDI is able to detect TMD-affected subjects with rheumatoid arthritis, with a statistically significant difference between affected and unaffected subjects [26–28].

Concurrent validity was also measured with Fonseca's anamnestic index (FAI), which is made up of 10 questions that can be answered with yes, no or sometimes, and these answers are scored 10, 0 or 5, respectively. This questionnaire classifies patients according to the affectation, with a total score between 0 and 100. The test categorises temporomandibular disorder as not affected when the score is between 0 and 15 points, mild affectation when the score is between 20 and 40 points, moderate affectation when the score is between 45 and 65 points and severe affectation when the score is between 70 and 100 points. The FAI has a Cronbach alpha of 0.826, an intraclass correlation coefficient of 0.937, a cut-off point of >35 points, a sensitivity of 83.33% and a specificity of 77.97% [29,30]. Similarly, the short version of Fonseca's anamnestic index (SFAI) was also considered; it is a five-question questionnaire that is answered and scored the same as the standard version of the FAI, and the questionnaire categorises patients as unaffected by TMD when the scores is between 0 and 15 points and as affected by TMD when the score is between 20 and 50 points. The SFAI has a sensitivity of 86% and a specificity of 95.5% based on a cut-off point of >17.5 [31].

Pain perception was evaluated by the Numerical Pain-Rating Scale (NPRS) test. The subjects indicate their perceived pain with a number between 0 (no pain) and 10 (the worst pain possible). This tool was used to quantify both the neck and the temporomandibular joint and is the pain assessment test preferred by Spanish-speaking patients. The test has a strong correlation with the Visual Analogue Scale (VAS) and the Four-category Verbal Rating Scale (VRS-4) instruments, with the NPRS being preferred by patients; the Kaiser–Meyer–Olkin (KMO) value is 0.85, with a Bartlett sphericity of <0.01, a landing factor of 0.95 and a lack of implementation percentage of <0.01% [32].

To evaluate the possibility of associated neck disability, the Neck Disability Index test was used; it is a 10-question survey, with answers being reported as a number between 0 and 5. For each question, a score of 0 refers to the total absence of disability, while a score of 5 refers to total disability. In this line, a total score between 0 and 5 indicates absence of disability, 5–14 points indicate low disability, 15–24 point indicates moderate disability and 35–50 points indicate great disability. Cronbach's alpha is 0.89, and the intraclass coefficient is 0.98, with a Pearson's correlation coefficient with the visual analogue pain scale of $r = 0.65$ and with the Northwick Park neck pain questionnaire of $r = 0.89$ [33].

The presence of vertigo and balance problems was assessed by the Dizziness Handicap Inventory (DHI). This questionnaire is composed of 25 questions that can be answered with yes, no or sometimes, scoring 4, 0 and 2 points, respectively. This questionnaire assesses physical, emotional and functional dimensions, each of which has an independent score in addition to the total score. There is a high correlation between each of the dimensions and the total score ($p < 0.01$); factorial analysis shows a structure formed by three components, and there is perfect correlation with the Dizziness Characteristics and Impact on Quality of Life (UCLA-DQ) (>0.75) [34–36].

Headache-associated symptoms were measured with the Headache Impact Test (HIT-6), which is an evaluation questionnaire consisting of six questions that can be answered with usual, almost always, sometimes, rarely and never, with a total score between

36 and 78 points. The correlation between the HIT-6 in different languages is high, it has high reliability, and its items are comparable [37].

Finally, the quality of life was assessed using the 12-item Short-Form Health Survey (SF-12). This questionnaire is the short version of the SF-36 and retains its self-administered form. It results in a Mental Component Summary score and a Physical Component Summary score (PCS-12), differentiating between the two components of the quality of life. The weights of the Spanish version of the SF-12 are similar to those of the original American version, with a correlation of >0.9. The questionnaire explains 91% of the variance of the SF-36 in the sum of the components, and the coefficient of internal consistency is 0.9 for the SF-36 and slightly lower for the SF-12 [38].

2.3. Statistical Analysis

Descriptive analysis was performed by calculating means and standard deviations for continuous variables and frequencies and percentages for categorical variables. The Kolmogorov–Smirnov test was used to verify the normality distribution of the continuous variables, and the Levene test was used to test the homoscedasticity of the samples. The confidence level was set at 95% ($p < 0.05$).

To test the agreement between the two raters for the total HCDI score, the intraclass correlation coefficient (ICC) of Shrout and Fleiss was used in a one-way random effects model of the absolute agreement type; it estimates the reliability of single ratings [39]. Reliability was considered poor when the ICC was <0.40, moderate when the ICC was between 0.40 and 0.75, substantial when the ICC was between 0.75 and 0.90 and excellent when the ICC was >0.90. From the ICC, the standard error of measurement (SEM) and the minimum detectable change (MDC) were calculated. The SEM was calculated as the baseline standard deviation (SD) (σ_{base}) minus the square root of (1-Rxx), where Rxx is the ICC. The MDC was quantified at the 95% confidence level (MDC95) from the SEM formula as follows: $MDC95 = 1.96 * \sigma_{base} * \sqrt{(1-ICC)}$, where 1.96 is the z-value corresponding to the 95% confidence interval (MDC95). The MDC provides a good tool for translating the ICC into units of change in the instrument. For measured agreement between two raters for the items, a weighted Kappa coefficient, weighted by quadratic weights, was used [40]. The agreement was considered null if Kappa was <0.00, insignificant if Kappa was between 0.00–0.20, discreet if Kappa was between 0.21–0.40, moderate if Kappa was between 0.41–0.60, substantial if Kappa was between 0.61–0.80 and almost perfect if Kappa was between 0.81–1.00 [41]. In addition, Bland–Altman charts were generated to evaluate the limits of agreement [42].

To analyse the concurrent validity of the HCDI with the FAI, NPRS, NDI, DHI, HIT-6 and SF-12, Pearson's correlation coefficient r was used. The correlation coefficient was considered strong if it was >0.50 and moderate if it was between 0.30 and 0.50 [43].

The ability of the HCDI to discriminate between TMD patients and healthy subjects was determined using receiver operating characteristic (ROC) curves. First, the classification of the subjects as TMD patients or healthy controls was carried out based on the diagnostic criteria of the DC/TMD protocol, and the total score obtained in the HCDI was evaluated as a variable. In the ROC curve, the fraction of true positives (sensitivity) was represented as a function of the fraction of false positives for different cut-off points. The area under the curve (AUC) was also calculated as a measure of the ability of the score to discriminate between the two diagnostic groups (TMD patients or healthy subjects). The AUC was considered statistically significant when the 95% confidence interval did not include 0.5 [44]. Values between 0.5 and 0.7 indicated low accuracy, values between 0.7 and 0.9 indicated good accuracy and values greater than 0.9 indicated high accuracy [45].

3. Results

In all, 158 people were contacted, but the final sample was composed of 107 participants (60 TMD patients and 47 healthy controls), as 51 did not meet the selection criteria or refused to participate. The sociodemographic and anthropometric characteristics of the sample are shown in Table 1.

Table 1. Anthropometric and sociodemographic characteristics of the sample and groups.

		All	$n = 107$	Healthy	$n = 47$	Temporomandibular Disorders (TMDs)	$n = 60$
Weight (kilograms)		72.83	17.05	77.86	19.22	68.90	14.07
Height (meters)		1.63	0.09	1.65	0.09	1.61	0.07
Body mass index		27.48	6.91	28.48	7.10	26.69	6.72
Age (years)		46.25	13.88	49.66	14.56	43.53	12.79
Sex	Female	83	77.6	27	57.45	56	93.3
	Male	24	22.4	20	42.55	4	6.7
Study level	Primary	19	17.8	12	25.53	7	11.7
	Secondary	52	48.6	25	53.19	27	45.0
	University	36	33.6	10	21.28	26	43.3
Physical activity	No	45	42.1	19	40.43	26	43.3
	Yes	62	57.9	28	59.57	34	56.7
Economic level	<€20.000	62	57.9	29	61.70	33	55.0
	>€20.000	45	42.1	18	38.30	27	45.0
Smoker	No	69	64.5	28	59.57	41	68.3
	Yes	13	12.1	6	12.77	7	11.7
	Occasional	12	11.2	6	12.77	6	10.0
	Ex-smoker	13	12.1	7	14.89	6	10.0
Drinker	No	38	35.5	19	40.43	19	31.7
	Regular drinker	6	5.6	3	6.38	3	5.0
	Occasional	63	58.9	25	53.19	38	63.3

3.1. Inter-Rater Reliability

Results showed a maximum weighted kappa value of 0.774 for item C and a minimum value of 0.426 for item A2. Based on these values, reliability ranged from moderate to substantial, while the total score of the scale reached an excellent degree of concordance of 0.905 (Table 2). Figure 1 shows the Bland–Altman plot. Table 3 shows concurrent validity of the Helkimo Clinical Dysfunction Index with other specific and generic instruments.

Table 2. Inter-rater concordance of the Helkimo items and the total score.

Measure	Value	95% Confidence Interval	Degree of Concordance
Item A1	0.62548	0.48243 to 0.76853	Substantial
Item A2	0.42641	0.20367 to 0.64916	Moderate
Item A3	0.51430	0.31876 to 0.70983	Moderate
Item A4	0.64430	0.52330 to 0.76529	Substantial
Item A	0.61987	0.49568 to 0.74407	Substantial
Item B	0.51661	0.37930 to 0.65391	Moderate
Item C	0.77395	0.66415 to 0.88375	Substantial
Item D	0.75750	0.65350 to 0.86149	Substantial
Item E	0.72116	0.60305 to 0.83926	Substantial
Total score	0.9053	0.8642 to 0.9345	Excellent

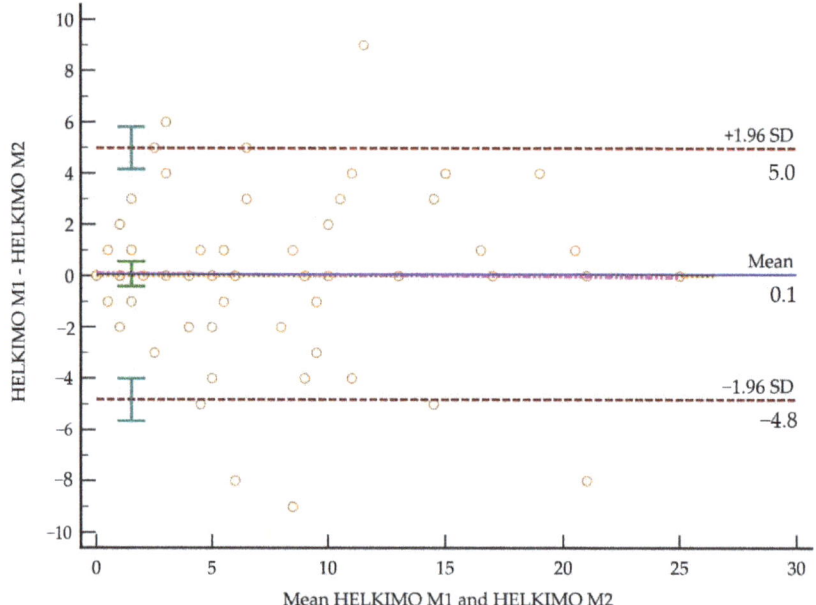

Figure 1. Limits of concordance by Bland–Altman plot.

Table 3. Concurrent validity of the Helkimo Clinical Dysfunction Index with other specific and generic instruments.

Variable	Pearson's r	p-Value	Correlation
Fonseca Anamnestic Index	0.692	<0.001	Strong
Short Form of the Fonseca Anamnestic Index	0.626	<0.001	Strong
Numerical Pain-Rating Scale Orofacial	0.777	<0.001	Strong
Numerical Pain-Rating Scale Neck Pain	0.302	0.002	Moderate
Neck Disability Index	0.265	0.006	Poor
Dizziness Handicap Inventory Functional	0.276	0.004	Poor
Dizziness Handicap Inventory Emotional	0.301	0.002	Moderate
Dizziness Handicap Inventory Physical	0.339	<0.001	Moderate
Dizziness Handicap Inventory Total	0.339	<0.001	Moderate
Headache Impact Test 6 items	0.187	0.054	Poor
Physical Component Summary SF-12	0.003	0.975	Poor
Mental Component Summary SF-12	−0.171	0.078	Poor

3.2. Validity and Accuracy of the TMD Diagnostic Ability

ROC curve analysis found an optimal cut-off point of more than 1 point in the HCDI score that showed a sensitivity of 86.67% with a specificity of 68.09% for the diagnosis of TMDs, making the DC/TMD protocol the gold standard (Table 4). This analysis showed an area under the curve (AUC) of 0.841 (Figure 2), which can be interpreted as good accuracy.

Table 4. Predictive values of the Helkimo Clinical Dysfunction Index (HCDI) total score by ROC curve analysis for the diagnosis of TMDs.

Sensitivity	95% CI	Specificity	95% CI	+LR	95% CI	-LR	95% CI	+PV	95% CI	-PV	95% CI
86.67%	75.4–94.1	68.09%	52.9–80.9	2.72	1.8–4.2	0.20	0.10–0.4	77.6	69.3–84.2	80.0	67.1–88.7

95% CI: 95% confidence interval; +LR: positive likelihood ratio; -LR: negative likelihood ratio; +PV: positive predictive value; -PV: negative predictive value.

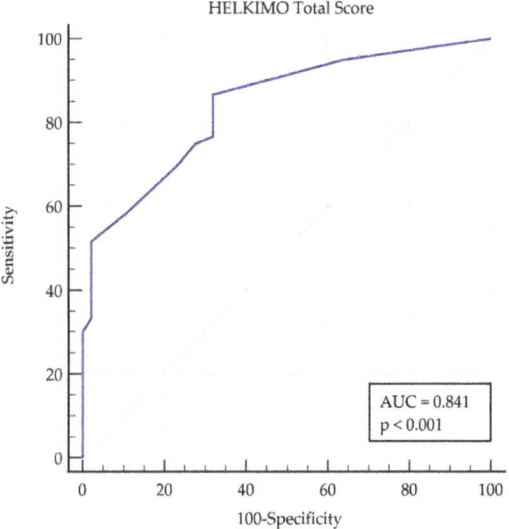

Figure 2. Receiver operating characteristic (ROC) curve plot showing the area under the curve (AUC).

4. Discussion

This study evaluated the clinimetric properties of the Helkimo Clinical Dysfunction Index. The data obtained suggested that it is a valid and reliable instrument for evaluating patients with TMD, determining the degree of severity of the condition and discriminating between affected and unaffected patients with TMD. In this study, a total sample of 107 patients was used (60 TMD patients and 47 healthy subjects), and all of them were evaluated by this test, which lasted approximately 4 min. The two groups were comparable, except that a higher proportion of females who suffered from TMD, which is a consistent observation among TMD studies [17,27]. This fact may have led to a reduction in the mean weight and height and a higher proportion of university-educated subjects among the female population [46].

Despite being a commonly used tool for TMD assessment [19], few authors have studied the HCDI in depth. In 1987, Van der Weele et al. conducted an argumentative analysis of the HCDI, studying the pertinence of the construction of such a test to evaluate patients with TMD according to the evidence of the moment. They concluded that there was insufficient scientific evidence to support the use of these items in a diagnostic test for TMD [28]. However, in the analysis of the current scientific evidence regarding the pertinence of the use of these items in a diagnostic test for TMD, there is a general consensus that supports their use, and no evidence casts doubt on it [19,47]. In 2007, Da Cunha et al. conducted a comparative study between the HCDI and the craniomandibular test. As in the present study, they found greater affectation of TMD among women, who represented 70% of the total sample of affected people in the study, and a mean age of 46 years in affected patients, which agrees with the mean age of 43 years observed in this study [27].

Oliveira de Santis et al. conducted the only study analysing the psychometric characteristics of the HCDI and the American Association of Orofacial Pain (AAOP) index in subjects aged between 6 and 18 years, using the DC/TMD protocol as a reference. The authors found a non-statistically significant difference between genders, a sensitivity of 53.40% and a specificity of 77.27% for the HCDI, as well as a low level of accordance between the test being considered and the gold standard [47]. Nonetheless, in the present study, the sensitivity obtained was 86.67%, while the specificity was 68.09%. These differences in the results may be due to the difference in age between samples (46.25 years old in our study, 8.18 years old in the one of Oliveira de Santis et al.), which could indicate that the HCDI is more useful for adults than children.

The present study had some limitations. First, the study sample had a higher proportion of women due to the higher proportion of women affected by TMD. Furthermore, although this study analysed the most common psychometric properties, we did not study the sensitivity to change or the ability to discriminate between different TMD populations. Additionally, this study was carried out on a sample of resident patients in a well-defined geographic location, which limits the generalisation of the results obtained.

5. Conclusions

The study shows that the HCDI is suitable for the diagnosis of TMD. The inter-observer concordance was between moderate and substantial for each of the items and excellent for the total score of the test. The HCDI has strong concurrent validity with the FAI, SFAI and NPRS orofacial assessment instruments; moderate validity with the NPRS neck pain assessment, emotional and physical facets and the total DHI value; and poor validity with respect to HIT-6 instruments, the mental and physical components of the SF-12 and the functional component of the DHI. The HCDI shows a sensitivity of 86.67%, a specificity of 68.09% and an AUC of 0.841 to predict the presence of TMD.

Author Contributions: All authors actively participated in the study and made substantial contributions to this article. Conceptualisation, R.A.-R., A.J.I.-V., C.M.S.-T., N.Z.-A. and R.L.-V.; methodology, N.Z.-A., Y.C.-C. and R.L.-V.; software, R.L.-V.; formal analysis, Y.C.-C. and R.L.-V.; investigation, R.A.-R., A.J.I.-V., C.M.S.-T., N.Z.-A., Y.C.-C., D.R.-A., E.O.-G. and R.L.-V.; data curation, R.A.-R., A.J.I.-V., C.M.S.-T. and R.L.-V.; writing—original draft preparation, R.A.-R., A.J.I.-V. and R.L.-V.; writing—review and editing A.J.I.-V. and R.L.-V.; visualisation and supervision, N.Z.-A., A.J.I.-V. and R.L.-V. All authors have read and agreed to the published version of the manuscript.

Funding: This research received no external funding.

Institutional Review Board Statement: The study was conducted according to the guidelines of the Declaration of Helsinki, and approved by the Ethics Committee of University of Jaen (internal code ABR.20/2.TFM; date of approval 27 April 2020).

Informed Consent Statement: Informed consent was obtained from all subjects involved in the study.

Data Availability Statement: Data available under request to corresponding author due to participants' consent.

Conflicts of Interest: The authors declare no conflict of interest.

References

1. Paduano, S.; Bucci, R.; Rongo, R.; Silva, R.; Michelotti, A. Prevalence of temporomandibular disorders and oral parafunctions in adolescents from public schools in Southern Italy. *Cranio J. Craniomandib. Pract.* **2020**, *38*, 370–375. [CrossRef]
2. Perez, C.V.; De Leeuw, R.; Okeson, J.P.; Carlson, C.R.; Li, H.F.; Bush, H.M.; Falace, D.A. The incidence and prevalence of temporomandibular disorders and posterior open bite in patients receiving mandibular advancement device therapy for obstructive sleep apnea. *Sleep Breath* **2013**, *17*, 323–332. [CrossRef] [PubMed]
3. Nieto Fernández-Pacheco, M.J. *Análisis de los Costes Producidos por una Incorrecta Derivación de Pacientes con Síndrome de Disfunción Temporomandibular*; Universidad Autónoma de Madrid: Madrid, Spain, 2017.
4. Ibi, M. Inflammation and temporomandibular joint derangement. *Biol. Pharm. Bull.* **2019**, *42*, 538–542. [CrossRef] [PubMed]
5. Minervini, G.; Lucchese, A.; Perillo, L.; Serpico, R.; Minervini, G. Unilateral superior condylar neck fracture with dislocation in a child treated with an acrylic splint in the upper arch for functional repositioning of the mandible. *Cranio J. Craniomandib. Pract.* **2017**, *35*, 337–341. [CrossRef] [PubMed]
6. Choi, J.; Oh, N.; Kim, I.K. A follow-up study of condyle fracture in children. *Int. J. Oral Maxillofac. Surg.* **2005**, *34*, 851–858. [CrossRef]
7. Suvinen, T.I.; Reade, P.C.; Kemppainen, P.; Könönen, M.; Dworkin, S.F. Review of aetiological concepts of temporomandibular pain disorders: Towards a biopsychosocial model for integration of physical disorder factors with psychological and psychosocial illness impact factors. *Eur. J. Pain* **2005**, *9*, 613. [CrossRef] [PubMed]
8. Fernández-de-las-Peñas, C.; Von Piekartz, H. Clinical reasoning for the examination and physical therapy treatment of temporomandibular disorders (TMD): A narrative literature review. *J. Clin. Med.* **2020**, *9*, 3686. [CrossRef]

9. Eberhard, D. The efficacy of anterior repositioning splint therapy studied by magnetic resonance imaging. *Eur. J. Orthod.* **2002**, *24*, 343–352. [CrossRef]
10. Minervini, G.; Nucci, L.; Lanza, A.; Femiano, F.; Contaldo, M.; Grassia, V. Temporomandibular disc displacement with reduction treated with anterior repositioning splint: A 2-year clinical and magnetic resonance imaging (MRI) follow-up. *J. Biol. Regul. Homeost. Agents* **2020**, *34*, 151–160. [PubMed]
11. Canter, H.I.; Kayikcioglu, A.; Aksu, M.; Mavili, M.E. Botulinum toxin in closed treatment of mandibular condylar fracture. *Ann. Plast. Surg.* **2007**, *58*, 474–478. [CrossRef]
12. Fayed, M.; El-Mangoury, N.; El-Bpkle, D.; Belal, A. Occlusal splint therapy and magnetic resonance imaging. *Worlf J. Orthod.* **2004**, *5*, 133–140.
13. Moccia, S.; Nucci, L.; Spagnuolo, C.; d'Apuzzo, F.; Piancino, M.G.; Minervini, G. Polyphenols as potential agents in the management of temporomandibular disorders. *Appl. Sci.* **2020**, *10*, 5305. [CrossRef]
14. Ting, J.; Li, J.; Zhen Kang, S. A primary research on the concomitant syntoms of temporomandibular joint pain. *Zhonghua Kou Qiang Yi Xue Za Zhi* **2005**, *40*, 219–222.
15. Katsoulis, K.; Bassetti, R.; Windecker Getaz, I.; Mericske Stern, R.; Katsoulis, J. Temporomandibular disorders/myoarthropathy of the masticatory system. *Res. Sci.* **2012**, *122*, 510–518.
16. Schiffman, E.; Ohrbach, R.; Truelove, E.; Look, J.; Anderson, G.; Goulet, J.-P.P.; List, T.; Svensson, P.; Gonzalez, Y.; Lobbezoo, F.; et al. Diagnostic criteria for temporomandibular disorders (DC/TMD) for clinical and research applications: Recommendations of the International RDC/TMD Consortium Network and Orofacial Pain Special Interest Group. *J. Oral Facial Pain Headache* **2014**, *28*, 6–27. [CrossRef]
17. Rani, S.; Pawah, S.; Gola, S.; Bakshi, M. Analysis of Helkimo index for temporomandibular disorder diagnosis in the dental students of Faridabad city: A cross-sectional study. *J. Indian Prosthodont. Soc.* **2017**, *17*, 48–52. [CrossRef]
18. Suhas, S.; Ramdas, S.; Lingam, P.; Naveen Kumar, H.; Sasidharan, A.; Aadithya, R. Assessment of temporomandibular joint dysfunction in condylar fracture of the mandible using the Helkimo index. *Indian J. Plast. Surg.* **2017**, *50*, 207–212. [CrossRef]
19. Nokar, S.; Sadighpour, L.; Shirzad, H.; Shahrokhi Rad, A.; Keshvad, A. Evaluation of signs, symptoms, and occlusal factors among patients with temporomandibular disorders according to Helkimo index. *Cranio J. Craniomandib. Pract.* **2019**, *37*, 383–388. [CrossRef]
20. Fu, K.; Ma, X.; Zhang, Z.; Tian, Y.; Zhou, Y.; Zhao, Y. Study on the use of temporomandibular joint dysfunction index in temporomandibular disorders-PubMed. *Zhonghua Kou Qiang Yi Xue Za Zhi* **2002**, *37*, 320–322.
21. John, M.; Zwijnenburg, A. Interobserver variability in assessment of signs of TMD-PubMed. *Int. J. Prosthodont.* **2001**, *14*, 265–270.
22. Abud, M.C.; Figueiredo, M.D.; dos Santos, M.B.F.; Consani, R.L.X.; Marchini, L. Correlation of prosthetic status with the GOHAI and TMD indices-PubMed. *Rest. Dent.* **2011**, *19*, 38–42.
23. Pocock, P.R.; Mamandras, A.H.; Bellamy, N. Evaluation of an anamnestic questionnaire as an instrument for investigating potential relationships between orthodontic therapy and temporomandibular disorders. *Am. J. Orthod. Dentofac. Orthop.* **1992**, *102*, 239–243. [CrossRef]
24. Hobart, J.C.; Cano, S.J.; Warner, T.T.; Thompson, A.J. What sample sizes for reliability and validity studies in neurology? *J. Neurol.* **2012**, *259*, 2681–2694. [CrossRef]
25. World Health Organization. *2013–2020 Global Action Plan for the Prevention and Control of Noncommunicable Diseases*; World Health Organization: Geneva, Switzerland, 2013.
26. Duinkerke, A.S.H.; Luteijn, F.; Bouman, T.K.; Jong, H.P. Reproducibility of a palpation test for the stomatognathic system. *Community Dent. Oral Epidemiol.* **1986**, *14*, 80–85. [CrossRef] [PubMed]
27. Da Cunha, S.C.; Nogueira, R.V.B.; Duarte, Â.P.; Vasconcelos, B.C.D.E.; Almeida, R.D.A.C. Análise dos índices de Helkimo e craniomandibular para diagnóstico de desordens temporomandibulares em pacientes com artrite reumatóide. *Braz. J. Otorhinolaryngol.* **2007**, *73*, 19–26. [CrossRef]
28. van der Weele, L.T.; Dibbets, J.M.H. Helkimo's index: A scale or just a set of symptoms? *J. Oral Rehabil.* **1987**, *14*, 229–237. [CrossRef]
29. Rodrigues-Bigaton, D.; de Castro, E.M.; Pires, P.F. Factor and Rasch analysis of the Fonseca anamnestic index for the diagnosis of myogenous temporomandibular disorder. *Braz. J. Phys. Ther.* **2017**, *21*, 120–126. [CrossRef] [PubMed]
30. Sánchez-Torrelo, C.; Zagalaz-Anula, N.; Alonso-Royo, R.; Ibáñez-Vera, A.; López-Collantes, J.; Rodríguez-Almagro, D.; Obrero-Gaitán, E.; Lomas-Vega, R. Transcultural adaptation and validation of the Fonseca Anamnestic Index in a Spanish population with temporomandibular disorders. *J. Clin. Med.* **2020**, *9*, 3230. [CrossRef] [PubMed]
31. Pires, P.F.; de Castro, E.M.; Pelai, E.B.; de Arruda, A.B.C.; Rodrigues-Bigaton, D. Analysis of the accuracy and reliability of the Short-Form Fonseca Anamnestic Index in the diagnosis of myogenous temporomandibular disorder in women. *Braz. J. Phys. Ther.* **2018**, *22*, 276–282. [CrossRef] [PubMed]
32. Jensen, M.P.; Castarlenas, E.; Roy, R.; Tomé Pires, C.; Racine, M.; Pathak, A.; Miró, J. The utility and construct validity of four measures of pain intensity: Results from a University-Based Study in Spain. *Pain Med.* **2019**, *20*, 2411–2420. [CrossRef]
33. Andrade Ortega, J.A.; Delgado Martínez, A.D.; Almécija Ruiz, R. Validation of a Spanish version of the Neck Disability Index. *Spine* **2010**, *35*, 85–89. [CrossRef] [PubMed]
34. Jacobson, G.P.; Newman, C.W. The Development of the Dizziness Handicap Inventory. *Arch. Otolaryngol. Head Neck Surg.* **1990**, *116*, 425–427. [CrossRef]

35. Perez, N.; Garmendia, I.; García-Granero, M.; Martin, E.; García-Tapia, R. Factor analysis and correlation between Dizziness Handicap Inventory and Dizziness Characteristics and Impact on Quality of Life Scales. *Acta Oto-Laryngol. Suppl.* **2001**, *545*, 145–154.
36. Pérez, N.; Garmendia, I.; Martín, E.; García-Tapia, R. Cultural adaptation of 2 questionnaires for health measurements in patients with vertigo. *Acta Otorrinolaringol. Esp.* **2000**, *51*, 572–580.
37. Martin, M.; Blaisdell, B.; Kwong, J.W.; Bjorner, J.B. The Short-Form Headache Impact Test (HIT-6) was psychometrically equivalent in nine languages. *J. Clin. Epidemiol.* **2004**, *57*, 1271–1278. [CrossRef] [PubMed]
38. Vilagut, G.; Valderas, J.M.; Ferrer, M.; Garin, O.; López-García, E.; Alonso, J. Interpretation of SF-36 and SF-12 questionnaires in Spain: Physical and mental components. *Med. Clin.* **2008**, *130*, 726–735. [CrossRef]
39. Shrout, P.E.; Fleiss, J.L. Intraclass correlations: Uses in assessing rater reliability. *Psychol. Bull.* **1979**, *86*, 420–428. [CrossRef] [PubMed]
40. Brenner, H.; Kliebsch, U. Dependence of weighted kappa coefficients on the number of categories. *Epidemiology* **1996**, *7*, 199–202. [CrossRef] [PubMed]
41. Landis, J.; Koch, G.G. The measurement of the observer agreement for categorial data. *Biometrics* **1977**, *33*, 159. [CrossRef] [PubMed]
42. Bland, J.; Altman, D.G. Measuring agreement in method comparison studies. *Stat. Methods Med. Res.* **1999**, *8*, 135–160. [CrossRef] [PubMed]
43. Cohen, J. *Statistical Power Analysis for the Behavioral Sciencies*, 2nd ed.; Hillsdale, N.J., Ed.; Lawrence Erlbaum Associates: New York, NY, USA, 1998; ISBN 0805802835.
44. Zweig, M.H.; Campbell, G. Receiver-operating characteristic (ROC) plots: A fundamental evaluation tool in clinical medicine. *Clin. Chem.* **1993**, *39*, 561–577. [CrossRef] [PubMed]
45. Swets, J. Measuring the accuracy of diagnostic information. *Science* **1988**, *240*, 1285–1293. [CrossRef] [PubMed]
46. Ministerio de Ciencia e Innovación de España Estadística de Estudiantes. Available online: https://www.ciencia.gob.es/portal/site/MICINN/menuitem.7eeac5cd345b4f34f09dfd1001432ea0/?vgnextoid=0930dd449de8b610VgnVCM1000001d04140aRCRD (accessed on 3 October 2020).
47. de Santis, T.O.; Motta, L.J.; Biasotto-Gonzalez, D.A.; Mesquita-Ferrari, R.A.; Fernandes, K.P.S.; de Godoy, C.H.L.; Alfaya, T.A.; Bussadori, S.K. Accuracy study of the main screening tools for temporomandibular disorder in children and adolescents. *J. Bodyw. Mov. Ther.* **2014**, *18*, 87–91. [CrossRef] [PubMed]

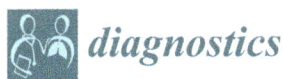

Article

Increased Risk of Migraine in Patients with Temporomandibular Disorder: A Longitudinal Follow-Up Study Using a National Health Screening Cohort

Soo-Hwan Byun [1,2], Chanyang Min [3], Dae-Myoung Yoo [3], Byoung-Eun Yang [1,2] and Hyo-Geun Choi [2,3,4,*]

1. Department of Oral & Maxillofacial Surgery, Dentistry, Hallym University College of Medicine, Anyang, Gyeonggi-do 14068, Korea; purheit@daum.net (S.-H.B.); face@hallym.ac.kr (B.-E.Y.)
2. Research Center of Clinical Dentistry, Hallym University Clinical Dentistry Graduate School, Chuncheon, Gangwon-do 24252, Korea
3. Hallym Data Science Laboratory, Hallym University College of Medicine, Anyang, Gyeonggi-do 14068, Korea; joicemin@naver.com (C.M.); ydm1285@naver.com (D.-M.Y.)
4. Department of Otorhinolaryngology-Head & Neck Surgery, Hallym University College of Medicine, Anyang, Gyeonggi-do 14068, Korea
* Correspondence: pupen@naver.com

Received: 11 August 2020; Accepted: 18 September 2020; Published: 20 September 2020

Abstract: Background: The aim of this study was to investigate the association between temporomandibular disorder (TMD) and migraine through a longitudinal follow-up study using population data from a national health screening cohort. Methods: This cohort study used data from the Korean National Health Insurance Service-Health Screening Cohort from 2002 to 2015. Of the 514,866 participants, 3884 TMD patients were matched at a 1:4 ratio with 15,536 control participants. Crude models and models adjusted for obesity, smoking, alcohol consumption, systolic blood pressure, diastolic blood pressure, fasting blood glucose, total cholesterol, and Charlson Comorbidity Index (CCI) scores were calculated. Chi-squared test, Kaplan–Meier analysis, and two-tailed log-rank test were used for statistical analysis. Stratified Cox proportional hazard models were used to assess hazard ratios (HR) and 95% confidence intervals (CIs) for migraine in both control groups. Results: The adjusted HR for migraine was 2.10 (95% CI: 1.81–2.44) in the TMD group compared to the control group, which was consistent in subgroup analyses according to age, sex, and Kaplan–Meier analysis. Conclusions: This study demonstrated that TMD patients have a higher risk of migraine. These results suggest that dentists can decrease the risk of migraine in TMD patients by managing TMD properly.

Keywords: migraine; TMD; Korean National Health Insurance Service; cohort; aura

1. Introduction

Temporomandibular disorder (TMD) is a collective term for comprehensive clinical symptoms related to the dysfunction of the temporomandibular joint (TMJ), masticatory muscles, and adjacent anatomic structures [1]. The etiology of TMD is multifactorial, including parafunctional habit, posture, and neurologic factors [2,3]. Mastication and other functions aggravate the condition, and most patients suffer from limited or asymmetric mouth opening. Related symptoms of TMD are headache, joint sounds (clicking, popping, and crepitus), and craniomaxillofacial pain [4]. TMD affects between 5–70% of Caucasians, and several studies have reported that maxillofacial pain is the major complaint of more than half of the consultations and up to 80% of dental appointments among adolescents [5,6]. Moreover, it was shown that clinicians feel incompetent in managing TMD, resulting in referrals to other clinicians [7].

Migraine usually occurs on one side of the head with throbbing pain or a pulsing sensation. The symptoms often occur with photosensitivity, vomiting, and nausea. Migraine can last for several hours, and it can interfere with normal activities. Medications could relieve some migraines and prevent them. Proper medications, combined with self-help solutions and healthier lifestyles, might help to manage this headache [8].

The International Classification of Headache Disorders (ICHD) has classified migraine into two types: with and without aura [9]. Based on the classification of ICHD-3, an aura must present with at least three of the following six symptoms: spreading gradually for more than 5 min, two or more symptoms occurring in succession, each individual aura symptom lasts 5–60 min, at least one aura symptom is unilateral, at least one aura symptom is positive, and the aura is accompanied or followed within 60 min by headache [9,10]. An aura is known as a warning sign prior to migraine for some patients. An aura can occur with visual disturbances, including blind spots, flashes of light, tingling on one side of the face, or difficulty speaking. Migraine with aura is considered to affect between one-fifth and one-third of those with migraine in the United States, an estimated 7.4–11.1 million people [11]. The pathophysiology of aura is widely known as cortical spreading depression (CSD) [12]. CSD is activated by slow depolarization in cortical neurons and glia, followed by hyperpolarization that moves across the cortex at a rate of 3–5 mm/min. It is accompanied by alterations in neurotransmitter release and ion homeostasis [13]. As greater energy is needed to restore homeostasis, this is accompanied by a rapid spike in cerebral blood flow [14].

A migraine without aura is the most common type of migraine, comprising approximately 75% of all migraines [9]. This type of migraine develops without aura, but it can present with various symptoms at its initial stages. According to ICHD-3, it lasts for 4–72 h and has at least two of the following headache characteristics: moderate-to-severe intensity, unilateral location, aggravation by physical activity, and pulsating quality [15]. One or more associated symptoms such as nausea/vomiting and photophobia/phonophobia would happen during the attack. In addition, attacks of a migraine without aura must not be attributable to another disorder.

Most painful symptoms are transient and are related to a specific lesion or disease that can be cured. Unfortunately, some types of pain are chronic, and chronic pain remains a public health issue [16]. Both TMD and migraine could be main causes of chronic pain in the orofacial area. Many patients with TMD have several comorbid conditions [17,18]. Moreover, previous studies of TMD patients have revealed that comorbid conditions are the reason for 50% of TMD patients requiring care for TMD symptoms, and for 20% of patients with long-term disability from their pain [19–21]. It is essential that any comorbid conditions and their influences on clinical outcomes are identified and evaluated by clinicians managing TMD patients [22].

Some studies have reported an association between TMD and migraine [8,23–26]. This association was thought to be induced by anatomic, neurologic, and emotional relationships. Previous studies reported that migraine is related to pain in the sinus, teeth, TMJ, and cervical areas [27–29]. However, most studies have been based on limited participants or subjective questionnaires [26,30].

The aim of this study was to investigate the association between TMD and migraine by conducting a longitudinal study using population data from a national health screening cohort. It was determined that patients with TMD have a greater risk of migraine than those without TMD.

2. Materials and Methods

2.1. Study Population

The ethics committee of Hallym University approved this study on 4 November 2019 (No. 2019-10-023). The need for written informed consent was waived by the Institutional Review Board.

All analyses adhered to the guidelines and regulations of the ethics committee. The details of the Korean National Health Insurance Service-Health Screening Cohort data have been described elsewhere [31].

2.2. Definition of Temporomandibular Disorder

TMD was defined if participants were diagnosed with the ICD (International Classification of Diseases)-10 code K07.6 (Temporomandibular joint disorders). For diagnostic accuracy, this study only selected participants who were treated ≥2 times for the diagnosis of TMD.

2.3. Definition of Migraine

Migraine was defined if participants were diagnosed with the ICD-10 code G43 (Migraine). For diagnostic accuracy, this study only selected participants who were treated ≥2 times for the diagnosis of migraine. Among them, migraine with aura was defined if participants were diagnosed with the ICD-10 code G43.1 (Migraine with aura).

2.4. Participant Selection

TMD patients were selected from 514,866 participants with 615,488,428 medical claim codes from 2002 to 2015 (n = 4627). The control group consisted of participants who were not diagnosed with TMD from 2002 to 2015 (n = 510,239). TMD patients were excluded if they had a 1-year washout period (n = 172). Control participants were excluded if they were diagnosed with the ICD-10 code K07.6 once (n = 6659). TMD patients were matched at a 1:4 ratio with control participants for age, sex, income, and region of residence; this was done randomly to prevent selection bias. In this study, we supposed that the matched participants were involved in the same date (index date). Participants who died before the index date and had a history of migraine before the index date were excluded. In the TMD group, 571 participants were excluded, and during matching, 488,044 control participants were excluded. As a result, 3884 TMD patients were matched at a 1:4 ratio with 15,536 control participants (Figure 1).

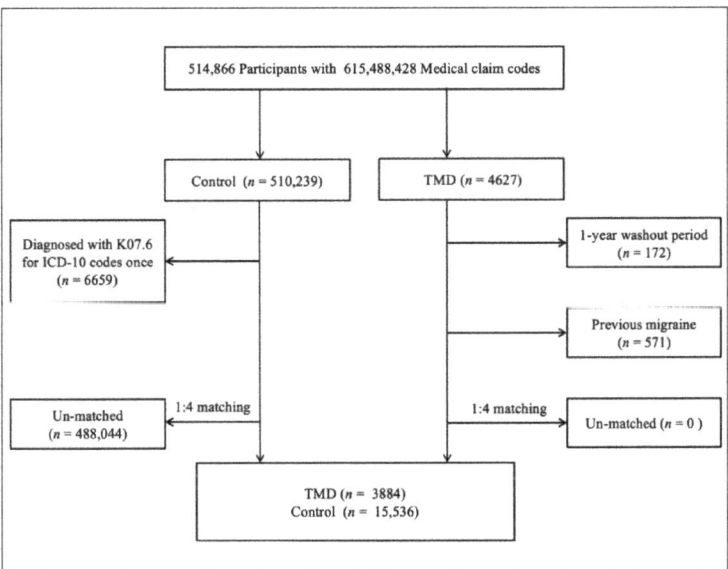

Figure 1. A schematic illustration of the participant selection process. Out of 514,866 participants, 3884 patients with temporomandibular disorder were matched at a 1:4 ratio with 15,536 control participants for age, sex, income, and region of residence. TMD, temporomandibular disorder; ICD-10, International Classification of Diseases, 10th edition.

2.5. Covariates

Age was categorized into ten groups ranging from 40–44 to 85+. Income groups were divided into five classes from lowest income (class 1) to highest (class 5) income. Regions of residence were grouped into urban and rural areas following our previous study [31].

Tobacco smoking, alcohol consumption, obesity based on body mass index (BMI, kg/m^2) [32,33], systolic blood pressure (BP), diastolic BP, fasting blood glucose, and total cholesterol were measured as described in our previous study [34]. The Charlson Comorbidity Index (CCI) was used to measure 17 comorbidities [35].

2.6. Statistical Analyses

Chi-squared tests were used to compare general characteristics between the TMD and control groups.

Stratified Cox proportional hazard models were used to assess the hazard ratios (HRs) and 95% confidence intervals (CIs) for migraine in the TMD group compared to the control group. In this analysis, crude (simple) and adjusted (for obesity, smoking, alcohol consumption, systolic BP, diastolic BP, fasting blood glucose, total cholesterol, and CCI scores) models were used. Age, sex, income, and region of residence were stratified. Additionally, this study calculated HRs with 95% CIs for migraine with and without aura in the TMD group compared to the control group.

A Kaplan–Meier analysis and the log-rank test were used to analyze the cumulative probability of migraine in the TMD group compared to the control group.

For subgroup analyses, this study divided participants by age and sex (<60 years old and ≥60 years old; males and females) and analyzed the crude and adjusted models. We additionally performed subgroup analyses of crude and adjusted HRs for migraine with and without aura in the TMD group compared to the control group (Tables S1 and S2).

Two-tailed analyses were performed, and significance was defined as p-values less than 0.05. SAS version 9.4 (SAS Institute, Cary, NC, USA) was used for statistical analyses.

3. Results

The general characteristics for age, sex, income, and region of residence were identical due to matching between the groups (Table 1), while those for obesity, smoking, alcohol consumption, BP, fasting blood glucose, total cholesterol, and CCI were different.

Table 1. General characteristics of participants.

Characteristics	Total Participants		
	TMD (n, %)	Control (n, %)	p-Value
Age (years old)			1.000
40–44	128 (3.3)	512 (3.3)	
45–49	403 (10.4)	1612 (10.4)	
50–54	626 (16.1)	2504 (16.1)	
55–59	629 (16.2)	2516 (16.2)	
60–64	538 (13.9)	2152 (13.9)	
65–69	595 (15.3)	2380 (15.3)	
70–74	512 (13.2)	2048 (13.2)	
75–79	319 (8.2)	1276 (8.2)	
80–84	107 (2.8)	428 (2.8)	
85+	27 (0.7)	108 (0.7)	

Table 1. Cont.

Characteristics	Total Participants		p-Value
	TMD (n, %)	Control (n, %)	
Sex			1.000
Male	1753 (45.1)	7012 (45.1)	
Female	2131 (54.9)	8524 (54.9)	
Income			1.000
1 (lowest)	598 (15.4)	2392 (15.4)	
2	505 (13.0)	2020 (13.0)	
3	626 (16.1)	2504 (16.1)	
4	800 (20.6)	3200 (20.6)	
5 (highest)	1355 (34.9)	5420 (34.9)	
Region of residence			1.000
Urban	1908 (40.1)	7632 (40.1)	
Rural	2850 (59.9)	11,400 (59.9)	
Obesity [†]			
Underweight	112 (2.9)	385 (2.5)	<0.001 *
Normal	1530 (39.4)	5601 (36.1)	
Overweight	1104 (28.4)	4171 (26.9)	
Obese I	1056 (27.2)	4885 (31.4)	
Obese II	82 (2.1)	494 (3.2)	
Smoking status			<0.001 *
Non-smoker	2923 (75.3)	11443 (73.7)	
Past smoker	485 (12.5)	1738 (11.2)	
Current smoker	476 (12.3)	2355 (15.2)	
Alcohol consumption			0.754
<1 time a week	2733 (70.4)	10,892 (70.1)	
≥1 time a week	1151 (29.6)	4644 (29.9)	
Systolic blood pressure			<0.001 *
<120 mmHg	1292 (33.3)	4704 (30.3)	
120–139 mmHg	1882 (48.5)	7508 (48.3)	
≥140 mmHg	710 (18.3)	3324 (21.4)	
Diastolic blood pressure			<0.001 *
<80 mmHg	1964 (50.6)	7306 (47.0)	
80–89 mmHg	1355 (34.9)	5540 (35.7)	
≥90 mmHg	565 (14.6)	2690 (17.3)	
Fasting blood glucose			0.001 *
<100 mg/dL	2540 (65.4)	9787 (63.0)	
100–125 mg/dL	1044 (26.9)	4297 (27.7)	
≥126 mg/dL	300 (7.7)	1452 (9.4)	
Total cholesterol			0.097
<200 mg/dL	2108 (54.3)	8288 (53.4)	
200–239 mg/dL	1294 (33.3)	5115 (32.9)	
≥240 mg/dL	482 (12.4)	2133 (13.7)	
CCI score			0.138
0	2630 (67.7)	10,594 (68.2)	
1	582 (15.0)	2254 (14.5)	
2	337 (8.7)	1206 (7.8)	
3	149 (3.8)	633 (4.1)	
≥4	186 (4.8)	849 (5.5)	
Migraine with/without aura	263 (6.8)	507 (3.3)	<0.001 *
Migraine without aura	253 (6.5)	476 (3.1)	<0.001 *
Migraine with aura	10 (0.3)	31 (0.2)	0.482

CCI, Charlson Comorbidity Index; TMD, temporomandibular disorder. * Chi-squared test, significance at $p < 0.05$.
[†] Obesity (body mass index, kg/m^2) was categorized as underweight (<18.5), normal (≥18.5 to <23), overweight (≥23 to <25), obese I (≥25 to <30), or obese II (≥30).

The adjusted HR for migraine was 2.10 (95% CI: 1.81–2.44) in the TMD group compared to the control group (Table 2). The results were consistent in subgroup analyses according to age and sex. These were also exhibited in the Kaplan–Meier analysis (Figure 2).

Table 2. Crude and adjusted hazard ratios (95% confidence interval) for migraine in temporomandibular disorder and control groups.

Characteristics	Hazard Ratios for Migraine			
	Crude [†]	p-Value	Adjusted [†,‡]	p-Value
Total participants (n = 19,420)				
TMD	2.12 (1.83–2.46)	<0.001 *	2.10 (1.81–2.44)	<0.001 *
Control	1.00		1.00	
Age < 60 years old, men (n = 4040)				
TMD	2.07 (1.34–3.19)	0.001 *	2.03 (1.31–3.14)	0.002 *
Control	1.00		1.00	
Age < 60 years old, women (n = 4890)				
TMD	1.92 (1.49–2.48)	<0.001 *	1.88 (1.46–2.44)	<0.001 *
Control	1.00		1.00	
Age ≥ 60 years old, men (n = 4725)				
TMD	2.24 (1.55–3.22)	<0.001 *	2.29 (1.58–3.31)	<0.001 *
Control	1.00		1.00	
Age ≥ 60 years old, women (n = 5765)				
TMD	2.30 (1.80–2.93)	<0.001 *	2.28 (1.78–2.91)	<0.001 *
Control	1.00		1.00	

CCI, Charlson Comorbidity Index; TMD, temporomandibular disorder. * Stratified Cox proportional hazard regression model, significance at $p < 0.05$. [†] Models were stratified by age, sex, income, and region of residence. [‡] The model was adjusted for obesity, smoking, alcohol consumption, systolic blood pressure, diastolic blood pressure, fasting blood glucose, total cholesterol, and CCI scores.

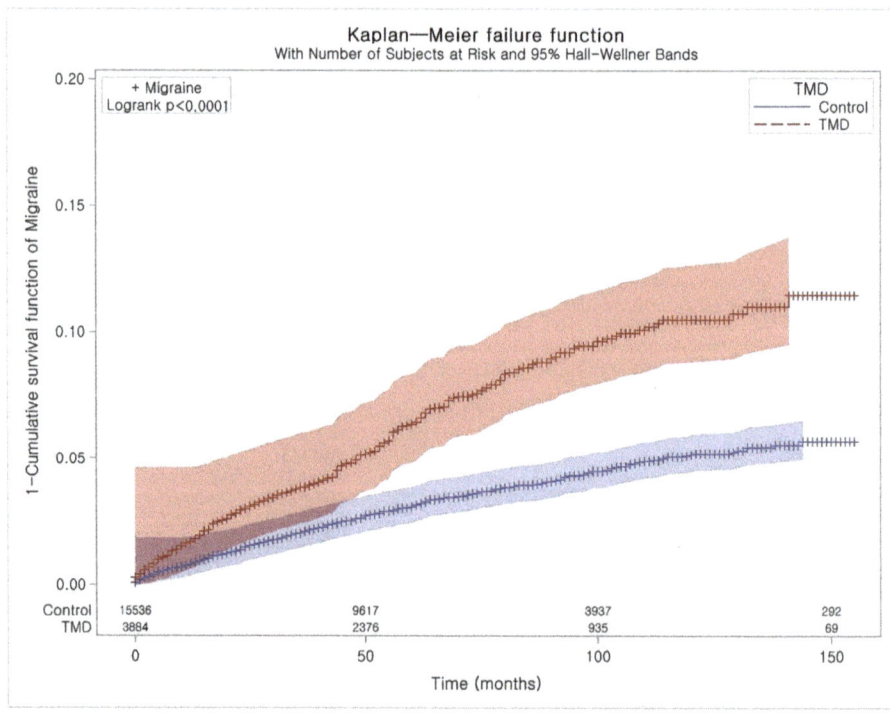

Figure 2. Kaplan–Meier curve of temporomandibular disorder with migraine with and without aura.

This study additionally analyzed the HRs for migraine with and without aura. The adjusted HR for migraine with aura did not reach statistical significance (Figure S1, Table S1). However, the adjusted HR for migraine without aura was significant in every subgroup (Figure S2, Table S2).

4. Discussion

Marklund et al. reported that subjects with TMD had a three-fold greater risk of developing frequent headaches during the 2-year longitudinal study. However, this study did not include a large population [36]. Lim et al. showed that subjects who developed TMD had more headaches compared with those who did not develop TMD and collected data by using a questionnaire [37].

The present study evaluated the association between TMD and migraine by calculating the adjusted HR of migraine after a diagnosis of TMD and used a large population-based dataset which was collected by dentists and physicians who performed objective examinations. The adjusted, statistically significant HR for migraine was 2.10 in the TMD group compared to the control group ($p < 0.001$). The results were consistent in subgroup analyses according to age and sex. These were also shown in the Kaplan–Meier analysis. These results demonstrated that the presence of TMD could increase the risk of migraine. The adjusted HR for migraine with aura did not reach statistical significance ($p > 0.05$). However, the adjusted HR for migraine without aura was significant in every subgroup ($p < 0.001$). These supplementary results could be due to an inaccurate statistical analysis. The association between TMD and migraine is known as a bidirectional link. Both diseases could induce the development of craniomaxillofacial allodynia during painful aggravation. This symptom is associated with peripheral and central sensitization. TMD could activate central sensitization and reduce the pain threshold in migraine [38]. In addition, parafunctional habits and associated painful TMD also could increase the risk for chronic migraine [39,40].

These diseases are related to the common nociceptive system. The preliminary neurons involved in migraine are linked to the first branch of the trigeminal nerve and to the trigeminocervical complex, and those involved in TMD are linked to the neurons of the third branches of the trigeminal nerve [24,41,42]. This nociceptive information converges toward the caudal nucleus of the trigeminal nerve, and from there the pathways of headache and TMD share specific central pathways involved in pain modulation, including the limbic system, brainstem nuclei, sensitive cortex, and thalamus [24]. Neurons in the trigeminal nucleus caudalis combine nociceptive input from intracranial and extracranial tissues and receive supraspinal facilitatory and inhibitory inputs [43]. The neurons integrate all these inputs, transmit the net results to the thalamus, and on to the cortex. Through this convergent point, migraine and TMD may influence each other [23].

Both conditions could share a similar genetic and hormonal basis. A previous study suggested that the association between TMD pain and migraine in women may be partially due to a modest shared genetic risk for both diseases [44]. Sex hormones, such as estrogen, may also control trigeminal nerve sensitization by modulating nociceptive mediators, such as calcitonin gene-related peptide (CGRP) [45]. The OPPERA (Orofacial Pain: Prospective Evaluation and Risk Assessment) study found a complex pattern of considerable changes in biopsychosocial function associated with changes in TMD status. Several biopsychosocial parameters improved among participants with chronic TMD despite pain persisting for years, suggesting considerable potential for ongoing coping and adaptation in response to persistent pain. These biopsychosocial factors could also influence the occurrence of migraine and mutual interaction between TMD and migraine [46].

Based on the results of the present study, clinicians could consider the possibility of improvement in migraine by the treatment of TMD. A few studies have suggested TMD treatment as a solution for migraine. Wright et al. reported that the headache disability score decreased by 17%, the consumption of analgesics was reduced by 18%, and headaches were reduced by 19%, with statistically significant differences, after TMD treatment [47]. Lim et al. showed that the treatment of TMD can improve frequent tension-type headaches associated with TMD secondary to problems of the TMJ [48].

This study had some advantages. First, the data were collected by trained and experienced dentists and physicians. Many previous studies were performed by researchers with questionnaires rather than clinicians [25,30,37,49]. Second, this study utilized a large population-based dataset, the Korean National Health Insurance Service-Health Screening Cohort, which was representative of the Korean population. There have been some studies about the association between TMD and migraine, but most of them were based on data from small populations [23,25,26,30,50]. Moreover, TMD participants were followed up for a maximum of 13 years. Third, various influential factors were adjusted to reduce surveillance bias. This study included multiple confounding factors, such as smoking, alcohol consumption, obesity, and hypertension. Lastly, both TMD and migraine are common conditions, so this study would have great clinical significance for clinicians.

This study also had some disadvantages. First, there were lower numbers of participants for subgroups through the matching procedure. Even though this study started with 514,866 participants, there were only 41 participants with migraine with aura. This may have led to inaccurate results in subgroup analyses. Second, we attempted to adjust for as many factors as possible. However, it was difficult to adjust for all factors, as not all factors were included in the dataset. Finally, the diagnosis of TMD was based on ICD-10. However, to provide the TMD phenotype of a patient population, more accurate criteria such as diagnostic criteria for temporomandibular disorders (DC/TMD) could be utilized. If the diagnosis was made by using standardized and validated criteria such as DC/TMD, the results of this study would be more trustworthy [51].

5. Conclusions

This study demonstrated that TMD patients have a higher risk of migraine. This suggests that dentists can decrease the risk of migraine in TMD patients by managing this condition properly.

However, this study did not show that all migraines could be prevented or treated by TMD treatment alone. This study simply showed that TMD could be an influential factor on migraine, so clinicians should be aware of the presence of TMD in migraine patients. If TMD symptoms are found in migraine patients, these symptoms must be managed. In addition, dentists should also determine the presence of migraine in TMD patients. If migraine is confirmed, patients should be referred to the neurology department for further evaluation and treatment.

Supplementary Materials: The following are available online at http://www.mdpi.com/2075-4418/10/9/724/s1, Figure S1: Subgroup analyses of crude and adjusted hazard ratios (95% confidence interval) for migraine with aura in temporomandibular disorder and control groups, Figure S2: Subgroup analyses of crude and adjusted hazard ratios (95% confidence interval) for migraine without aura in temporomandibular disorder and control groups, Table S1: Subgroup analyses of crude and adjusted hazard ratios (95% confidence interval) for migraine with aura in temporomandibular disorder and control groups, Table S2: Subgroup analyses of crude and adjusted hazard ratios (95% confidence interval) for migraine without aura in temporomandibular disorder and control groups.

Author Contributions: Conceptualization, S.-H.B. and H.-G.C.; data curation, C.M. and H.-G.C.; formal analysis, C.M. and H.-G.C.; funding acquisition, H.-G.C.; investigation, S.-H.B. and H.-G.C; methodology, C.M. and H.-G.C.; project administration, H.-G.C.; resources, D.-M.Y. and B.-E.Y.; software, S.-H.B. and D.-M.Y.; supervision, S.-H.B., B.-E.Y., and H.-G.C.; validation, S.-H.B. and H.-G.C.; writing—original draft, S.-H.B.; writing—review and editing, S.-H.B. All authors have read and agreed to the published version of the manuscript.

Funding: This work was supported in part by a research grant (NRF-2018-R1D1A1A0-2085328) from the National Research Foundation (NRF) of Korea and the Hallym University Research Fund (HURF). This work was supported by the Korea Medical Device Development Fund grant funded by the Korea government (the Ministry of Science and ICT; the Ministry of Trade, Industry, and Energy; the Ministry of Health & Welfare, Republic of Korea; and the Ministry of Food and Drug Safety).

Conflicts of Interest: The authors declare no conflict of interest.

References

1. Fernandes, G.; Franco, A.L.; Siqueira, J.T.T.; Gonçalves, D.A.D.G.; Camparis, C.M. Sleep bruxism increases the risk for painful temporomandibular disorder, depression and non-specific physical symptoms. *J. Oral Rehabil.* **2012**, *39*, 538–544. [CrossRef] [PubMed]
2. Ramírez, L.M.; Ballesteros, L.E.; Sandoval, G.P. [Otological symptoms among patients with temporomandibular joint disorders]. *Rev. Médica Chile* **2008**, *135*, 1582–1590.
3. Kang, J.-H. Effects on migraine, neck pain, and head and neck posture, of temporomandibular disorder treatment: Study of a retrospective cohort. *Arch. Oral Boil.* **2020**, *114*, 104718. [CrossRef] [PubMed]

4. Motghare, V.; Kumar, J.; Kamate, S.; Kushwaha, S.; Anand, R.; Gupta, N.; Gupta, B.; Singh, I. Association Between Harmful Oral Habits and Sign and Symptoms of Temporomandibular Joint Disorders Among Adolescents. *J. Clin. Diagn. Res.* **2015**, *9*, ZC45–ZC48. [CrossRef]
5. Chaudhari, P.K.; Verma, S.K.; Maheshwari, S. Etiological factors of temporomandibular joint disorders. *Natl. J. Maxillofac. Surg.* **2012**, *3*, 238–239. [CrossRef]
6. Okeson, J.P. Temporomandibular disorders in children. *Pediatr. Dent.* **1989**, *11*, 325–329.
7. Christidis, N.; Ndanshau, E.L.; Sandberg, A.; Tsilingaridis, G. Prevalence and treatment strategies regarding temporomandibular disorders in children and adolescents—A systematic review. *J. Oral Rehabil.* **2019**, *46*, 291–301. [CrossRef]
8. Graff-Radford, S.B. Temporomandibular Disorders and Headache. *Dent. Clin. North Am.* **2007**, *51*, 129–144. [CrossRef]
9. Vgontzas, A.; Burch, R. Episodic Migraine With and Without Aura: Key Differences and Implications for Pathophysiology, Management, and Assessing Risks. *Curr. Pain Headache Rep.* **2018**, *22*, 78. [CrossRef]
10. Olesen, J.D. International Classification of Headache Disorders. *Lancet Neurol.* **2018**, *17*, 396–397. [CrossRef]
11. Buse, D.C.; Loder, E.W.; Gorman, J.A.; Stewart, W.F.; Reed, M.L.; Fanning, K.M.; Serrano, D.; Lipton, R.B. Sex Differences in the Prevalence, Symptoms, and Associated Features of Migraine, Probable Migraine and Other Severe Headache: Results of the American Migraine Prevalence and Prevention (AMPP) Study. *Headache J. Head Face Pain* **2013**, *53*, 1278–1299. [CrossRef] [PubMed]
12. Krivánek, J. Spreading cortical depression and acetylcholinesterase activity in rat cerebral cortex. *Physiol. Bohemoslov.* **1972**, *21*, 163–169. [PubMed]
13. Sugaya, E.; Takato, M.; Noda, Y. Neuronal and glial activity during spreading depression in cerebral cortex of cat. *J. Neurophysiol.* **1975**, *38*, 822–841. [CrossRef] [PubMed]
14. Shinohara, M.; Dollinger, B.; Brown, G.; Rapoport, S.; Sokoloff, L. Cerebral glucose utilization: Local changes during and after recovery from spreading cortical depression. *Science* **1979**, *203*, 188–190. [CrossRef] [PubMed]
15. Hansen, J.M.; Charles, A.C. Differences in treatment response between migraine with aura and migraine without aura: Lessons from clinical practice and RCTs. *J. Headache Pain* **2019**, *20*, 96. [CrossRef]
16. Giordano, J.; Schatman, M.E. A crisis in chronic pain care: An ethical analysis. Part three: Toward an integrative, multi-disciplinary pain medicine built around the needs of the patient. *Pain Physician* **2008**, *11*, 775–784.
17. De Leeuw, R.; Klasser, G.D.; Albuquerque, R.J. Are female patients with orofacial pain medically compromised? *J. Am. Dent. Assoc.* **2005**, *136*, 459–468. [CrossRef]
18. Lim, P.F.; Maixner, W.; Khan, A.A. Temporomandibular disorder and comorbid pain conditions. *J. Am. Dent. Assoc.* **2011**, *142*, 1365–1367. [CrossRef]
19. Fernández-De-Las-Peñas, C.; Galán-Del-Río, F.; Fernández-Carnero, J.; Pesquera, J.; Arendt-Nielsen, L.; Svensson, P. Bilateral Widespread Mechanical Pain Sensitivity in Women with Myofascial Temporomandibular Disorder: Evidence of Impairment in Central Nociceptive Processing. *J. Pain* **2009**, *10*, 1170–1178. [CrossRef]
20. Popescu, A.; LeResche, L.; Truelove, E.L.; Drangsholt, M.T. Gender differences in pain modulation by diffuse noxious inhibitory controls: A systematic review. *Pain* **2010**, *150*, 309–318. [CrossRef]
21. Velly, A.M.; Look, J.O.; Carlson, C.; Lenton, P.A.; Kang, W.; Holcroft, C.A.; Fricton, J.R. The effect of catastrophizing and depression on chronic pain—A prospective cohort study of temporomandibular muscle and joint pain disorders. *Pain* **2011**, *152*, 2377–2383. [CrossRef] [PubMed]
22. Mercuri, L.G. Temporomandibular Joint Disorder Management in Oral and Maxillofacial Surgery. *J. Oral Maxillofac. Surg.* **2017**, *75*, 927–930. [CrossRef] [PubMed]
23. Gonçalves, D.A.D.C.; Camparis, C.M.; Speciali, J.G.; Franco, A.L.; Castanharo, S.M.; Bigal, M.E. Temporomandibular Disorders Are Differentially Associated with Headache Diagnoses. *Clin. J. Pain* **2011**, *27*, 611–615. [CrossRef] [PubMed]
24. Speciali, J.G.; Dach, F. Temporomandibular Dysfunction and Headache Disorder. *Headache J. Head Face Pain* **2015**, *55*, 72–83. [CrossRef] [PubMed]
25. Gil-Martínez, C.C.-L.A.; Navarro-Fernández, G.; Mangas-Guijarro, M.Á.; Lara-Lara, M.; López-López, A.; Fernández-Carnero, J.; La Touche, R. Comparison Between Chronic Migraine and Temporomandibular Disorders in Pain-Related Disability and Fear-Avoidance Behaviors. *Pain Med.* **2017**, *18*, 2214–2223. [CrossRef]

26. Florencio, L.L.; Oliveira, A.S.; Carvalho, G.F.; Dach, F.; Bigal, M.E.; Fernández-De-Las-Peñas, C.; Grossi, D.B. Association between Severity of Temporomandibular Disorders and the Frequency of Headache Attacks in Women with Migraine: A Cross-Sectional Study. *J. Manip. Physiol. Ther.* **2017**, *40*, 250–254. [CrossRef] [PubMed]
27. Cady, R.; Schreiber, C.; Farmer, K.; Sheftell, F. Primary Headaches: A Convergence Hypothesis. *Headache J. Head Face Pain* **2002**, *42*, 204–216. [CrossRef]
28. Graff-Radford, S.B. Headache problems that can present as toothache. *Dent. Clin. North. Am.* **1991**, *35*, 155–170.
29. Kaniecki, R.G. Migraine and tension-type headache: An assessment of challenges in diagnosis. *Neurology* **2002**, *58*, S15–S20. [CrossRef]
30. Gonçalves, D.A.D.G.; Bigal, M.E.; Jales, L.C.; Camparis, C.M.; Speciali, J.G. Headache and Symptoms of Temporomandibular Disorder: An Epidemiological Study. *Headache J. Head Face Pain* **2010**, *50*, 231–241. [CrossRef]
31. Kim, S.Y.; Min, C.; Oh, D.J.; Choi, H.-G. Tobacco Smoking and Alcohol Consumption Are Related to Benign Parotid Tumor: A Nested Case-Control Study Using a National Health Screening Cohort. *Clin. Exp. Otorhinolaryngol.* **2019**, *12*, 412–419. [CrossRef] [PubMed]
32. Yoon, J.L.; Cho, J.J.; Park, K.M.; Noh, H.-M.; Park, Y. Diagnostic Performance of Body Mass Index Using the Western Pacific Regional Office of World Health Organization Reference Standards for Body Fat Percentage. *J. Korean Med. Sci.* **2015**, *30*, 162–166. [CrossRef] [PubMed]
33. Anuurad, E.; Shiwaku, K.; Nogi, A.; Kitajima, K.; Enkhmaa, B.; Shimono, K.; Yamane, Y. The New BMI Criteria for Asians by the Regional Office for the Western Pacific Region of WHO are Suitable for Screening of Overweight to Prevent Metabolic Syndrome in Elder Japanese Workers. *J. Occup. Health* **2003**, *45*, 335–343. [CrossRef] [PubMed]
34. Choi, H.G.; Min, C.; Lee, C.H.; Kim, S.Y. The Relation of Sudden Sensorineural Hearing Loss in Pediatric Patients With Recurrent Otitis Media. *Otol. Neurotol.* **2020**, *41*, 836. [CrossRef]
35. Quan, H.; Li, B.; Couris, C.M.; Fushimi, K.; Graham, P.; Hider, P.; Januel, J.-M.; Sundararajan, V. Updating and Validating the Charlson Comorbidity Index and Score for Risk Adjustment in Hospital Discharge Abstracts Using Data From 6 Countries. *Am. J. Epidemiol.* **2011**, *173*, 676–682. [CrossRef]
36. Marklund, S.; Wiesinger, B.; Wänman, A. Reciprocal influence on the incidence of symptoms in trigeminally and spinally innervated areas. *Eur. J. Pain* **2010**, *14*, 366–371. [CrossRef]
37. Lim, P.F.; Smith, S.B.; Bhalang, K.; Slade, G.D.; Maixner, W. Development of Temporomandibular Disorders Is Associated With Greater Bodily Pain Experience. *Clin. J. Pain* **2010**, *26*, 116–120. [CrossRef]
38. Grossi, D.B.; Lipton, R.; Napchan, U.; Grosberg, B.; Ashina, S.; Bigal, M. Temporomandibular disorders and cutaneous allodynia are associated in individuals with migraine. *Cephalalgia* **2009**, *30*, 425–432. [CrossRef]
39. Manfredini, D.; Winocur, E.; Guarda-Nardini, L.; Paesani, D.; Lobbezoo, F. Epidemiology of bruxism in adults: A systematic review of the literature. *J. Orofac. Pain* **2013**, *27*, 99–110. [CrossRef]
40. Didier, H.A.; Marchetti, A.; Giannì, A.B.; Tullo, V.; Di Fiore, P.; Peccarisi, C.; D'Amico, D.; Bussone, G.; Marchetti, C. Study of parafunctions in patients with chronic migraine. *Neurol. Sci.* **2014**, *35*, 199–202. [CrossRef]
41. Boening, K.; Wieckiewicz, M.; Paradowska-Stolarz, A.; Wiland, P.; Shiau, Y.-Y. Temporomandibular Disorders and Oral Parafunctions: Mechanism, Diagnostics, and Therapy. *BioMed Res. Int.* **2015**, *2015*, 1–2. [CrossRef] [PubMed]
42. Paparo, F.; Fatone, F.M.G.; Ramieri, V.; Cascone, P. Anatomic relationship between trigeminal nerve and temporomandibular joint. *Eur. Rev. Med. Pharmacol. Sci.* **2008**, *12*, 15–18. [PubMed]
43. Olesen, J.D. Clinical and pathophysiological observations in migraine and tension-type headache explained by integration of vascular, supraspinal and myofascial inputs. *Pain* **1991**, *46*, 125–132. [CrossRef]
44. Plesh, O.; Noonan, C.; Buchwald, D.; Goldberg, J.; Afari, N. Temporomandibular disorder-type pain and migraine headache in women: A preliminary twin study. *J. Orofac. Pain* **2012**, *26*, 91–98. [PubMed]
45. Gupta, S.; McCarson, K.E.; Welch, K.; Berman, N.E. Mechanisms of Pain Modulation by Sex Hormones in Migraine. *Headache J. Head Face Pain* **2011**, *51*, 905–922. [CrossRef] [PubMed]
46. Sauro, K.M.; Becker, W.J. The Stress and Migraine Interaction. *Headache J. Head Face Pain* **2009**, *49*, 1378–1386. [CrossRef]

47. Wright, E.F.; Clark, E.G.; Paunovich, E.D.; Hart, R.G. Headache Improvement through TMD Stabilization Appliance and Self-management Therapies. *CRANIO®* **2006**, *24*, 104–111. [CrossRef]
48. Ekberg, E.; Vallon, D.; Nilner, M. Treatment outcome of headache after occlusal appliance therapy in a randomised controlled trial among patients with temporomandibular disorders of mainly arthrogenous origin. *Swed. Dent. J.* **2002**, *26*, 115–124.
49. Fernandes, G.; Arruda, M.A.; Bigal, M.E.; Camparis, C.M.; Gonçalves, D.A.D.G. Painful Temporomandibular Disorder Is Associated With Migraine in Adolescents: A Case-Control Study. *J. Pain* **2019**, *20*, 1155–1163. [CrossRef]
50. Monticone, M.; Rocca, B.; Abelli, P.; Tecco, S.; Geri, T.; Gherlone, E.F.; Luzzi, D.; Testa, M. Cross-cultural adaptation, reliability and validity of the Italian version of the craniofacial pain and disability inventory in patients with chronic temporomandibular joint disorders. *BMC Oral Health* **2019**, *19*, 244. [CrossRef]
51. Schiffman, E.; Ohrbach, R.; Truelove, E.; Look, J.; Anderson, G.; Goulet, J.-P.; List, T.; Svensson, P.; Gonzalez, Y.; Lobbezoo, F.; et al. Diagnostic Criteria for Temporomandibular Disorders (DC/TMD) for Clinical and Research Applications: Recommendations of the International RDC/TMD Consortium Network* and Orofacial Pain Special Interest Group†. *J. Oral Facial Pain Headache* **2014**, *28*, 6–27. [CrossRef] [PubMed]

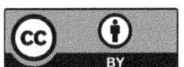

© 2020 by the authors. Licensee MDPI, Basel, Switzerland. This article is an open access article distributed under the terms and conditions of the Creative Commons Attribution (CC BY) license (http://creativecommons.org/licenses/by/4.0/).

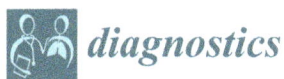

Article

Electromyography-Guided Adjustment of an Occlusal Appliance: Effect on Pain Perceptions Related with Temporomandibular Disorders. A Controlled Clinical Study

Simona Tecco [1,*], Vincenzo Quinzi [2], Alessandro Nota [1], Alessandro Giovannozzi [3], Maria Rosaria Abed [3] and Giuseppe Marzo [2]

1. Faculty of Medicine, Vita-Salute San Raffaele University, I.R.C.C.S. San Raffaele Hospital, 20132 Milano, Italy; nota.alessandro@hsr.it
2. Department of Life, Health and Environmental Sciences, University of L'Aquila, 67100 L'Aquila, Italy; vincenzo.quinzi@univaq.it (V.Q.); giuseppe.marzo@cc.univaq.it (G.M.)
3. Private Practice, 00040 Roma, Italy; alegiovannozzi@gmail.com (A.G.); simtecc@tin.it (M.R.A.)
* Correspondence: tecco.simona@hsr.it

Citation: Tecco, S.; Quinzi, V.; Nota, A.; Giovannozzi, A.; Abed, M.R.; Marzo, G. Electromyography-Guided Adjustment of an Occlusal Appliance: Effect on Pain Perceptions Related with Temporomandibular Disorders. A Controlled Clinical Study. *Diagnostics* **2021**, *11*, 667. https://doi.org/10.3390/diagnostics11040667

Academic Editor: Timo Sorsa

Received: 15 March 2021
Accepted: 6 April 2021
Published: 8 April 2021

Publisher's Note: MDPI stays neutral with regard to jurisdictional claims in published maps and institutional affiliations.

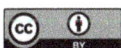

Copyright: © 2021 by the authors. Licensee MDPI, Basel, Switzerland. This article is an open access article distributed under the terms and conditions of the Creative Commons Attribution (CC BY) license (https://creativecommons.org/licenses/by/4.0/).

Abstract: Background: The purpose of this study is to evaluate the effect of an electromyography-guided adjustment of an occlusal appliance on the management of Temporomandibular disorder-related pain. Methods: Data from 40 adult patients (20 males and 20 females), who underwent treatment with occlusal appliances, were recorded. A total of 20 appliances were adjusted according to electromyographic data (group 1), while the others were adjusted by a clinical conventional procedure (group 2). Muscle pain to palpation, pain during articular movements and headache were recorded by a VAS score (from 0 to 100) before the beginning of treatment (T0), at T1 (4 weeks) and T2 (8 weeks). Results: Results showed a reduction of pain in both groups, with a better trend for group 1, where better results were achieved at T1 and maintained stability at T2, with an improved mean value regarding all parameters studied. After 8 weeks, only small recurrences started to occur in muscle pain to palpation in group 2. Conclusions: An occlusal appliance seems to be able to achieve a clinical improvement of Temporomandibular disorder (TMD)-related pain and headache, independently from the adjustment procedure adopted. However, the use of a surface electromyographic activity of masticatory muscles (sEMG) device as an aid in the calibration procedure seems to allow a better trend because the improvement of symptoms was obtained before, after the first four weeks, with an improvement in percentages of all the variables investigated. While the conventional procedure obtained later the improvement.

Keywords: occlusal appliance; electromyography; temporomandibular joint disorders; muscle pain; removable appliance

1. Introduction

Temporomandibular disorders (TMDs) are a heterogeneous group of clinical dysfunctions involving the masticatory muscles and/or temporomandibular joints (TMJ) and associated structures (American Association of Dental research. Policy Statement on TDM. March 2010—reaffirmed 2015—http://www.iadr.org/AADR/About-Us/Policy-Steatments/Science-Policy/Temporomandibular-Disorders-TMD, accessed on 1 February 2021). TMDs are the most prevalent orofacial pain condition, among inflammation (e.g., sinusitis), vascular compression (e.g., vascular migraines), other disorders of the musculoskeletal, neurological and/or neuropathic involvement (e.g., trigeminal neuralgia), and idiopathic trigeminal pain [1].

In general, TMD is believed to affect anywhere between 5 and 15% of adults in the population [2]. Interestingly, there is evidence that the prevalence of TMD appears to be increased in recent years [2].

TMDs are diffused in males and females with a prevalence of female gender, and are also observed in the pediatric and adolescent population (about 11% was reported) [2].

To date, the main guidelines on TMDs management are provided by the American Association of Dental Research (AADR), which read verbatim as follows: "The signs and symptoms associated with these disorders are diverse, and may include difficulties with chewing, speaking, and other orofacial functions. They also are frequently associated with acute or persistent pain, and the patients often suffer from other painful disorders (comorbidities)".

TMDs are classified from painless clicking of the joint (Stage I) to severe degenerative bony changes (Stage V) [2]. In some cases, a patient is diagnosed with multiple diagnoses, and often those diagnoses may change as the disease progresses or resolves.

Chewing problems include intra-articular sounds, reduced range of motion of the lower jaw, pain and discomfort pressing the area around TMJ, or masticatory muscles.

Some signs and symptoms resolve spontaneously even without treatment, whereas others persist for years despite all treatment options having been exhausted [2].

Treatments include the use of occlusal appliances, sometimes surgical procedures as arthrocentesis, cognitive behavioral therapy for muscle parafunction, and other various treatments involving other specialists (physiotherapy, for example) [2].

Again, today, occlusal appliances are the most widely used intraoral devices for the management of pain, due to the reversibility of the procedure [3]. The desired outcomes of reversible therapy with occlusal appliances are essentially a reduction in the Algic component, masticatory muscle relaxation and, hopefully, reduction of headache [4]. Therefore, TMDs are also associated with the presence of intra-articular sounds (clicks) and occlusal splint often reduces their frequency because of its capability to re-establish immediately the normal condyle/disk relationship [2,5].

Therefore, the success of reversible therapy on pain appears to be paramount for long-term rehabilitation [6]. According to the literature, however, there is a lack of clarity regarding the management of occlusal appliances by the clinicians, due to different existing protocols for their adjustment. For example, Wiens (2016) has shown the technical advances over time, but did not reflect a desired clinical outcome [7]. An optimum adjustment should include point-like homogeneous contact points on the appliance, all distributed on the dental arch. The clinical effect of the occlusal appliance should be an improvement of signs and symptoms.

Undoubtedly, it is worth mentioning that the clinical effects of occlusal appliances for the different types of disorders may suffer from the role played by the practitioner itself during the clinical conventional procedure of its adjustment [7,8].

One of the emerging digital procedures for the adjustment of intraoral appliances or prostheses is based on the analysis of surface electromyographic activity of masticatory muscles (sEMG), which monitor the synergistic action of muscles in order to evaluate their balanced function [8,9]. This approach is based on data that highlight how symmetry in the electromyographic activity of the masticatory muscles is necessary for oral [9,10] as well as functional rehabilitation [11]. However, on these digitized procedures, there are no studies that have evaluated the results from a clinical and symptomatological point of view (on pain).

Thus, the purpose of this observational study was to analyze the effects of an electromyography-guided adjustment of an occlusal appliance on muscular pain comparing it with a standard procedure in a control group.

2. Materials and Methods

The present observational protocol was approved by the Ethics Committee of the University of L'Aquila, Italy (Document DR206/2013, dated 10 January 2014). Data from a sample of 40 subjects, 20 males and 20 females, aged between 20 and 30 years old (average 25 years), who were going to receive an occlusal appliance for the management of TMD at George Eastman Dental Hospital in Rome (Italy) were selected for the present study. All the patients complained of muscle tension headache, associated with masticatory muscle pain to palpation, as well as pain during mandibular movements. None of them was affected by disc displacement, or degenerative joint disease. All patients were treated with an individualized 1.5 mm thick occlusal appliance, made of a heat-cured acrylic resin (Duran®, Scheu-Dental Technology, Iserlohn, Germany), applied in their lower jaw (Figure 1).

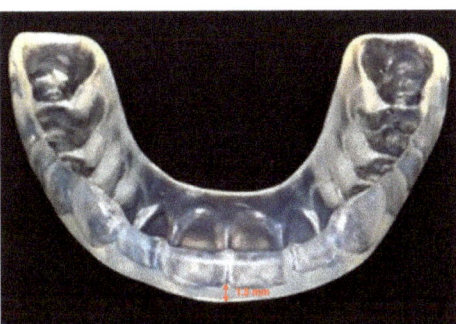

Figure 1. Individualized 1.5 mm thick occlusal appliance, made of a heat-cured acrylic resin (Duran®, Scheu-Dental Technology, Iserlohn, Germany).

In the study group (the study group) (20 patients) the calibration was performed by achieving a condition of muscular balance and relaxation according to sEMG data, whereas in the control group (the control group) (20 patients) it was performed by a standard procedure aimed to achieve homogeneous point-shaped dental contacts on the appliance [12]. The patients were instructed to wear the appliance 22 h per day, removing it only for meals and were treated by the same expert operator (the author A.G.) In the study group, sEMG was performed using TEETHAN® (Teethan S.p.a. Garbagnate Milanese, Milan, Italy) a 4-channel wireless electromyograph, featuring surface electrodes placed at the level of the masseter muscles and anterior temporalis muscle [13,14]. All patients underwent clinical follow up during the subsequent weeks, and painful muscles at palpation, pain arising during mandibular function (functional pain) and headache, were recorded by using the VAS scale, on a range of scores from 0 to 100. Follow-ups were scheduled after 4 weeks (T1) and after 8 weeks (T2) from in the initial phase.

Data Handling and Statistical Analyses

The sample size was evaluated a priori by performing analysis for estimating the minimum number of subjects to achieve a statistical power of 80% with alpha 0.05 on the comparison between groups for the primary outcome. The results showed that a minimum of 18 subjects per group was required. Applying the Shapiro–Wilk W test normal distribution of data was confirmed for the variables muscular pain at palpation (Shapiro–Wilk W = 0.95; $p = 0.14$) and headache (Shapiro–Wilk W = 0.96; $p = 0.19$). Differently, for functional complaints, data did not show a normal distribution (Shapiro–Wilk W = 0.92; $p = 0.008$). Descriptive statistics for the variables muscular pain at palpation and headache included mean and standard deviation. While functional pain was described as median with 25th and 75th percentiles. In order to analyze the variables of muscular pain at palpation and headache, a *t*-test for independent samples was performed to analyze the differences between the groups at each time point while a one-way ANOVA test was adopted to analyze the significance of changes over time. When significant, a post-hoc Tukey test was employed to further illuminate the statistically significant differences. For the variable of functional pain, the Friedman test and the Wilcoxon signed rank test were used to evaluate intra-groups differences; while the Mann–Whitney test was adopted to evaluate between groups differences at T0, T1 and T2. Statistical analyses were performed with the software StatPlus Pro for MAC (build 7.3.3.0/Core v7.3.32; AnalystSoft Inc., 2020, Walnut, CA, USA). For each test, p was set at 0.05 level.

3. Results

Table 1 reports descriptive statistics for the variables muscular pain at palpation and headache. Table 2 reports descriptive statistics for the variable functional pain.

Table 1. Descriptive statistic for muscular pain at palpation and headache. VAS scores mean ± standard deviation (SD).

	Test Group			Control Group		
	T0 Mean ± SD	T1 Mean ± SD	T2 Mean ± SD	T0 Mean ± SD	T1 Mean ± SD	T2 Mean ± SD
VAS (Muscular Pain at Palpation)	54 ± 20.2	15 ± 8.29	13 ± 9.36	60 ± 25.17	24 ± 22.61	34 ± 28.82
VAS (Headache)	35 ± 15.44	11 ± 9.76	11.4 ± 9.13	44 ± 17.18	38 ± 16.08	22 ± 16.13

Table 2. Descriptive statistic for functional pain. VAS scores, median, 25th and 75th percentiles.

	Test Group			Control Group		
	T0 Median (25th and 75th p.le)	T1 Median (25th and 75th p.le)	T2 Median (25th and 75th p.le)	T0 Median (25th and 75th p.le)	T1 Median (25th and 75th p.le)	T2 Median (25th and 75th p.le)
VAS (Functional Pain)	29.5 (18.75–48.5)	10 * (5–20.25)	12.5 (8.75–22.25)	52.5 (26.5–66.25)	25 (10–56.25)	9 (3.75–11.25)

$* p < 0.05$.

3.1. Muscular Pain at Palpation

At T0, VAS score averaged 54 in group 1 and 60 in group 2 (range: 10–90 for the whole sample), without any statistically significant difference between the two groups. While at T2, a significantly lower mean VAS score was observed in the study group respect to the control group (mean difference = −21; 95% C.I. = −43.04–1.04; t = 3.22; $p < 0.05$) (Figure 2).

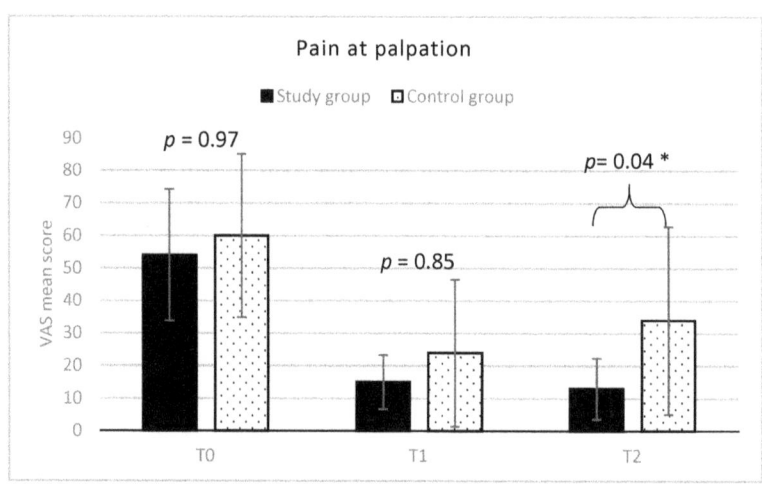

Figure 2. Muscle pain at palpation (mean VAS scores and SD) in the two groups. * indicates between groups statistically significant differences ($p < 0.05$).

Considering the trend of the variable in each group over time, VAS significantly decreased at T1 in the test group, achieving a mean value of 15 (T0-T1 mean difference = 39;

95% C.I. = 16.95–61.04; t = 5.99; $p < 0.01$), and it remained almost stable at T2, with a mean value of 13 (T0-T2 mean difference = 41; 95% C.I. = 18.95–63.04; t = 6.29; $p < 0.01$) (Figure 3).

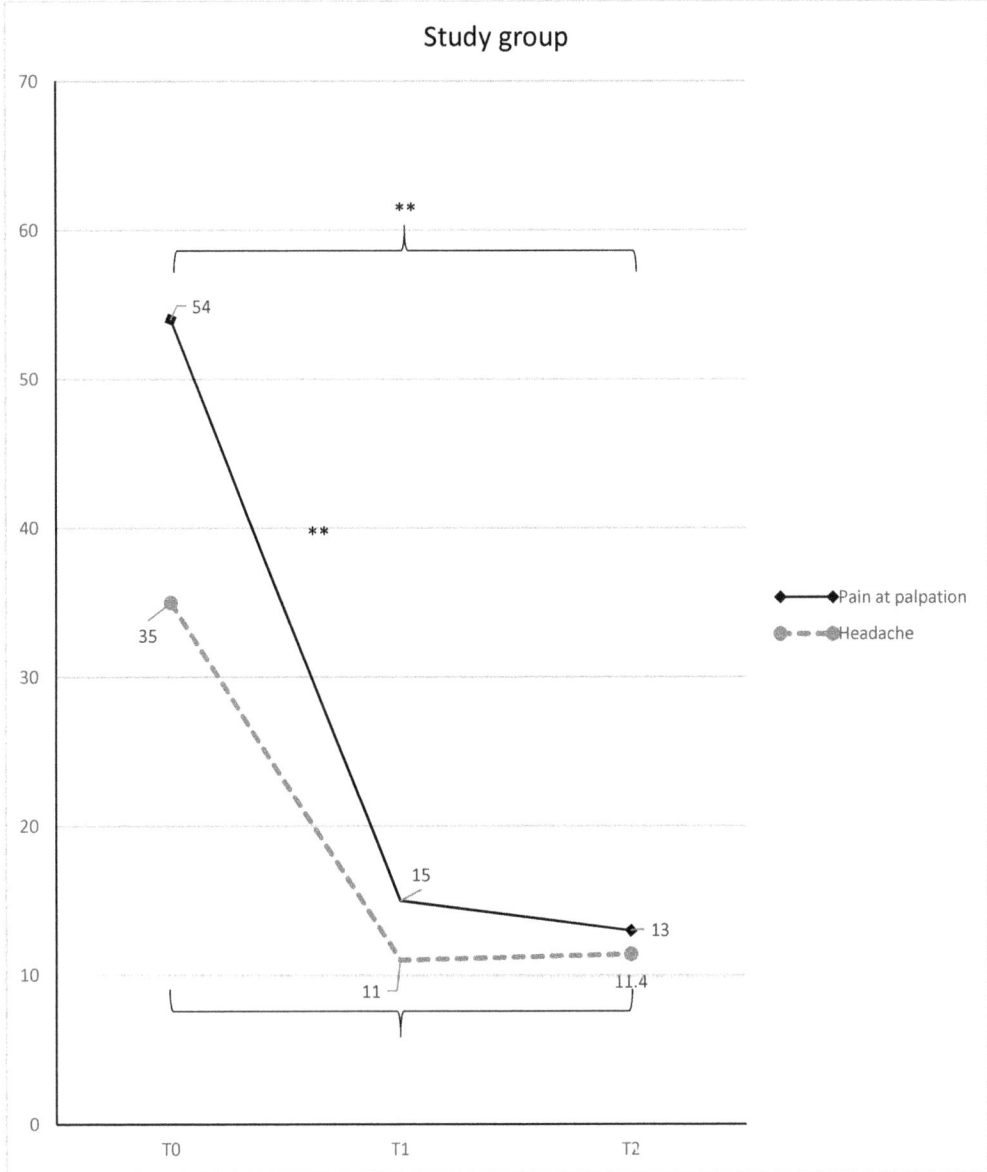

Figure 3. Muscle pain at palpation and headache (mean VAS scores and SD) in the study group, with statistically significant differences overtime (* = $p < 0.05$; ** = $p < 0.01$).

In the control group, it scored from 60 to 24 at T1 (T0-T1 mean difference = 36; 95% C.I. = 13.95–58.04; t = 5.53; $p < 0.01$), and 34 at T2 (T0-T2 mean difference = 26; 95% C.I. = 3.95–48.04; t = 3.99; $p < 0.01$) (Figure 4).

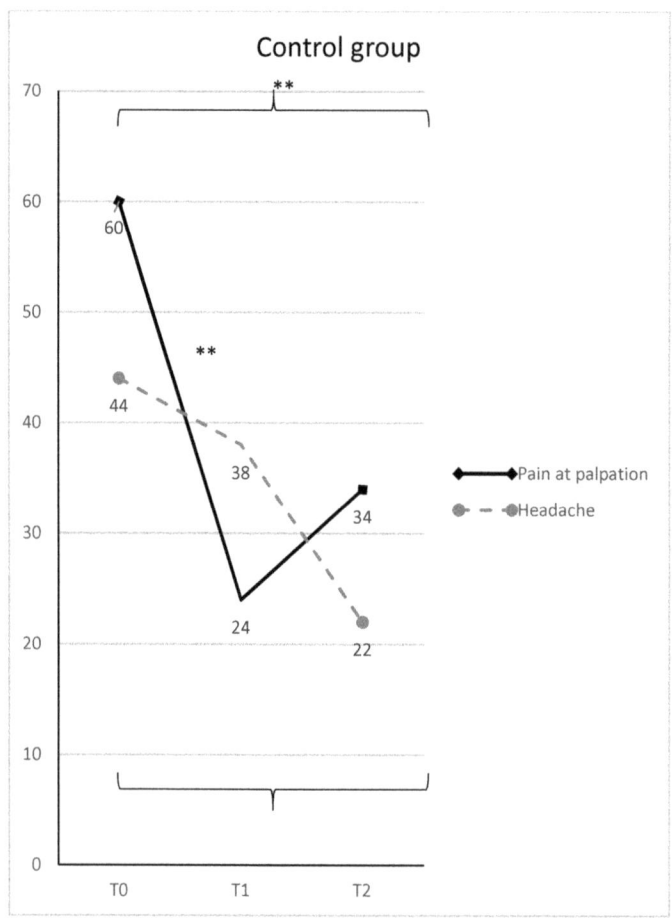

Figure 4. Muscle pain at palpation and headache (mean VAS scores and SD) in the control group, with statistically significant differences overtime (* = $p < 0.05$; ** = $p < 0.01$).

3.2. Functional Pain

At T0, the median VAS score in the study group 29.5, and it was 52.5 in the control group, (range: 10–90 for the whole sample), without any statistically significant difference between the two groups. At T1 the study group showed a statistically significant lower VAS score, with respect to the control group (Mann–Whitney U = 282,000; $p = 0.026$) (Table 2). No statistically significant differences were observed at T2. Considering the trend over time, the study group experimented with a statistically significant reduction of pain over time, from T0 to T1 (Wilcoxon ranks z = −3.82; $p < 0.01$); and from T0 to T2 (Wilcoxon ranks z = −3.57; $p < 0.01$) (Figure 5).

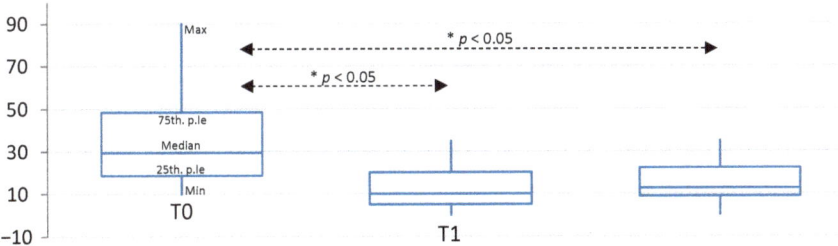

Figure 5. Box plots represent median, 25th and 75th percentiles of VAS scores for functional pain in the study group over time. * indicates statistically significant differences, $p < 0.05$.

The control group showed a statistically significant decrease of VAS score from T0 to T1 (Wilcoxon ranks $z = -3.40$; $p < 0.01$); from T0 to T2 (Wilcoxon ranks $z = -3.74$; $p < 0.01$); and from T1 to T2 (Wilcoxon ranks $z = -3.04$; $p < 0.01$) (Figure 6).

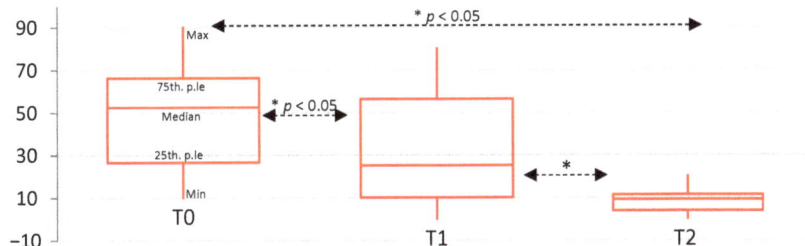

Figure 6. Box plots represent median, 25th and 75th percentiles of VAS scores for functional pain in the control group over time. * indicates statistically significant differences, $p < 0.05$.

3.3. Muscular Tension Headache

The trend of headache VAS score for both the groups, at any stage, is depicted in Figure 7.

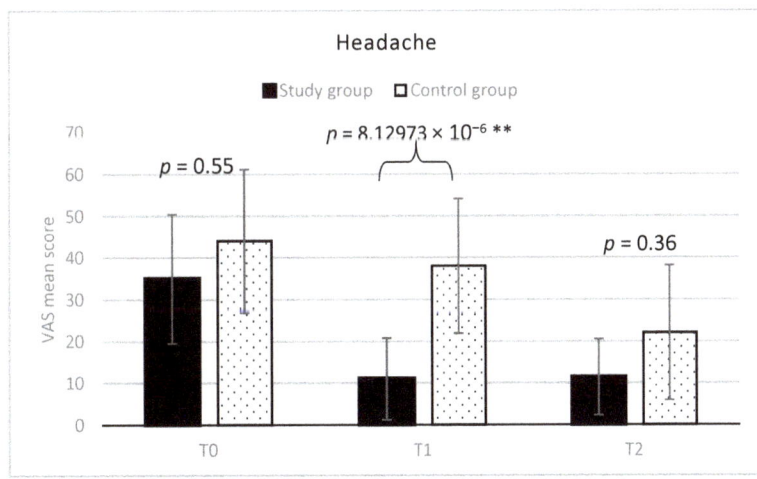

Figure 7. Headache at palpation (mean VAS scores and SD) in the two groups. ** indicates between groups statistically significant differences ($p < 0.01$).

At T0, VAS averaged 35 in group 1, and 44 in group 2 (range: 10–70 for the whole sample) without any statistically significant difference between the two groups. At T1, the study group showed a significantly lower mean VAS score, respect to the control group (mean difference = 27; 95% C.I. = 42.34–11.65; t = 5.95; $p < 0.01$). However, there was not any statistically significant difference between the two groups at T2. Considering the trend over time, VAS significantly decreased in the study group till a value of 11 (mean difference T0-T1 = 24; 95% C.I. = 8.65–39.34; t = 5.29; $p = 0.0001$) and remained almost stable at T2 (mean difference T0-T2 = 23; 95% C.I. = 8.25–38.94; t = 5.20; $p = 0.0001$) (Figure 3). Differently, in the control group VAS scores decreased overtime more slowly and became 38 at T1, and 22 at T2 (T0-T2 mean difference = 22; 95% C.I. = 6.65–37.34; t = 4.85; $p = 0.00059$) (Figure 4). The percentages of VAS score improvement for all the considered variables in the two groups are reported for both the groups in Table 3.

Table 3. Intra-group differences expressed in percentage for both the groups.

	Group 1			Group 2		
	T0-T1	T1-T2	T0-T2	T0-T1	T1-T2	T0-T2
Muscular Pain at Palpation	−72.22%	−13.32%	−75.92%	−60.00%	+41.66%	−43.33%
Headache	−68.57%	+3.63%	−67.42%	−13.63%	−42.10%	−50%
Functional Pain	−66.66%	+25%	−58.33%	−36.00%	−62.5%	−76%

4. Discussion

This observational study was aimed to compare the effect of occlusal appliances adjusted with sEMG aid (the study group) versus the conventional adjustment procedure (the control group) in the management of TMDs related pain.

The comparison of the VAS scores between the two groups showed some improvements for both groups. However, it seems that there was a better trend for the study group, respect to the control group. For the study group, the improvement of symptoms was obtained after the first four weeks (T0-T1 difference), with an improvement in percentages of all the variables investigated. While the control group showed a slightly different trend after the first four weeks of treatment, with a lower improvement (in percentage) than the study group. In addition, the control subjects showed a recurrence of light symptoms as shown by the score obtained for muscle palpation after the first four weeks, between T1 and T2, but results indicate that there was a statistically significant improvement of this variable from T0 to T2. Overall, in conclusion, between T1 and T2 there were positive results, for both the groups, according to all the other variables.

Thus, the present observations confirm that the most common and widespread therapy procedure for TMDs consisting of the use of occlusal appliances, is useful in controlling the pain related to altered muscular activity [7,8]. Thus, the present findings seem to support the principle that occlusal appliances could be able to maintain a primary role in the symptomatic treatment of TMD patients, allowing a change in the distribution of joint load vectors and relaxation of muscle fibers.

The TMJ is located near a major nerve in the face, which is at the center of a network of nerves that connect throughout the face, head and neck. So when the TMJ is affected, pain can spread throughout the face, head and neck (the eyes, ears, mouth, forehead, cheeks, tongue, teeth and throat). Even the muscles of the neck can be involved.

TMDs are diffused in males and females with a prevalence of female gender [15]. They are also observed in the pediatric and adolescent population, (about 11% was reported) [2] in which they were related also to poor cervical posture, [16] and in some cases occlusal appliances were also referend to influence the general mandibular posture [17]. Diagnosis is made through an anamnestic questionnaire and clinical exam with palpation [18].

For the study group, the best results were obtained after the first four weeks (T0-T1 difference), with an improvement in percentages of all the variables investigate: in particular, muscular pain at palpation improved by 72.2%, headache by 68.5% and functional pain by 66.6%, with statistically significant differences. The control group showed a slightly different trend after the first four weeks of treatment, with a lower improvement (in percentage) than the study group: muscular pain at palpation improved by 60%, headache by 13% and functional pain by 36%. In the control group, headache showed an improvement later than other symptoms, as results indicate that there was a statistically significant improvement of this variable from T0 to T2 in group 2. After the first four weeks, between T1 and T2, there was a recurrence of light symptoms as shown by the score obtained by the control group for muscle palpation (41% worsening between T1 and T2) (Figure 4). Overall, between T1 and T2, there were positive results for both the groups, according to all the other variables. It can be concluded from the present data that the general outcome was an overall improvement for both groups between T0 and T2.

The results observed in the study group, where the occlusal appliance adjustment was aided by sEMG, seem to suggest that a better adjustment of the appliance was performed, helping the clinician to increase the predictability in the balance of the bilateral contacts of the occlusal appliance, as previously suggested [19–22]. The use of electromyography to adjust an occlusal splint is only one of the techniques that can be used for the adjustment of an occlusal splint, so the present results cannot be generalized for all the other technique.

Multiple designs are available, such as hard, soft, and anterior repositioning splint. At present, there is no consensus on which design is superior, as results from different studies are equivocal in terms of the efficacy of different designs of occlusal splints [2].

It should be considered that the traditional procedure applied in the control group, without using any digital equipment, could bring results more dependent on the practitioner's expertise. The worsening percentage for muscle pain to palpation, registered between T1 and T2 in group 2 may be justified by the fact that, after an initial unlocking of the occlusion and subsequent improvement of the symptomatology, the modified occlusion could have determined the onset of new symptoms. For this reason, occlusal appliances are generally preferred and recommended against irreversible treatments, as modifying the occlusion in the long term could expose the patient to the risk of recurrence of symptomatology. On the other hand, the sEMG seems a useful method for improving the quality and predictability of the appliance adjustment, even though it also requires a learning curve for its use.

5. Conclusions

An occlusal appliance seems to be able to achieve a clinical improvement of TMDs related pain and headache, independently from the adjustment procedure adopted.

However, the use of an sEMG device as an aid in the calibration procedure seems to allow a better trend because the improvement of symptoms was obtained before and after the first four weeks, with an improvement in percentages of all the variables investigated. Meanwhile, the conventional procedure was obtained later than the improvement.

Future studies will clarify the effects of other material-based appliances or adjustment procedures for clinics.

Author Contributions: Conceptualization, S.T., A.G. and A.N.; methodology, S.T., A.G., M.R.A., A.N.; validation, S.T., A.N., V.Q. and G.M.; formal analysis, S.T. and A.N.; investigation, A.G. and M.R.A.; resources, A.G. and M.R.A.; data curation, S.T. and A.N.; writing—original draft preparation, S.T., A.G. and A.N.; writing—review and editing, S.T. and A.N.; supervision, S.T. and V.Q.; project administration, V.Q. and G.M.; All authors have read and agreed to the published version of the manuscript.

Funding: This research received no external funding.

Institutional Review Board Statement: The study was conducted according to the guidelines of the Declaration of Helsinki and approved by the Institutional Review Board (or Ethics Committee) of the University of L'Aquila, but approval was waived for this study, due to retrospective construction.

Informed Consent Statement: Informed consent was obtained from all subjects involved in the study. Written informed consent has been obtained from the patients to publish this paper.

Data Availability Statement: The data that support the findings of this study are available from the University of L'Aquila, but restrictions apply to the availability of these data, which were used under license for the current study, and so are not publicly available. Data are however available from the authors upon reasonable request and with permission of the University of L'Aquila partner.

Acknowledgments: The authors acknowledge Ettore Accivile for clinical support.

Conflicts of Interest: The authors declare no conflict of interest.

References

1. Manfredini, D.; Perinetti, G.; Stellini, E.; Di Leonardo, B.; Guarda-Nardini, L. Prevalence of Static and Dynamic Dental Malocclusion features in Subgroups of Temporomandibular Disorder Patients: Implications for the Epidemiology of the TMD-Occlusion Association. *Quintessence Int.* **2015**, *46*, 341–349. [PubMed]
2. Li, D.T.S.; Leung, Y.Y. Temporomandibular Disorders: Current Concepts and Controversies in Diagnosis and Management. *Diagnostics* **2021**, *11*, 459. [CrossRef] [PubMed]
3. Ferreira, F.M.; Cézar Simamoto-Júnior, P.; Soares, C.J.; Ramos, A.M.d.A.M.; Fernandes-Neto, A.J. Effect of Occlusal Splints on the Stress Distribution on the Temporomandibular Joint Disc. *Braz. Dent. J.* **2017**, *28*, 324–329. [CrossRef]
4. Bender, S.D. Orofacial Pain and Headache: A Review and Look at the Commonalities. *Curr. Pain Headache Rep.* **2014**, *18*, 400. [CrossRef] [PubMed]
5. Tecco, S.; Festa, F.; Salini, V.; Epifania, E.; D'Attilio, M. Treatment of Joint Pain and Joint Noises Associated with a Recent TMJ Internal Derangement: A Comparison of an Anterior Repositioning Splint, a Full-Arch Maxillary Stabilization Splint, and an Untreated Control Group. *Cranio* **2004**, *22*, 209–219. [CrossRef] [PubMed]
6. Magnusson, T.; Egermarki, I.; Carlsson, G.E. A Prospective Investigation Over Two Decades on Signs and Symptoms of Temporomandibular Disorders and Associated Variables. A Final Summary. *Acta Odontol. Scand.* **2005**, *63*, 99–109. [CrossRef]
7. Wiens, J.P. A Progressive Approach for the Use of Occlusal Devices in the Management of Temporomandibular Disorders. *Gen. Dent.* **2016**, *64*, 29–36.
8. Klasser, G.D.; Greene, C.S. Oral Appliances in the Management of Temporomandibular Disorders. *Oral Surg. Oral Med. Oral Pathol. Oral Radiol. Endod.* **2009**, *107*, 212–223. [CrossRef] [PubMed]
9. Ferrario, V.F.; Sforza, C. Coordinated Electromyographic Activity of the Human Masseter and Temporalis Anterior Muscles During Mastication. *Eur. J. Oral Sci.* **1996**, *104*, 511–517. [CrossRef]
10. Tecco, S.; Cattoni, F.; Darvizeh, A.; Bosco, F.; Sanci, V.; Nota, A.; Gastaldi, G.; Gherlone, E.F. Evaluation of Masticatory Muscle Function Using Digital versus Traditional Techniques for Mockup Fabrication: A Controlled Prospective Study. *Appl. Sci.* **2020**, *10*, 6013. [CrossRef]
11. Tecco, S.; Mummolo, S.; Marchetti, E.; Tetè, S.; Campanella, V.; Gatto, R.; Gallusi, G.; Tagliabue, A.; Marzo, G. sEMG Activity of Masticatory, Neck, and Trunk Muscles During the Treatment of Scoliosis with Functional Braces. A Longitudinal Controlled Study. *J. Electromyogr. Kinesiol.* **2011**, *21*, 885–892. [CrossRef] [PubMed]
12. Al-Rafah, E.M.; Alammari, M.R.; Banasr, F.H. The efficacy of bilateral balanced and canine guidance occlusal splints in the treatment of temporomandibular joint disorder. *Oral Health Dent. Manag.* **2014**, *13*, 536–542.
13. Vieira de Silva, C.A.; da Silva, M.A.M.R.; Melchior, M.d.O.; de Felício, C.M.; Sforza, C.; Tartaglia, G.M. Treatment for TMD with Occlusal Splint and Electromyographic Control: Application of the FARC Protocol in a Brazilian Population. *Cranio* **2012**, *30*, 218–226. [CrossRef] [PubMed]
14. Ciuffolo, F.; Manzoli, L.; Ferritto, A.L.; Tecco, S.; D'Attilio, M.; Festa, F. Surface Electromyographic Response of the Neck Muscles to Maximal Voluntary Clenching of the Teeth. *J. Oral Rehabil.* **2005**, *32*, 79–84. [CrossRef] [PubMed]
15. Tecco, S.; Nota, A.; Caruso, S.; Primozic, J.; Marzo, G.; Baldini, A.; Gherlone, E.F. Temporomandibular Clinical Exploration in Italian Adolescents. *Cranio* **2019**, *37*, 77–84. [CrossRef] [PubMed]
16. Tecco, S.; Caputi, S.; Festa, F. Evaluation of Cervical Posture Following Palatal Expansion: A 12-Month Follow-Up Controlled Study. *Eur. J. Orthod.* **2007**, *29*, 45–51, Erratum in: *Eur. J. Orthod.* **2008**, *30*, 110. [CrossRef] [PubMed]
17. Tecco, S.; Polimeni, A.; Saccucci, M.; Festa, F. Postural Loads During Walking After an Imbalance of Occlusion Created with Unilateral Cotton Roll. *BMC Res Notes.* **2010**, *25*, 3–141. [CrossRef]
18. Schiffman, E.; Ohrbach, R.; Truelove, E.; Look, J.; Anderson, G.; Goulet, J.P.; List, T.; Svensson, P.; Gonzalez, Y.; Lobbezoo, F.; et al. Orofacial Pain Special Interest Group, International Association for the Study of Pain. Diagnostic Criteria for Temporomandibular Disorders (DC/TMD) for Clinical and Research Applications: Recommendations of the International RDC/TMD Consortium Network* and Orofacial Pain Special Interest Group†. *J. Oral Facial Pain Headache* **2014**, *28*, 6–27. [CrossRef]
19. Baldini, A.; Tecco, S.; Cioffi, D.; Rinaldi, A.; Longoni, S. Gnatho-Postural Treatment in an Air Force Pilot. *Aviat. Space Environ. Med.* **2012**, *83*, 522–526. [CrossRef] [PubMed]
20. Ferrario, V.F.; Tartaglia, G.M.; Galletta, A.; Grassi, G.P.; Sforza, C. The Influence of Occlusion on Jaw and Neck Muscle Activity: A Surface EMG study in Healthy Young Adults. *J. Oral Rehabil.* **2006**, *33*, 341–348. [CrossRef]

21. Sforza, C.; Rosati, R.; De Menezes, M.; Musto, F.; Toma, M. EMG Analysis of Trapezius and Masticatory Muscles: Experimental Protocol and Data Reproducibility. *J. Oral Rehabil.* **2011**, *38*, 648–654. [CrossRef] [PubMed]
22. De Felício, C.M.; Ferreira, C.L.P.; Medeiros, A.P.M.; Rodrigues Da Silva, M.A.M.; Tartaglia, G.M.; Sforza, C. Electromyographic Indices, Orofacial Myofunctional Status and Temporomandibular Disorders Severity: A Correlation Study. *J. Electromyogr. Kinesiol.* **2012**, *22*, 266–272. [CrossRef] [PubMed]

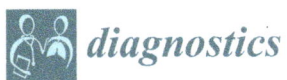

Article

Electromyographic Patterns of Masticatory Muscles in Relation to Active Myofascial Trigger Points of the Upper Trapezius and Temporomandibular Disorders

Grzegorz Zieliński [1], Aleksandra Byś [1], Jacek Szkutnik [2], Piotr Majcher [1] and Michał Ginszt [1,*]

1 Department of Rehabilitation and Physiotherapy, Medical University of Lublin, 20-093 Lublin, Poland; grzegorz.zielinski@umlub.pl (G.Z.); aleksandra.bys@umlub.pl (A.B.); piotr.majcher@umlub.pl (P.M.)
2 Department of Functional Masticatory Disorders, Medical University of Lublin, 20-093 Lublin, Poland; zakladzaburzen@umlub.pl
* Correspondence: michal.ginszt@umlub.pl; Tel.: +48-81-448-6780

Abstract: The presented study aimed to analyze and compare the electromyographic patterns of masticatory muscles in subjects with active myofascial trigger points (MTrPs) within upper trapezius, patients with temporomandibular disorders (TMDs) and healthy adults. Based on the diagnostic criteria of MTrPs according to Travell & Simons and the Research Diagnostic Criteria for Temporomandibular Disorders, 167 people were qualified for the study. Subjects were divided into 3 groups: with active MTrPs in the upper trapezius, with diagnosed temporomandibular disorders (TMDs) and healthy adults. Measurements of the bioelectric activity of the temporalis anterior (TA) and masseter muscle (MM) were carried out using the BioEMG III ™. Based on statistical analysis, significantly lower values of TA resting activity were observed among controls in comparison to MTrPs (1.49 µV vs. 2.81 µV, $p = 0.00$) and TMDs (1.49 µV vs. 2.97 µV, $p = 0.01$). The POC index values at rest differed significantly between MTrPs and TMDs (86.61% vs. 105%, $p = 0.04$). Controls presented different electromyographic patterns within AcI in comparison to both MTrPs (4.90 vs. -15.51, $p = 0.00$) and TMDs (4.90 vs. -16.49, $p = 0.00$). During clenching, the difference between MTrPs and TMDs was observed within MVC TA (91.82% vs. 116.98%, $p = 0.02$). TMDs showed differences within AcI in comparison to both MTrPs group (-42.52 vs. 20.42, $p = 0.01$) and controls (-42.52 vs. 3.07, $p = 0.00$). During maximum mouth opening, differences between MTrPs and TMDs were observed within the bioelectric activity of masseter muscle (16.45 µV vs. 10.73 µV, $p = 0.01$), AsI MM (0.67 vs. 11.12, $p = 0.04$) and AcI (13.04 vs. -3.89, $p = 0.01$). Both the presence of MTrPs in the upper trapezius and TMDs are related to changes in electromyographic patterns of masticatory muscles.

Keywords: electromyography; temporalis anterior; masseter muscle; myofascial pain; myofascial trigger points; trapezius

Citation: Zieliński, G.; Byś, A.; Szkutnik, J.; Majcher, P.; Ginszt, M. Electromyographic Patterns of Masticatory Muscles in Relation to Active Myofascial Trigger Points of the Upper Trapezius and Temporomandibular Disorders. *Diagnostics* **2021**, *11*, 580. https://doi.org/10.3390/diagnostics11040580

Academic Editors: Daniel Fried and Luis Eduardo Almeida

Received: 23 February 2021
Accepted: 20 March 2021
Published: 24 March 2021

Publisher's Note: MDPI stays neutral with regard to jurisdictional claims in published maps and institutional affiliations.

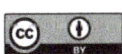

Copyright: © 2021 by the authors. Licensee MDPI, Basel, Switzerland. This article is an open access article distributed under the terms and conditions of the Creative Commons Attribution (CC BY) license (https://creativecommons.org/licenses/by/4.0/).

1. Introduction

Myofascial trigger points (MTrPs) are defined as hyperactive points located in the tense area of the skeletal muscle or its fascia. MTrPs are associated with the development of myofascial pain syndrome (MPS), causing local or referred pain [1]. The compression stimulation of MTrPs may induce a local pain sensation or a referred pain response [2]. The development of MTrPs may be caused by the accumulation of microtraumas within the muscle or its direct injury [1,3]. Muscle overload and consequently the formation of MTrPs, is the result of prolonged or repeated low-amplitude muscle contractions, eccentric contractions and maximal or submaximal muscle contractions [3,4]. Moreover, MTrPs can arise as a result of nutrient deficiencies, hormonal disorders or muscle imbalances [4], fatigue and even viral infections [2,5]. The pathology mentioned above may be related to tissue hypoxia processes in the MTrPs environment [6] when the concentration of inflammatory mediators increases near MTrPs [7]. The above factors may lead to increased nociceptor activity, which results in increased pain response [8]. It is estimated that the prevalence of MPS in clinical populations varies widely, ranging from 9% to 85% [9].

The temporomandibular joint (TMJ) is a bilateral joint composed of the temporal bone's articular surface and the head of the mandible [10]. TMJ is separated into two synovial joint cavities by an articular disc, allowing a smooth articulation between the mandibular condyle and the articular eminence. Moreover, the TMJ disc increases the contact area between opposing articulating surfaces, distributing lower stresses to a larger surface area in the joint [11]. The anterior portion of the TMJ disc is attached to the joint capsule, articular eminence, anterior condyle and the lateral pterygoid's upper area. The posterior portion attaches superiorly to the temporal bone and inferiorly to the posterior condyle. Several ligaments, TMJ disc, articular capsule and masticatory muscles stabilize the TMJ and manage the TMJ forces [12]. Both TMJ dysfunction and abnormalities within masticatory muscles may lead to Temporomandibular Disorders (TMDs). TMDs affect the TMJ, masticatory muscles and/or surrounding tissues and are mainly characterized by pain, acoustic symptoms and limited, incorrect or parafunctional muscle activity [13]. The most common conditions comprising TMDs are myofascial pain, disc displacements and TMJ arthritides [13]. In addition, MPS associated with the presence of MTrPs accounts for approximately 45% of all reported cases of TMDs [14]. Moreover, TMDs significantly reduced life quality and are recognized by the World Health Organization as the third most common dental disease [15,16]. The American National Institute of Dental and Craniofacial Research estimates that TMDs affect 5 to 12% of the population, more often women than men [17]. However, TMDs' etiology is multifactorial and still unclear, with some suggesting that due to their association with other somatic syndromes, TMDs may be part of the same phenomenon [18].

The phenomenon of referred pain is the subject of discussion concerning the stomatognathic system disorders. However, the mechanisms causing this phenomenon have not been clearly explained [19]. Trigger points in the upper trapezius have been associated with tension-type headache episodes [20]. Therefore, through the mechanism of referred pain, MTrPs in the upper trapezius may be responsible for developing pain within the masticatory muscles. The association between TMDs and disorders within cervical spine muscles remaining unclear and there are just several studies confirming the relationship between MTrPs in the cervical muscles and TMDs [21]. Previous reports indicate the coexistence of MTrPs in the neck muscles in patients with TMDs [14,19,22]. However, according to the authors' knowledge, there is a lack of studies that have analyzed the relationship between active MTrPs of the trapezius muscle and the masticatory muscle activity. Thus, the presented study aimed to determine, analyze and compare electromyographic patterns of masticatory muscles in relation to active MTrPs of the upper trapezius and TMDs. Based on the above-mentioned interactions between MTrPs in cervical spine muscles and the occurrence of TMDs, we hypothesize that MTrPs within the upper trapezius significantly influence the activity of the masticatory muscles. We also assume that the electromyographic patterns of masticatory muscles in individuals with MTrPs within trapezius and TMDs patients will differ from healthy individuals.

2. Materials and Methods

The study was carried out in accordance with the recommendations of the Helsinki Declaration and with the consent of the Bioethical Commission of the Medical University of Lublin (approval number KE-0254/346/2016, date of approval 23.11.2016). All participants were informed about the aim of the study and have given written consent for the research.

The inclusion criteria used in the presented study were: age range 18–35 years, good or very good general health status according to the RDC/TMD questionnaire, the presence of active MTrPs in the upper trapezius and absence of any type of TMDs (MTrPs group), presence of pain-related TMDs based on the Research Diagnostic Criteria for Temporomandibular Disorders RDC/TMD [23] without MTrPs in the upper trapezius (TMDs group) and absence of TMDs and active and/or latent MTrPs in the head and neck muscles (control group).

The diagnostic of pain-related TMDs was performed by an experienced dentist with a specialization in dental prosthetics. The TMDs group included only patients with masticatory muscle disorders diagnosed with myalgia—myofascial pain. Patients with temporomandibular joint disorders (e.g., joint pain, disc disorders, joint diseases), other masticatory muscle dysfunctions (e.g., contracture, tendonitis, myositis, spasm, hypertrophy), fibromyalgia, headaches attributed to TMD and coronoid hyperplasia were excluded from the presented study [24].

The presence of active MTrPs within the upper trapezius was established by the following diagnostic criteria according to Travell and Simons [2].

- the presence of a taut band within the above-mentioned muscle;
- presence of a tender nodule within the taut band;
- recognizing pain as previously felt under pressure from a taut band;
- the appearance of radiating pain under pressure.

The following exclusion criteria were used: skin diseases in the head and neck area, neurological disorders in the head and neck area, neoplastic diseases (regardless of type and location), head and neck injuries within the last 6 months before the examination, surgical treatment in the area of head and neck in the last 6 months before the examination, class II and III according to Angle's classification, class I malocclusions patients, open bite, having an orthodontic appliance, lack of four support zones in dental arches, lack of more than four teeth within both dental arches and possession of dental prostheses (regardless of type). After applying the above criteria, 167 people (age 26 ± 8 years) were divided into three groups: 60 in the MTrPs group, 47 in the TMDs group and 60 controls (Table 1).

Table 1. General characteristics of participants.

	MTrPs Group	TMDs Group	Control Group	p Value MTrPs vs. TMDs	p Value MTrPs vs. Controls	p Value TMDs vs. Controls
N	60	47	60	1.00	1.00	1.00
Female	42	33	42	1.00	1.00	1.00
Male	18	14	18	1.00	1.00	1.00
Age	23 ± 3	33 ± 1	23 ± 3	0.00 *	1.00	0.00 *

* Significant difference.

In the next stage, an electromyographic examination was carried out, which was always performed in the morning hours (9 am–11 am) to reduce the impact of the daily bioelectric variability of muscles on the results. The subjects sat on the dental chair, the head rested on the headrest and the torso was perpendicular to the ground. The lower limbs were straight, relaxed and parallel. Before electrode placement, the skin was cleansed with a 90% ethyl alcohol solution to reduce electrode–skin impedance. Ag/AgCl electrodes (SORIMEX, Poland) with a diameter of 30 mm and a conductive surface of 16 mm were used. The placement of the surface electrodes was performed following the Surface Electromyography for Non-invasive Assessment of Muscles (SENIAM) project [25]. The surface electrodes were placed on o the temporalis anterior (TA) and the superficial part of the masseter muscle (MM) in accordance with the course of the muscle fibers, according to the placement technique described by Ferrario et al. [26]. The reference electrode was placed on the forehead (Figure 1). An 8-channel BioEMG III^{TM} surface electromyography apparatus with BioPak Measurement System (BioResearch Associates, Inc. Milwaukee, WI, USA) was used for the study.

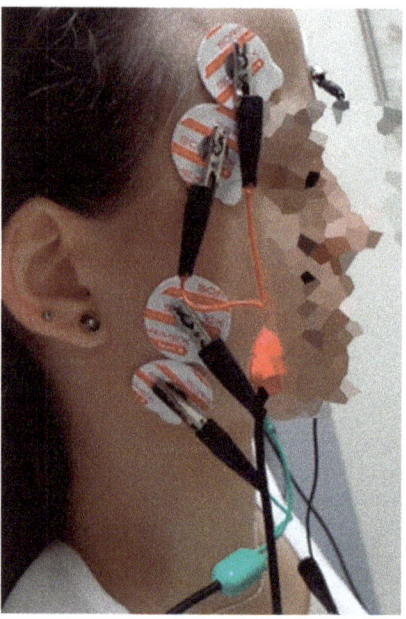

Figure 1. Electrodes placement during the electromyographic examination.

The activity of the masticatory muscles (TA, MM) was recorded in the following protocol: during resting mandibular position (10 s), during maximum voluntary clenching (three clenches of 3 s, each with a 2-s break), during maximum voluntary clenching on dental cotton rollers (three clenches of 3 s, with a 2-s break) and during maximum mouth opening (three abductions of 3 s, with a 2-s rest between) [27,28].

The electromyographic signals were amplified and purified from 99% of the noise scale on a linear scale using the BioPak digital NoiseBuster filter.

Based on the bioelectric data obtained, the following indices were calculated according to standardized protocols:

- MCV (maximum voluntary contraction) based on the formula [28]:

$$MCV = [\text{voluntary teeth clenching}/\text{voluntary teeth clenching on cotton rollers}] \times 100\%$$

- POC (percentage overlapping coefficient) based on the formula [29]:

$$POC = [(MM_{right} + TA_{right})/(MM_{left} + TA_{left})] \times 100\%$$

- AsI (asymmetry index) based on the formula [30]

$$ASI = [(RMS_{right} - RMS_{left})/(RMS_{right} + RMS_{left})] \times 100$$

- AcI (activity index) based on the formula [30]:

$$ACI = [(RMS_{masseter} - RMS_{temporal})/(RMS_{masseter} + RMS_{temporal})] \times 100$$

- TC (torque) based on the formula [31]:

$$TC = [(TA_{right} + MM_{left}) - (TA_{left} + MM_{right})] \times 100\%$$

The checklist developed by the Strengthening the Reporting of Observational Studies in Epidemiology (STROBE) initiative was used to assess the methodological quality of the presented study [32]. IBM SPSS Statistics 21 software was used for statistical analysis. First, the normality of the distribution of variables was verified using the Shapiro-Wilk test and the Kolmogorov–Smirnov test (with Lillierfors correction). All the distributions were abnormal; therefore, the Kruskal—Wallis test was used. The significance level was set at 0.05. When there were significant differences between the analyzed groups, the post-hoc test was applied (Dunn's Test).

3. Results

3.1. General Characteristics of Participants

There were no significant differences in the number of participants and gender between study groups and controls. Post-hoc analysis showed considerable age differences between the TMDs and the rest of the groups (MTrPs group and controls) (Table 1).

There were significant differences in the mandibular range of motion (ROM) between TMDs group vs. controls and TMDs vs. MTrPs. TMDs presented a decrease within the maximum comfortable pain-free opening (MCO), maximum mouth opening (MMO) and protrusion compared to other groups. Moreover, statistical analysis showed differences in the right lateral excursion (RLE) between the TMDs and controls. The mean mandibular ROM values were similar between MTrPs and controls (Table 2).

Table 2. Comparison of the mean values (± SD) of mandibular range of motion during maximum comfortable pain-free opening (MCO), maximum mouth opening (MMO), right lateral excursion (RLE), left lateral excursion (LLE) and protrusion between groups.

	MTrPs Group	TMDs Group	Control Group	p Value MTrPs vs. TMDs	p Value MTrPs vs. Controls	p Value TMDs vs. Controls
MCO (mm)	50.13 ± 7.38	35.13 ± 13.08	51.13 ± 6.12	0.00 *	1.00	0.00 *
MMO (mm)	51.22 ± 7.49	42.51 ± 11.05	51.57 ± 6.10	0.00 *	1.00	0.00 *
RLE (mm)	9.00 ± 2.54	7.62 ± 3.52	9.17 ± 2.82	0.18	1.00	0.03 *
LLE (mm)	9.50 ± 2.61	8.34 ± 3.60	9.27 ± 3.21	0.20	1.00	0.43
Protrusion (mm)	7.48 ± 2.49	5.15 ± 2.59	7.60 ± 2.61	0.00 *	1.00	0.00 *

* Significant difference.

3.2. Electromyographic Analysis of Resting Masticatory Muscle Activity

Based on statistical analysis, significantly lower values of TA resting activity were observed among controls in comparison to MTrPs (Controls: 1.49 µV vs. MTrPs: 2.81 µV; $p = 0.00$) and TMDs (Controls: 1.49 µV vs. TMDs: 2.97 µV; $p = 0.01$), as presented in Table 2. The values of POC index at rest differed significantly between MTrPs and TMDs (MTrPs: 86.61% vs. TMDs: 105%; $p = 0.04$). Significant differences in electromyographic patterns between MTrPs and the other groups were also observed for the AsI TA (MTrPs: −14.72 vs. TMDs: −1.48 and Controls: −4.48; $p = 0.00$ and $p = 0.01$, respectively) and TC (MTrPs: −90.43% vs. TMDs: 0.28% and Controls: −3.67%; $p = 0.02$ and $p = 0.03$, respectively). Controls presented different electromyographic patterns within AcI in comparison to both MTrPs (Controls: 4.90 vs. MTrPs: −15.51; $p = 0.00$) and TMDs (Controls: 4.90 vs. TMDs: −16.49; $p = 0.00$) (Table 3).

Table 3. Comparison of the mean values (± SD) of resting bioelectric activity of temporalis anterior (TA), masseter muscle (MM) and electromyographic indices between groups.

		MTrPs Group	TMDs Group	Control Group	p Value MTrPs vs. TMDs	p Value MTrPs vs. Controls	p Value TMDs vs. Controls
Rest	TA (µV)	2.81 ± 1.23	2.97 ± 2.42	1.49 ± 0.51	0.14	0.00 *	0.00 *
	MM (µV)	2.05 ± 1.03	1.81 ± 1.25	1.72 ± 0.83	0.10	0.32	1.00
	POC (%)	86.61 ± 26.78	105.00 ± 40.60	95.92 ± 21.88	0.04 *	0.07	1.00
	AsI TA	−14.72 ± 20.60	−1.48 ± 21.31	−4.48 ± 12.13	0.00 *	0.01 *	1.00
	AsI MM	−1.04 ± 19.27	−0.19 ± 20.62	−2.09 ± 16.27	1.00	1.00	1.00
	AcI R	−7.93 ± 27.87	−15.69 ± 32.81	5.70 ± 23.47	0.84	0.02 *	0.00 *
	AcI L	−21.20 ± 28.13	−16.77 ± 33.07	3.43 ± 23.47	0.97	0.00 *	0.00 *
	AcI	−15.51 ± 25.30	−16.49 ± 31.48	4.90 ± 22.42	1.00	0.00 *	0.00 *
	TC (%)	−90.43 + 191.56	0.28 ± 2.28	−3.67 ± 76.13	0.02 *	0.03 *	1.00

* Significant differences ($p < 0.05$) between groups (Kruskal-Wallis test).

3.3. Electromyographic Analysis of Masticatory Muscle Activity during Clenching

During clenching, difference between MTrPs and TMDs was observed within bioelectric activity of masseter muscle (MTrPs: 120.43 µV vs. TMDs: 68.30 µV; $p = 0.00$) and MVC TA (MTrPs: 91.82% vs. TMDs: 116.98%; $p = 0.02$). Moreover, differences between TMDs and controls were obserwed within bioelectric activity of TA (TMDs: 89.56 µV vs. Controls: 118.37 µV; $p = 0.03$) and MM (TMDs: 68.3 µV vs. Controls: 133.63 µV; $p = 0.00$). In addition, TMDs showed differences within AcI in comparison to both MTrPs group (TMDs: −42.52 vs. MTrPs: 20.42; $p = 0.01$) and controls (TMDs: −42.52 vs. Controls: 3.07; $p = 0.00$) (Table 4).

Table 4. Comparison of the mean values (± SD) of bioelectric activity of temporalis anterior (TA), masseter muscle (MM) and electromyographic indices between groups during clenching.

		MTrPs Group	TMDs Group	Control Group	p Value MTrPs vs. TMDs	p Value MTrPs vs. Controls	p Value TMDs vs. Controls
Clenching	TA (µV)	110.22 ± 63.79	89.56 ± 52.39	118.37 ± 63.77	0.29	0.99	0.03 *
	MM (µV)	120.43 ± 91.15	68.30 ± 46.58	133.63 ± 86.03	0.00 *	0.49	0.00 *
	MVC TA (%)	91.82 ± 38.94	116.98 ± 77.34	103.09 ± 42.94	0.02 *	0.32	0.69
	MCV MM (%)	68.95 ± 31.17	77.34 ± 39,59	76.29 ± 32.37	0.67	0.56	1.00
	POC (%)	96.79 ± 33.09	105.51 ± 43.01	97.89 ± 31.02	0.51	1.00	1.00
	AsI TA	−11.47 ± 63.56	−1.22 ± 48.56	−4.47 ± 15.65	0.37	0.07	1.00
	AsI MM	1.44 ± 5.44	1.27 ± 25.64	−1.31 ± 21.33	1.00	1.00	1.00
	AcI R	0.72 ± 28.91	−14.46 ± 26.65	4.12 ± 27.40	0.03 *	1.00	0.00 *
	AcI L	−5.54 ± 28.67	−15.69 ± 34,62	1.09 ± 29.48	0.15	0.61	0.01 *
	AcI	20.42 ± 100.33	−42.52 ± 74.05	3.07 ± 26.23	0.01 *	1.00	0.00 *
	TC (%)	−18.40 ± 68.96	−344.47 ± 4458.64	−14.41 ± 65.91	1.00	1.00	1.00

* Significant differences ($p < 0.05$) between groups (Kruskal-Wallis test).

3.4. Electromyographic Analysis of Masticatory Muscle Activity during Maximum Mouth Opening

During maximum mouth opening, differences between MTrPs and TMDs were observed within the bioelectric activity of masseter muscle (MTrPs: 16.45 µV vs. TMDs: 10.73 µV; $p = 0.01$), AsI MM (MTrPs: 0.67 vs. TMDs: 11.12; $p = 0.04$), AcI R (MTrPs: 14.35 vs. TMDs: −0.23; $p = 0.03$), AcI L (MTrPs: 11.32 vs. TMDs: −11.06; $p = 0.00$) and AcI (MTrPs: 13.04 vs. −3.89; $p = 0.01$). Moreover, TMDs showed differences within AcI L in comparison to controls (TMDs: −11.06 vs. Controls: 7.65; $p = 0.02$) (Table 5). In terms of other indices, the differences between the studied groups did not reach the assumed significance level (Tables 3–5).

Table 5. Comparison of the mean values (± SD) of bioelectric activity of temporalis anterior (TA), masseter muscle (MM) and electromyographic indices between groups during maximum mouth opening.

		MTrPs Group	TMDs Group	Control Group	p Value MTrPs vs. TMDs	p Value MTrPs vs. Controls	p Value TMDs vs. Controls
Maximum mouth opening	TA (µV)	10.54 ± 7.25	9.71 ± 7.89	8.41 ± 6.63	0.48	0.21	1.00
	MM (µV)	16.45 ± 15.01	10.73 ± 13.37	11.94 ± 14.28	0.01 *	0.33	0.31
	POC (%)	103.49 ± 33.75	135.39 ± 108.85	104.08 ± 32.01	0.17	1.00	0.34
	AsI TA	−2.05 ± 20.10	−0.82 ± 24.49	−0.38 ± 18.97	1.00	1.00	1.00
	AsI MM	0.67 ± 19.50	11.12 ± 28.02	1.27 ± 19.56	0.04 *	1.00	0.12
	AcI R	14.35 ± 24.11	−0.23 ± 36.07	9.60 ± 23.68	0.03 *	1.00	0.28
	AcI L	11.32 ± 26.61	−11.06 ± 31.34	7.65 ± 28.98	0.00 *	1.00	0.02 *
	AcI	13.04 ± 22.63	−3.89 ± 32.12	8.90 ± 24.46	0.01 *	1.00	0.08
	TC (%)	145.17 ± 1141.30	422.55 ± 2474.46	116.17 ± 860.95	0.53	1.00	0.63

* Significant differences ($p < 0.05$) between groups (Kruskal–Wallis test).

4. Discussion

The referred pain induced from active MTrPs in the neck muscles shared a similar pain pattern as spontaneous TMDs [19]. Thus, MTrPs in the upper trapezius may be responsible for the development of pain within the masticatory muscles. However, the association between TMDs and disorders within trapezius remaining unclear. Thus, the presented study aimed to determine, analyze and compare electromyographic patterns of masticatory muscles in relation to active MTrPs of the upper trapezius and TMDs. To our knowledge, this is the first study to evaluate electromyographic patterns of masticatory muscles in relation to active myofascial trigger points of the upper trapezius and temporomandibular disorders. We hypothesized that MTrPs within the upper trapezius significantly influence the activity of the masticatory muscles. We also assumed that the electromyographic patterns of masticatory muscles in the group with MTrPs within trapezius and TMDs patients would be different from healthy individuals.

During the electromyographic examination, significantly higher values of resting activity within temporalis anterior were observed among both MTrPs and TMDs patients in comparison to healthy individuals. The above-mentioned association was not observed within masseter muscle. Moreover, the differences within the distribution of resting muscle activity between the temporalis anterior and the masseter muscle significantly influenced activity index values in both studied groups. Both MTrPs and TMDs patients showed negative (−). AcI values, compared to healthy individuals whose AcI values were slightly positive (+). Negative values of AcI among MTrPs and TMDs indicate the predominance of the temporalis anterior during rest, in contrast to healthy controls with slight positive AcI values (masseter muscle advantage). However, the electromyographic patterns of teeth clenching differ significantly between MTrPs and TMDs patients regarding the activity index. The positive values of AcI during clenching showed the predominance of masseter muscle activity among individuals with active MTrPs within trapezius, unlike TMDs patients with negative values of AcI, indicating the predominance of the temporalis anterior during clenching tasks. In addition, the MVC index within the TA was significantly lower in MTrPs patients than in TMDs and healthy participants. Different electromyographic patterns between TMDs and MTrPs were also observed during maximum mouth opening in terms of bioelectric activity of the masseter muscle, as well as AsI MM and AcI indices.

The above changes in the masticatory muscle activity seem to be related to the integrated pain adaptation model, which assumes a new muscle activation strategy to maintain homeostasis [33]. The presented model postulates that the key factor in maintaining homeostasis may be the need to minimize the generation of further pain at rest or during movement. Thus, changes in the electromyographic patterns of masticatory muscles may be associated with the presence of pain due to active MTrPs. Previous studies indicate the association between the active MTrPs within masticatory muscles, increased muscle activity during rest and a decrease in sEMG values during teeth clenching [34–36]. The above-mentioned association may be linked with TA resting activity obtained in our work, both in TMDs and MTrPs groups, showing a similar resting activity pattern in both groups of patients.Note, however, that the AcI values differed significantly between MTrPs and TMDs during clenching tasks. The predominance of TA muscle activity in TMDs patients could be caused by reducing contraction patterns within the MM, which seems to be confirmed in the Mapelli et al. study [37]. However, the MTrPs group presented an entirely different electromyographic pattern with decreased temporalis anterior activity, both during teeth clenching and maximum mouth opening. We suspect that this altered pattern may be related to the occurrence of active MTrPs in the trapezius muscle, which, as a result of a referred pain mechanism, alters TA activity. Our suppositions seem to be in line with the referred pain patterns presented by Travell and Simons, in which the temporal area is one of the most commonly painful regions raised from MTrPs located in the upper trapezius [38]. As, based on our data, we cannot directly confirm this mechanism, we should treat this as a supposition and future studies should test if this mechanism is true.

Our hypothesis that MTrPs within the upper trapezius significantly influence the masticatory muscle activity seems to be confirmed in the presented research. This notion is in line with the results of previous findings showing the relationship between MTrPs in the upper trapezius and tension-type headache episodes [20,39–43]. In addition, the presence of bilateral pain hypersensitivity in the trigeminal region in patients with idiopathic neck pain was observed in La Touche et al. study, which suggests a sensitization process of the trigeminocervical nucleus [44]. Moreover, a study conducted by De-la-Llave-Rincon et al. suggests that chronic pain in the cervical region influences the formation of latent trigger points in the masticatory muscles [45]. The relationship between the masticatory muscles and the pain within the cervical area seems to be confirmed by Testa et al. [46]. In the above-mentioned study, patients with chronic pain in the cervical spine region presented the altered distribution of the electromyographic patterns within masticatory muscles during clenching. The authors also suggest that changes in the activity of the masticatory muscles observed in patients with cervical spine pain patterns may affect the development of TMDs.

Our assumption that the electromyographic patterns of masticatory muscles in the group with MTrPs within trapezius and in TMDs patients will be different from healthy individuals seems to be justified by obtained results. However, we cannot clearly explain the significant differences observed between MTrPs and TMD within the electromyographic patterns, which requires further research.The presented study has several limitations. Firstly, the diagnostics criteria for TMDs were changed to DC/TMD in 2014. However, there is no validated Polish version of the DC/TMD so far. Therefore, we used the clinical examination based on the Axis-I protocol of the RDC/TM. Moreover, the Axis I section of the RDC/TMD form is widely used in the current literature in high-impact journals [47–50]. Secondly, the study sample consists of young adults aged 18 to 35. Thus, future research should include a population with an expanded age range.

5. Conclusions

Both the presence of MTrPs in the upper trapezius and TMDs are related to changes in electromyographic patterns of masticatory muscles. Future research is needed to explain the above differences and underlying mechanisms.

Author Contributions: Conceptualization, G.Z., A.B. and M.G.; data curation, G.Z., A.B. and M.G.; investigation, G.Z., A.B., J.S. and M.G., methodology, M.G. and G.Z.; project administration, P.M. and M.G.; resources, P.M. and J.S.; supervision, M.G.; writing—original draft, G.Z., A.B. and M.G.; writing—review and editing, M.G. All authors have read and agreed to the published version of the manuscript.

Funding: This research received no external funding.

Institutional Review Board Statement: The study was conducted according to the guidelines of the Declaration of Helsinki, and approved by the Bioethical Commission of the Medical University of Lublin (approval number KE-0254/346/2016, date of approval 23.11.2016).

Informed Consent Statement: Informed consent was obtained from all subjects involved in the study.

Data Availability Statement: The data presented in this study are available on request from the corresponding author.

Acknowledgments: We acknowledge support from the Medical University of Lublin for Open Access Publishing.

Conflicts of Interest: The authors declare no conflict of interest.

References

1. Bron, C.; Dommerholt, J.D. Etiology of Myofascial Trigger Points. *Curr. Pain Headache Rep.* **2012**, *16*, 439–444. [CrossRef]
2. Simons, D.G.; Travel, J.G.; Simons, L.S.; Cummings, B.D. *Myofascial Pain and Dysfunction: The Trigger Point Manual*, 2nd ed.; Lippincott Williams & Wilkins: Philadelphia, PA, USA, 1998.
3. Gerwin, R. Myofascial Pain Syndrome: Here We Are, Where Must We Go? *J. Musculoskelet. Pain* **2010**, *18*, 329–347. [CrossRef]
4. Zhuang, X.; Tan, S.; Huang, Q. Understanding of Myofascial Trigger Points. *Chin. Med. J.* **2014**, *127*, 4271–4277. [PubMed]
5. Simons, D.G. Review of Enigmatic MTrPs as a Common Cause of Enigmatic Musculoskeletal Pain and Dysfunction. *J. Electromyogr. Kinesiol.* **2004**, *14*, 95–107. [CrossRef]
6. Pal, U.S.; Kumar, L.; Mehta, G.; Singh, N.; Singh, G.; Singh, M.; Yadav, H.K. Trends in Management of Myofacial Pain. *Natl. J. Maxillofac. Surg.* **2014**, *5*, 109–116. [CrossRef]
7. Shah, J.P.; Thaker, N.; Heimur, J.; Aredo, J.V.; Sikdar, S.; Gerber, L. Myofascial Trigger Points Then and Now: A Historical and Scientific Perspective. *PM&R* **2015**, *7*, 746–761.
8. Pinho-Ribeiro, F.A.; Verri, W.A.; Chiu, I.M. Nociceptor Sensory Neuron-Immune Interactions in Pain and Inflammation. *Trends Immunol.* **2017**, *38*, 5–19. [CrossRef]
9. Bourgaize, S.; Newton, G.; Kumbhare, D.; Srbely, J. A Comparison of the Clinical Manifestation and Pathophysiology of Myofascial Pain Syndrome and Fibromyalgia: Implications for Differential Diagnosis and Management. *J. Can. Chiropr. Assoc.* **2018**, *62*, 26–41. [PubMed]
10. Runci Anastasi, M.; Centofanti, A.; Arco, A.; Vermiglio, G.; Nicita, F.; Santoro, G.; Cascone, P.; Anastasi, G.P.; Rizzo, G.; Cutroneo, G. Histological and Immunofluorescence Study of Discal Ligaments in Human Temporomandibular Joint. *J. Funct. Morphol. Kinesiol.* **2020**, *5*, 90. [CrossRef]
11. Kubein-Meesenburg, D.; Fanghänel, J.; Ihlow, D.; Lotzmann, U.; Hahn, W.; Thieme, K.M.; Proff, P.; Gedrange, T.; Nägerl, H. Functional State of the Mandible and Rolling-Gliding Characteristics in the TMJ. *Ann. Anat.* **2007**, *189*, 393–396. [CrossRef]
12. Cuccia, A.M.; Caradonna, C.; Caradonna, D. Manual Therapy of the Mandibular Accessory Ligaments for the Management of Temporomandibular Joint Disorders. *J. Am. Osteopath. Assoc.* **2011**, *111*, 102–112. [PubMed]
13. Durham, J.; Wassell, R. Recent Advancements in Temporomandibular Disorders (TMDs). *Rev. Pain* **2011**, *5*, 18–25. [CrossRef]
14. Poluha, R.L.; Grossmann, E.; Iwaki, L.C.V.; Uchimura, T.T.; Santana, R.G.; Iwaki, L. Myofascial Trigger Points in Patients with Temporomandibular Joint Disc Displacement with Reduction: A Cross-Sectional Study. *J. Appl. Oral Sci.* **2018**, *26*, e20170578. [CrossRef] [PubMed]
15. Rener-Sitar, K.; Celebić, A.; Mehulić, K.; Petricević, N. Factors Related to Oral Health Related Quality of Life in TMD Patients. *Coll. Antropol.* **2013**, *37*, 407–413.
16. Ey-Chmielewska, H.; Teul, I.; LorkowskI, J. Functional disorders of the temporomandibular joints as a factor responsible for sleep apnoea. *Ann. Acad. Med. Stetin.* **2014**, *60*, 65–68.
17. Facial Pain | National Institute of Dental and Craniofacial Research. Available online: https://www.nidcr.nih.gov/research/data-statistics/facial-pain (accessed on 22 January 2021).
18. Ohrbach, R.; Dworkin, S.F. Five-Year Outcomes in TMD: Relationship of Changes in Pain to Changes in Physical and Psychological Variables. *Pain* **1998**, *74*, 315–326. [CrossRef]
19. Fernández-de-Las-Peñas, C.; Galán-Del-Río, F.; Alonso-Blanco, C.; Jiménez-García, R.; Arendt-Nielsen, L.; Svensson, P. Referred Pain from Muscle Trigger Points in the Masticatory and Neck-Shoulder Musculature in Women with Temporomandibular Disoders. *J. Pain* **2010**, *11*, 1295–1304. [CrossRef]
20. Alonso-Blanco, C.; de-la-Llave-Rincón, A.I.; Fernández-de-las-Peñas, C. Muscle Trigger Point Therapy in Tension-Type Headache. *Expert Rev. Neurother.* **2012**, *12*, 315–322. [CrossRef]
21. Olivo, S.A.; Bravo, J.; Magee, D.J.; Thie, N.M.R.; Major, P.W.; Flores-Mir, C. The Association between Head and Cervical Posture and Temporomandibular Disorders: A Systematic Review. *J. Orofac. Pain* **2006**, *20*, 9–23.
22. Alonso-Blanco, C.; Fernández-de-las-Peñas, C.; de-la-Llave-Rincón, A.I.; Zarco-Moreno, P.; Galán-del-Río, F.; Svensson, P. Characteristics of Referred Muscle Pain to the Head from Active Trigger Points in Women with Myofascial Temporomandibular Pain and Fibromyalgia Syndrome. *J. Headache Pain* **2012**, *13*, 625–637. [CrossRef]

23. Osiewicz, M.A.; Lobbezoo, F.; Loster, B.W.; Wilkosz, M.; Naeije, M.; Ohrbach, R. Research Diagnostic Criteria for Temporomandibular Disorders (RDC/TMD): The Polish Version of a Dual-Axis System for the Diagnosis of TMD.* RDC/TMD Form. *Open J. Stomatol.* **2013**, *66*, 576–649. [CrossRef]
24. Peck, C.C.; Goulet, J.-P.; Lobbezoo, F.; Schiffman, E.L.; Alstergren, P.; Anderson, G.C.; de Leeuw, R.; Jensen, R.; Michelotti, A.; Ohrbach, R.; et al. Expanding the Taxonomy of the Diagnostic Criteria for Temporomandibular Disorders. *J. Oral Rehabil.* **2014**, *41*, 2–23. [CrossRef]
25. Hermens, H.J.; Freriks, B.; Disselhorst-Klug, C.; Rau, G. Development of Recommendations for SEMG Sensors and Sensor Placement Procedures. *J. Electromyogr. Kinesiol.* **2000**, *10*, 361–374. [CrossRef]
26. Ferrario, V.F.; Sforza, C.; Miani, A.; D'Addona, A.; Barbini, E. Electromyographic Activity of Human Masticatory Muscles in Normal Young People. Statistical Evaluation of Reference Values for Clinical Applications. *J. Oral Rehabil.* **1993**, *20*, 271–280. [CrossRef] [PubMed]
27. Wieczorek, A.; Loster, J.; Loster, B.W. Relationship between Occlusal Force Distribution and the Activity of Masseter and Anterior Temporalis Muscles in Asymptomatic Young Adults. *Biomed Res. Int.* **2012**, *2013*, e354017. [CrossRef]
28. De Felício, C.M.; Sidequersky, F.V.; Tartaglia, G.M.; Sforza, C. Electromyographic Standardized Indices in Healthy Brazilian Young Adults and Data Reproducibility. *J. Oral Rehabil.* **2009**, *36*, 577–583. [CrossRef]
29. Vozzi, F.; Favero, L.; Peretta, R.; Guarda-Nardini, L.; Cocilovo, F.; Manfredini, D. Indexes of Jaw Muscle Function in Asymptomatic Individuals with Different Occlusal Features. *Clin. Exp. Dent. Res.* **2018**, *4*, 263–267. [CrossRef]
30. Wieczorek, A.; Loster, J.E. Activity of the Masticatory Muscles and Occlusal Contacts in Young Adults with and without Orthodontic Treatment. *BMC Oral Health* **2015**, *15*, 116. [CrossRef]
31. Ferrario, V.F.; Tartaglia, G.M.; Galletta, A.; Grassi, G.P.; Sforza, C. The Influence of Occlusion on Jaw and Neck Muscle Activity: A Surface EMG Study in Healthy Young Adults. *J. Oral Rehabil.* **2006**, *33*, 341–348. [CrossRef]
32. Von Elm, E.; Altman, D.G.; Egger, M.; Pocock, S.J.; Gøtzsche, P.C.; Vandenbroucke, J.P. STROBE Initiative The Strengthening the Reporting of Observational Studies in Epidemiology (STROBE) Statement: Guidelines for Reporting Observational Studies. *J. Clin. Epidemiol.* **2008**, *61*, 344–349. [CrossRef]
33. Peck, C.; Murray, G.; Gerzina, T. How Does Pain Affect Jaw Muscle Activity? The Integrated Pain Adaptation Model. *Aust. Dent. J.* **2008**, *53*, 201–207. [CrossRef]
34. Ginszt, M.; Zieliński, G.; Berger, M.; Szkutnik, J.; Bakalczuk, M.; Majcher, P. Acute Effect of the Compression Technique on the Electromyographic Activity of the Masticatory Muscles and Mouth Opening in Subjects with Active Myofascial Trigger Points. *Appl. Sci.* **2020**, *10*, 7750. [CrossRef]
35. Pietropaoli, D.; Ortu, E.; Giannoni, M.; Cattaneo, R.; Mummolo, A.; Monaco, A. Alterations in Surface Electromyography Are Associated with Subjective Masticatory Muscle Pain. *Pain Res. Manag.* **2019**, *2019*, 6256179. [CrossRef]
36. Manfredini, D.; Cocilovo, F.; Favero, L.; Ferronato, G.; Tonello, S.; Guarda-Nardini, L. Surface Electromyography of Jaw Muscles and Kinesiographic Recordings: Diagnostic Accuracy for Myofascial Pain. *J. Oral Rehabil.* **2011**, *38*, 791–799. [CrossRef]
37. Mapelli, A.; Zanandréa Machado, B.C.; Giglio, L.D.; Sforza, C.; De Felício, C.M. Reorganization of Muscle Activity in Patients with Chronic Temporomandibular Disorders. *Arch. Oral Biol.* **2016**, *72*, 164–171. [CrossRef]
38. Simons, D.G.; Travell, J.G.; Simons, L.S. *Travell & Simons' Myofascial Pain and Dysfunction: The Trigger Point Manual*, 2nd ed.; Williams & Wilkins: Baltimore, MD, USA, 1999.
39. Couppé, C.; Torelli, P.; Fuglsang-Frederiksen, A.; Andersen, K.V.; Jensen, R. Myofascial Trigger Points Are Very Prevalent in Patients with Chronic Tension-Type Headache: A Double-Blinded Controlled Study. *Clin. J. Pain* **2007**, *23*, 23–27. [CrossRef]
40. Alonso-Blanco, C.; Fernández-de-las-Peñas, C.; Fernández-Mayoralas, D.M.; de-la-Llave-Rincón, A.I.; Pareja, J.A.; Svensson, P. Prevalence and Anatomical Localization of Muscle Referred Pain from Active Trigger Points in Head and Neck Musculature in Adults and Children with Chronic Tension-Type Headache. *Pain Med.* **2011**, *12*, 1453–1463. [CrossRef]
41. Fernández-de-las-Peñas, C.; Fernández-Mayoralas, D.M.; Ortega-Santiago, R.; Ambite-Quesada, S.; Palacios-Ceña, D.; Pareja, J.A. Referred Pain from Myofascial Trigger Points in Head and Neck-Shoulder Muscles Reproduces Head Pain Features in Children with Chronic Tension Type Headache. *J. Headache Pain* **2011**, *12*, 35–43. [CrossRef]
42. Fernández-de-Las-Peñas, C.; Cuadrado, M.L.; Pareja, J.A. Myofascial Trigger Points, Neck Mobility, and Forward Head Posture in Episodic Tension-Type Headache. *Headache* **2007**, *47*, 662–672. [CrossRef]
43. Fernández-de-Las-Peñas, C.; Ge, H.-Y.; Arendt-Nielsen, L.; Cuadrado, M.L.; Pareja, J.A. Referred Pain from Trapezius Muscle Trigger Points Shares Similar Characteristics with Chronic Tension Type Headache. *Eur. J. Pain* **2007**, *11*, 475–482. [CrossRef]
44. La Touche, R.; Fernández-de-Las-Peñas, C.; Fernández-Carnero, J.; Díaz-Parreño, S.; Paris-Alemany, A.; Arendt-Nielsen, L. Bilateral Mechanical-Pain Sensitivity over the Trigeminal Region in Patients with Chronic Mechanical Neck Pain. *J. Pain* **2010**, *11*, 256–263. [CrossRef]
45. De-la-Llave-Rincon, A.I.; Alonso-Blanco, C.; Gil-Crujera, A.; Ambite-Quesada, S.; Svensson, P.; Fernández-de-Las-Peñas, C. Myofascial Trigger Points in the Masticatory Muscles in Patients with and without Chronic Mechanical Neck Pain. *J. Manip. Physiol. Ther.* **2012**, *35*, 678–684. [CrossRef]
46. Testa, M.; Geri, T.; Gizzi, L.; Falla, D. High-Density EMG Reveals Novel Evidence of Altered Masseter Muscle Activity During Symmetrical and Asymmetrical Bilateral Jaw Clenching Tasks in People With Chronic Nonspecific Neck Pain. *Clin. J. Pain* **2017**, *33*, 148–159. [CrossRef]

47. Ohlmann, B.; Waldecker, M.; Leckel, M.; Bömicke, W.; Behnisch, R.; Rammelsberg, P.; Schmitter, M. Correlations between Sleep Bruxism and Temporomandibular Disorders. *J. Clin. Med.* **2020**, *9*, 611. [CrossRef] [PubMed]
48. Pihut, M.; Górnicki, M.; Orczykowska, M.; Zarzecka, E.; Ryniewicz, W.; Gala, A. The Application of Radiofrequency Waves in Supportive Treatment of Temporomandibular Disorders. *Pain Res. Manag.* **2020**, *2020*, 6195601. [CrossRef] [PubMed]
49. Eraslan, R.; Kılıç, K.; Etöz, M.; Soydan, D. The Evaluation of Agreement between High-Frequency Ultrasonography and Research Diagnostic Criteria for the Diagnosis of Temporomandibular Joint Internal Derangements. *J. Indian Prosthodont. Soc.* **2020**, *20*, 387–393. [CrossRef] [PubMed]
50. Rehm, D.D.; Progiante, P.S.; Pattussi, M.P.; Pellizzer, E.P.; Grossi, P.K.; Grossi, M.L. Sleep Disorders in Patients with Temporomandibular Disorders (TMD) in an Adult Population-Based Cross-Sectional Survey in Southern Brazil. *Int. J. Prosthodont.* **2020**, *33*, 9–13. [CrossRef] [PubMed]

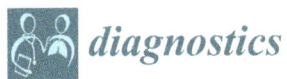

Article

Temporomandibular Joint Osseous Morphology of Class I and Class II Malocclusions in the Normal Skeletal Pattern: A Cone-Beam Computed Tomography Study

Xiao-Chuan Fan [1,†], Lin-Sha Ma [1,†], Li Chen [2], Diwakar Singh [3], Xiaohui Rausch-Fan [3,*] and Xiao-Feng Huang [1,*]

1. Department of Stomatology, Beijing Friendship Hospital, Capital Medical University, Beijing 100050, China; foxtail_09@hotmail.com (X.-C.F.); malinthe@yeah.net (L.-S.M.)
2. Department of Orthodontics, Beijing Stomatological Hospital & School of Stomatology, Capital Medical University, Beijing 100050, China; lydiach323@ccmu.edu.cn
3. Clinical Research Center, Division of Conservative Dentistry and Periodontology, School of Dentistry, Medical University of Vienna, 1090 Vienna, Austria; dentistdiwakarsingh@gmail.com

* Correspondence: xiaohui.rausch-fan@meduniwien.ac.at (X.R.-F.); huangxf1998@163.com (X.-F.H.)

† These authors contributed equally to this work.

Abstract: (1) Background—The aim of the present study was to evaluate the correlation between the temporomandibular joint (TMJ) osseous morphology of normal skeletal pattern individuals with different dental malocclusions by using cone-beam computed tomography (CBCT). (2) Methods—The CBCT images of bilateral TMJs in 67 subjects with skeletal class I and average mandibular angle (26 males and 41 females, age range 20–49 years) were evaluated in this study. The subjects were divided into class I, class II division 1, and class II division 2 according to the molar relationship and retroclination of the maxillary incisors. Angular and linear measurements of TMJ were evaluated and the differences between the groups were statistically analyzed. (3) Results—Intragroup comparisons showed statistical differences for articular eminence inclination, the width of the glenoid fossa, the ratio of the width of the glenoid fossa to the depth of the glenoid fossa, the condylar angle, and the intercondylar angle between the malocclusion groups. The measurements of the glenoid fossa shape showed no significant difference between the left and right sides. Females showed more differences in the morphological parameters of TMJ between the three malocclusion groups than the males. (4) Conclusion—The present study revealed differences in the TMJ osseous morphology between dental class I and class II malocclusions in the normal skeletal pattern.

Keywords: temporomandibular joint; cone-beam computed tomography; malocclusions; articular eminence inclination

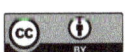

1. Introduction

The temporomandibular joint (TMJ) is one of the most complex joints in the human body. It is formed by the condyle of the mandibular, the inferior component of the joint, and the glenoid fossa forming the superior component of the joint, which is located at the inferior aspect of the squamous part of the temporal bone [1,2]. The joint cavity is separated into the upper and lower compartments by the articular disk, which is made of avascular and aneural dense fibrous connective tissue [3]. The unique anatomy of the TMJ allows for the hinging movement of the mandible and is therefore considered a ginglymoid joint. It can also provide gliding movements and is therefore also an arthrodial joint; thus, it is technically considered a compound joint.

Form and function are considered to be closely linked, and it follows that the osseous morphology of the TMJ might be related to the dynamic balance of mandibular functions in three dimensions. During the mandibular movement, the condyle-disk complex process slides over the posterior slope of the articular eminence. The inclination of articular eminence dictates the path of condylar movement, as well as the degree of rotation of the articular disk over the condyle [4,5]. For patients with a steeper articular eminence, the condyle is forced to move more inferior and the disk rotates more prominent when protruding or opening. This may lead the mandible to move more vertically during the functional movement [6]. It is reported that a patient with steeper articular eminence is more likely to develop internal dysfunctions, such as anterior disk displacements, than a patient with a flatter articular eminence [7,8].

The articular eminence is sometimes described as the anterior limit of the glenoid fossa. The quantitative evaluation of the articular eminence morphology can be assessed using the inclination, length, and height, where the articular eminence inclination (AEI) is defined as the angle formed by the articular eminence and the horizontal reference plane, which may be the Frankfort horizontal (FH) plane, the true horizontal line, the anterior nasal spine to the posterior nasal plane (ANS–PNS), or the occlusal plane [4,9–11]. The normal value of the AEI in adults has been reported to be 30 to 60 degrees. This angle is not only related to physiological factors, such as age, gender, tooth inclination, dental arch morphology, and the facial growth pattern [4,12–14], but also pathological factors, including occlusion change, TMJ osteoarthritis, internal derangements, and posterior tooth loss [15–18].

A thorough understanding of the morphology and anatomical features of the TMJ is crucial such that we can distinguish the normal condition from the abnormal variant. It is reported that the surface of the structural features of the glenoid fossa may take part in remodeling and reconfiguring following the mechanical and functional conditions to which the adjacent structures are subjected [19]. Some authors suggested that changing the relationship between the upper and lower dentition may lead to right-to-left-side differences in masticatory muscles, which affect the relative relationship of the condyle and glenoid fossa [20,21]. The effect of occlusal factors on the morphology of the temporomandibular joint remains to be clarified. Based on this context, we hypothesized that the discrepancy of the occlusion relationship may be an independent factor that affects the morphology of the TMJ. Thus, the purpose of the present study was to evaluate the correlation between the TMJ osseous morphology of the normal skeletal pattern individuals with different dental malocclusion by using cone-beam computed tomography (CBCT).

2. Materials and Methods

2.1. Data Collection and Grouping

The present study was performed at the Department of Stomatology, Beijing Friendship Hospital, Capital Medical University, and it was approved by the Ethical Committee of Beijing Friendship Hospital (approval number 2021-P2-008-01, updated on 1 February 2021). High-resolution CBCT imaging volumes were obtained from examinations that were previously conducted for orthodontic purposes between January 2019 to December 2020; therefore, they had no connection to the present study.

The age of the patients in the sample selected for the study needed to be no less than 20 years old. The sagittal skeletal relationship was defined using the ANB angle (ANB), Frankfurt horizontal–mandibular plane angle (FH–MP), and sella–nasion to gnathion–gonion angle (SN–GnGo), which were measured from the lateral cephalograms that were automatically reconstructed and generated using the QR-NNT Viewer version 5.6 software program (Quantitative Radiology, Verona, Italy). The participants included were limited to skeletal class I with an average mandibular angle, which was defined as $0.7° \leq ANB \leq 4.7°$, $21.2° \leq FH–MP \leq 33.4°$, $27.3° \leq SN–GnGo \leq 37.7°$ [22]. The exclusion criteria were as follows: (1) evidence of temporomandibular disorders (TMDs) in a clinical or imaging examination; (2) previous history of orthodontics or TMJ treatment; (3) craniofacial syndrome or anomalies, such as cleft lip and palate; (4) systemic diseases, such as rheumatic arthritis and rheumatoid arthritis; (5) deciduous or missing teeth, except third molars; (6) asymmetric molar relationship or class III molar relationship from the plaster models before treatment; (7) fracture or other pathologies in the region of the TMJs, such as anomalies, tumors, ankylosis, or degenerative changes; (8) poor image quality. After applying the inclusion and exclusion criteria, 67 patients (26 males and 41 females, age range 20–49 years) were included and recorded bilaterally; in total, 134 TMJs were evaluated.

The included samples were divided into three groups: class I (CI), class II division 1 (CII-1), and class II division 2 (CII-2). The assignment to each group was done based on the molar relationship on the patient's plaster models before treatment, and the class II groups were then divided according to the retroclination of the maxillary incisors. The interval between the model making and CBCT taking should be less than 1 week. Each study group was then subdivided according to gender and left or right side.

2.2. Simple Size Calculation

Based on our preliminary data, we got a minimum detectable difference value of 5, and we calculated the sample size using the Power Analysis and Sample Size software version 11.0 (PASS, NSCC, LLC, Kaysville, Utah, USA) in the present study. Considering a study with a two-tailed hypothesis, for an α value of 0.05, a β value of 0.2, and a statistical power of 80%, the minimum sample size was computed to be 38 subjects per group.

2.3. Acquisition of CBCT Images

The CBCT scans were performed using a New Tom 5G version FP (Quantitative Radiology, Verona, Italy) flat-panel-based CBCT machine with a field of view of 18×16 cm. The scanner operated with a maximum output of 110 kV and 5 mAs, exposure time of 3.6 s, and a voxel size of 0.15 mm. The patients with teeth in the maximum intercuspation position were placed in a horizontal position according to the laser indicators and we ensured that the Frankfort horizontal plane was perpendicular to the flat panel of the device in order to obtain a consistent orientation of sagittal images. All CBCT scans were obtained under the same scanning conditions by the same experienced oral radiologist with the same device.

2.4. Measurements

The CBCT examination results were analyzed using the QR-NNT Viewer version 5.6 software program, which was the proprietary software of the New Tom 5G CBCT system. Before the quantitative evaluation, a secondary calibration was performed to ensure the Frankfort plane was held parallel to the horizontal plane on the sagittal reference view. The CBCT data were also spatially oriented by aligning the anterior and posterior nasal spine on the axial reference view. Digital reconstruction was then conducted in the TMJ regions.

On the axial view, the slice of the condylar processes that had the widest mediolateral extent on both sides of TMJ was used to measure the angulation of the condyles, which involved two variables:

(1) Condylar angle (CA): the angle between the long axis (the line passing through the medial and lateral pole of the condyle) of the left or right condyle and the midsagittal plane in the axial view (Figure 1).

(2) Intercondylar angle (IA): the angle between the long axis of the right and left condyles in the axial view (Figure 2).

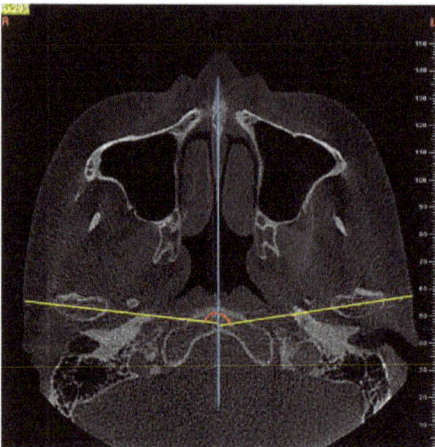

Figure 1. The measurement of condylar angle (CA) on the axial slice. The angle between the long axis of the condyle (yellow line) and the midsagittal plane (blue line) was measured.

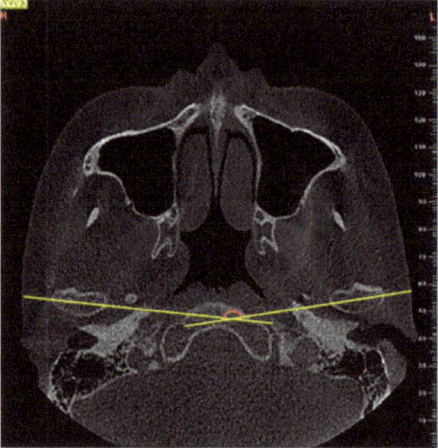

Figure 2. The measurement of intercondylar angle (IA) on the axial slice. The angle between the long axis of the left and right condyle (yellow line) was measured.

The chosen slice was also used as the reference view for the secondary reconstruction of the sagittal slices [13], on which a line parallel to the long axis of the condylar process was drawn and sagittal images were reconstructed with a 0.5 mm slice interval and a 0.5 mm thickness. The following variables were calculated on the central sagittal slice of the TMJ:

(1) AEI using the best-fit line method (AEI-BFL): the angle between the tangent line drawn to the posterior slope of the articular eminence and a line parallel to the FH plane (Figure 3).

(2) AEI using the top-roof line method (AEI-TRL): the angle between the "top-roof line" of the articular eminence (the line connecting the crest point of the articular eminence and the roof of the glenoid fossa) and a line parallel to the FH plane (Figure 4).

(3) Width of the glenoid fossa (GFW): the distance between the crest point of the articular eminence and the posterior part of the glenoid process.

(4) Depth of the glenoid fossa (GFD): the perpendicular distance between the highest point of the glenoid fossa and the GFW line (the line passing through the crest point of the articular eminence and the posterior part of the glenoid process) (Figure 5).

(5) Ratio of the GFW to the GFD (GFW/GFD).

(6) Height of the articular eminence (AEH): the perpendicular distance between the highest point of the glenoid fossa and the line parallel to the FH plane through the crest point of the articular eminence (Figure 6).

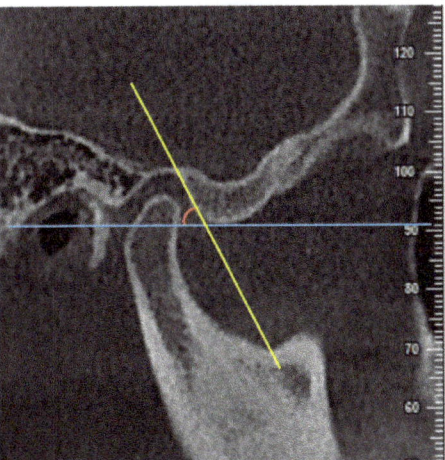

Figure 3. The measurement of articular eminence inclination (AEI) using the best-fit line method (AEI-BFL) on the central sagittal slice. The angle between the tangent line drawn to the posterior slope of the articular eminence (yellow line) and a line parallel to the Frankfort horizontal (FH) plane (blue line) was measured.

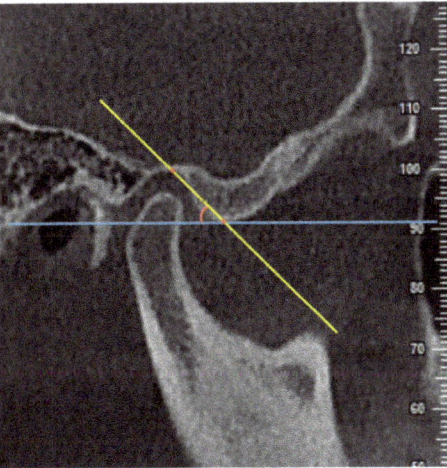

Figure 4. The measurement of AEI using the top-roof line method (AEI-TRL) on the central sagittal slice. The angle between the "top-roof line (the line connecting the crest point of the articular eminence and the roof of the glenoid fossa)" (yellow line) and a line parallel to the FH plane (blue line) was measured.

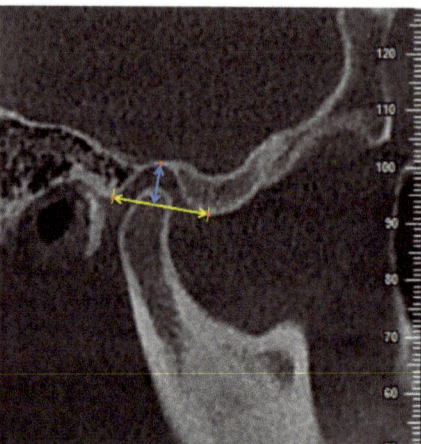

Figure 5. The measurement of the width of the glenoid fossa (GFW) and depth of the glenoid fossa (GFD) on the central sagittal slice. The distance between the crest point of the articular eminence and the posterior part of the glenoid process was measured as the GFW (yellow arrow) and the perpendicular distance between the highest point of the glenoid fossa and the GFW line was measured as the GFD (blue arrow).

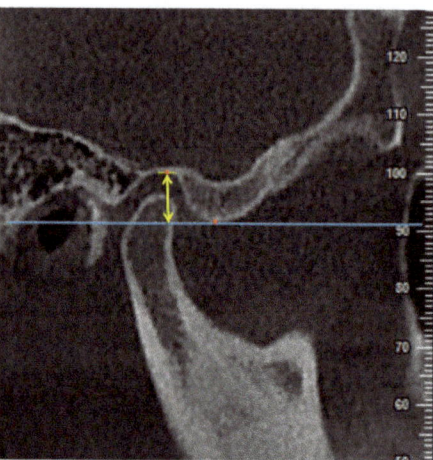

Figure 6. The measurement of the height of the articular eminence (AEH) on the central sagittal slice. The perpendicular distance between the line parallel to the FH plane through the crest point of the articular eminence (blue line) and the highest point of the glenoid fossa was measured (yellow arrow).

The measurements and angles evaluated on both the axial and central sagittal slices were obtained according to the methods mentioned by İlgüy, Park, Sümbüllü, and Paknahad [13,23–25]. All the assessments were performed independently by two operators (X.-C.F. and L.-S.M.) and the mean of the results was used for the statistical analysis.

2.5. Measurements Precision

To test the reliability of the measurements, 30 joints (10 joints from each group) were randomly selected from the collected samples and measured twice with a 1-week interval by the same operators (X.-C.F. and L.-S.M.). The first and the second series of measurements were compared using a paired *t*-test to check for systematic error at a significance level of $p < 0.05$. The random errors were assessed using the intraclass correlation coefficient (ICC) [26].

2.6. Statistical Analysis

All the variables were analyzed using the Statistical Package for Social Sciences software version 20.0 (SPSS, IBM, New York, NY, USA). The one-way analysis of variance (ANOVA) followed by the Bonferroni multiple comparisons test was used to analyze the statistical differences between three malocclusion groups. A paired *t*-test and an independent sample *t*-test were applied to determine the possible differences between the left–right sides and the genders in the same malocclusion group, respectively. A *p*-value < 0.05 was considered statistically significant.

3. Results

3.1. Error of the Study

The paired *t*-test showed no statistically significant differences between the data obtained from the different operators and double measurements from the same operator at a significant level of 0.05. The ICC for intra-operators (operator 1: $r = 0.981$–0.987; operator 2: $r = 0.875$–0.912) and inter-operators ($r = 0.871$–0.901) showed excellent agreement and good reliability for all the measures analyzed.

3.2. Descriptive Statistics of Age and Basic Measurements of the Skeletal Pattern

A total of 67 high-resolution CBCT imaging volumes with skeletal class I (mean ANB angle of $3.44 \pm 1.05°$) and average mandibular angle (mean FH–MP of $26.52 \pm 3.76°$ with a mean SN–GnGo of $33.22 \pm 3.35°$) were collected. The mean age of the participants of the present study was 27.91 ± 6.94 years. The means and standard deviations for age and the angular measurements of the skeletal pattern for the different malocclusion groups are presented in Table 1. The intergroup results showed that there were no statistically significant differences between the three malocclusion groups.

Table 1. Descriptive statistics of age and the basic measurements of the skeletal patterns.

Variable	Total ($N = 67$)		Class I ($n = 24$)		Class II-1 ($n = 20$)		Class II-2 ($n = 23$)		F-Value	p-Value
	Mean ± SD	Range	Mean ± SD	Range	Mean ± SD	Range	Mean ± SD	Range		
Age (year)	27.91 ± 6.94	20–49	27.00 ± 5.56	20–40	27.50 ± 8.52	20–49	29.22 ± 6.84	20–45	0.642	0.530
ANB (°)	3.44 ± 1.05	1.1–4.9	3.10 ± 1.07	1.1–4.6	3.41 ± 0.97	1.4–4.7	3.84 ± 1.02	1.6–4.9	3.125	0.051
FH–MP (°)	26.52 ± 3.76	21.2–33.3	26.58 ± 4.15	21.2–33.2	26.43 ± 3.12	22.0–33.1	26.53 ± 4.00	21.2–33.3	0.009	0.991
SN–GnGo (°)	33.22 ± 3.35	27.4–37.7	33.06 ± 3.43	27.4–37.6	33.43 ± 2.88	28.3–37.6	33.21 ± 3.75	27.4–37.7	0.066	0.937

ANB: ANB angle; FH–MP: Frankfurt horizontal–mandibular plane angle; SN–GnGo: sella-nasion to gnathion-gonion angle.

3.3. Measurements of the Temporomandibular Joint According to Malocclusion

The distributions of the TMJ osseous morphology measurements in the three malocclusion groups are summarized in Table 2. By using the one-way ANOVA, all the angular and linear measurements showed significant differences between the three groups, except for the GFD and AEH ($p < 0.05$). The Bonferroni multiple comparisons test further showed that the AEI found using the best-fit line method of class II division 2 was significantly higher than the class II division 1 ($p = 0.017$), followed by the class I AEI ($p = 0.000$). However, the difference was not obvious between the class II division 1 and class II division 2 ($p = 1.000$) for the AEI found using the top-roof methods. The widths of the glenoid fossa of the three groups were 17.37 ± 1.60 mm (C-I), 16.86 ± 1.40 mm (CII-1), and 16.59 ± 1.28 mm (CII-2). The indicators of the GFW and GFW/GFD only presented differences between the class I and the class II division 2 groups. As for the measurements of the condyle on the axial slice, the condylar and intercondylar angles of the class II division 2 group were lower than the other two groups (Table 3).

Table 2. Measurements of the temporomandibular joint osseous morphology according to the malocclusion.

Variable	Class I			Class II-1			Class II-2			F-Value	p-Value
	n	Mean ± SD	Range	n	Mean ± SD	Range	n	Mean ± SD	Range		
AEI-BFL (°)	48	52.56 ± 7.01	39.7–68.7	40	62.06 ± 5.85	49.1–75.6	46	66.43 ± 8.30	47.5–82.7	45.799	0.000 **
AEI-TRL (°)	48	38.16 ± 5.43	29.4–48.4	40	42.21 ± 5.45	32.5–55.7	46	42.84 ± 4.86	32.7–52.8	10.929	0.000 **
GFW (mm)	48	17.37 ± 1.60	13.8–21.0	40	16.86 ± 1.40	14.8–19.7	46	16.59 ± 1.28	14.1–19.3	3.615	0.030 *
GFD (mm)	48	5.92 ± 1.08	3.9–8.4	40	6.09 ± 0.95	3.7–8.1	46	6.40 ± 0.96	3.9–8.5	2.760	0.067
GFW/GFD	48	3.01 ± 0.49	2.14–4.19	40	2.83 ± 0.47	2.09–4.03	46	2.63 ± 0.33	2.16–3.67	8.843	0.000 **
AEH (mm)	48	7.15 ± 1.30	5.1–10.4	40	7.53 ± 0.93	5.0–10.2	46	7.45 ± 1.22	4.8–10.3	1.270	0.284
CA (°)	48	73.94 ± 5.71	59.8–85.5	40	73.64 ± 7.17	55.8–86.1	46	69.87 ± 6.31	58.0–84.1	5.775	0.004 **
IA (°)	24	147.87 ± 10.34	125.9–168.1	20	147.29 ± 13.29	114.4–165.4	23	139.01 ± 12.03	114.4–168.1	3.96	0.024 *

AEI-BFL: AEI found using the best-fit line method; AEI-TRL: AEI found using the top-roof line method; GFW: width of the glenoid fossa; GFD: depth of the glenoid fossa; GFW/GFD: ratio of the GFW to the GFD; AEH: height of the articular eminence; CA: condylar angle; IA: intercondylar angle; *: p-value < 0.05; **: p-value < 0.01.

Table 3. Bonferroni test results for the measurements of the temporomandibular joint for the three malocclusion groups.

Variable	CI to CII-1		CI to CII-2		CII-1 to CII-2	
	Mean Difference (I–J)	p-Value	Mean Difference (I–J)	p-Value	Mean Difference (I–J)	p-Value
AEI-BFL	−9.4975	0.000 **	−13.8658	0.000 **	−4.3683	0.017 *
AEI-TRL	−4.0496	0.001 **	−4.6831	0.000 **	−0.6335	1.000
GFW	0.5138	0.289	0.7818	0.028 *	0.2680	1.000
GFD	−0.01692	1.000	−0.4813	0.065	−0.3122	0.458
GFW/GFD	0.18000	0.163	0.37549	0.000 **	0.19549	0.116
AEH	−0.3729	0.421	−0.2936	1.000	0.0793	1.000
CA	0.2929	1.000	4.0680	0.007 **	3.7751	0.021 *
IA	0.58583	1.000	8.86214	0.039 *	8.27630	0.079

CI: class I; CII-1: class II division 1; CII-2: class II division 2; AEI-BFL: AEI found using the best-fit line method; AEI-TRL: AEI found using the top-roof line method; GFW: width of the glenoid fossa; GFD: depth of the glenoid fossa; GFW/GFD: ratio of the GFW to the GFD; AEH: height of the articular eminence; CA: condylar angle; IA: intercondylar angle; *: p-value < 0.05; **: p-value < 0.01.

3.4. Descriptive Statistics of the Measurements of the TMJ According to the Left and Right Side

Table 4 lists the mean values and standard deviations of the TMJ morphology measurements for the left and right sides of the three malocclusion groups. According to the paired t-test, only the variables of GFW/GFD and CA in the class II division 1 group and CA in the class II division 2 group showed significant differences ($p < 0.05$).

Table 4. Descriptive statistics of the measurements of the temporomandibular joint according to the left and right sides for the three malocclusion groups.

Variable	Class I (n = 24)			Class II-1 (n = 20)			Class II-2 (n = 23)		
	Left Side	Right Side	p-Value	Left Side	Right Side	p-Value	Left Side	Right Side	p-Value
AEI-BFL (°)	52.78 ± 6.27	52.34 ± 7.83	0.710	62.95 ± 6.50	61.17 ± 5.14	0.246	65.82 ± 7.44	67.04 ± 9.22	0.346
AEI-TRL (°)	38.23 ± 6.05	38.09 ± 4.86	0.821	43.29 ± 6.22	41.14 ± 4.46	0.098	42.97 ± 4.29	42.72 ± 5.47	0.739
GFW (mm)	17.21 ± 1.68	17.53 ± 1.53	0.232	16.95 ± 1.45	16.76 ± 1.37	0.337	16.56 ± 1.25	16.61 ± 1.33	0.824
GFD (mm)	5.74 ± 1.01	6.10 ± 1.15	0.084	5.92 ± 1.05	6.27 ± 0.83	0.099	6.34 ± 1.07	6.47 ± 0.87	0.518
GFW/GFD	3.07 ± 0.50	2.95 ± 0.48	0.128	2.94 ± 0.48	2.72 ± 0.43	0.024 *	2.67 ± 0.37	2.60 ± 0.28	0.393
AEH (mm)	7.22 ± 1.34	7.09 ± 1.29	0.616	7.67 ± 0.96	7.38 ± 0.89	0.234	7.48 ± 1.14	7.41 ± 1.32	0.725
CA (°)	73.09 ± 5.64	74.78 ± 5.77	0.083	72.08 ± 7.20	75.21 ± 6.96	0.010 **	68.07 ± 5.93	71.67 ± 6.28	0.001 **

AEI-BFL: AEI found using the best-fit line method; AEI-TRL: AEI found using the top-roof line method; GFW: width of the glenoid fossa; GFD: depth of the glenoid fossa; GFW/GFD: ratio of the GFW to the GFD; AEH: height of the articular eminence; CA: condylar angle; IA: intercondylar angle; *: p-value < 0.05; **: p-value < 0.01

3.5. Descriptive Statistics of the Measurements of the TMJ According to Gender

The differences between the male and female participants of the same occlusion pattern are shown in Table 5. No statistically significant differences were observed between both genders among three malocclusion groups except for the two angular variables of the condyle in the class I group and the GFW/GFD ratio of the class II division 1 group.

Table 5. Descriptive statistics of the measurements of the temporomandibular joint according to gender among the three malocclusion groups.

Variable	Class I			Class II-1			Class II-2		
	Male (n = 22/11)	Female (n = 26/13)	p-Value	Male (n = 14/7)	Female (n = 26/13)	p-Value	Male (n = 16/8)	Female (n = 30/15)	p-Value
AEI-BFL (°)	53.14 ± 5.90	52.08 ± 7.92	0.608	60.95 ± 5.24	62.66 ± 6.17	0.386	64.40 ± 5.21	67.51 ± 9.46	0.158
AEI-TRL (°)	37.96 ± 4.67	38.33 ± 6.08	0.816	43.21 ± 6.19	41.67 ± 5.05	0.399	42.45 ± 4.31	43.05 ± 5.19	0.693
GFW (mm)	17.26 ± 1.61	17.46 ± 1.61	0.679	16.36 ± 1.27	17.12 ± 1.41	0.099	16.73 ± 1.33	16.51 ± 1.26	0.597
GFD (mm)	6.14 ± 1.07	5.74 ± 1.08	0.209	6.36 ± 1.04	5.94 ± 0.88	0.183	6.69 ± 0.84	6.25 ± 1.00	0.135
GFW/GFD	2.87 ± 0.38	3.13 ± 0.55	0.070	2.62 ± 0.35	2.94 ± 0.48	0.032 *	2.52 ± 0.23	2.69 ± 0.35	0.081
AEH (mm)	7.30 ± 1.39	7.03 ± 1.24	0.489	7.40 ± 0.67	7.59 ± 1.04	0.538	7.59 ± 1.14	7.37 ± 1.27	0.554
CA (°)	70.64 ± 5.53	76.72 ± 4.24	0.000 **	72.07 ± 5.99	74.49 ± 7.70	0.315	69.49 ± 6.65	70.07 ± 6.22	0.769
IA (°)	141.28 ± 9.89	153.45 ± 7.38	0.002 **	144.14 ± 8.12	148.98 ± 15.43	0.453	136.9 ± 13.19	140.13 ± 11.69	0.552

AEI-BFL: AEI found using the best-fit line method; AEI-TRL: AEI found using the top-roof line method; GFW: width of the glenoid fossa; GFD: depth of the glenoid fossa; GFW/GFD: ratio of the GFW to the GFD; AEH: height of the articular eminence; CA: condylar angle; IA: intercondylar angle; *: p-value < 0.05; **: p-value < 0.01.

A comparison of the three malocclusion groups according to gender using one-way ANOVA followed by the Bonferroni multiple comparisons is illustrated in Table 6. The AEI evaluated using two methods presented significant differences between different malocclusion groups in both genders ($p < 0.05$). In addition, the indicators of GFW, GFW/GFD, CA, and IA showed more intergroup differences in females than in males.

Table 6. Statistical summary of the measurements of the temporomandibular joint according to malocclusion in different genders.

Variable	Male				Female				
	F-Value	p-Value			F-Value	p-Value			
		CI to CII-1	CI to CII-2	CII-1 to CII-2		CI to CII-1	CI to CII-2	CII-1 to CII-2	
AEI-BFL (°)	20.840 **	0.000 **	0.000 **	0.238	26.337 **	0.000 **	0.000 **	0.082	
AEI-TRL (°)	6.001 **	0.011 *	0.027 *	1.000	5.430 **	0.090	0.005 **	1.000	
GFW (mm)	1.784	0.216	0.783	1.000	3.178 *	1.000	0.047 *	0.344	
GFD (mm)	1.444	1.000	0.287	1.000	1.872	1.000	0.178	0.766	
GFW/GFD	5.549 **	0.096	0.008 **	1.000	6.177 **	0.473	0.002 **	0.144	
AEH (mm)	0.307	1.000	1.000	1.000	1.459	0.281	0.890	1.000	
CA (°)	0.689	1.000	1.000	0.739	8.376 **	0.597	0.000 **	0.029 *	
IA (°)	0.897	1.000	1.000	0.602	4.546 *	1.000	0.017 *	0.174	

CI: class I; CII-1: class II division 1; CII-2: class II division 2; AEI-BFL: AEI found using the best-fit line method; AEI-TRL: AEI found using the top-roof line method; GFW: width of the glenoid fossa; GFD: depth of the glenoid fossa; GFW/GFD: ratio of the GFW to the GFD; AEH: height of the articular eminence; CA: condylar angle; IA: intercondylar angle; *: p-value < 0.05; **: p-value < 0.01.

4. Discussion

TMJ is a region with high anatomical complexity, whereas the clinical examination can only provide us with very limited information because it is hard to precisely reveal the internal environment. Taking this restriction into consideration, various radiographic methods were selected to evaluate the morphology of the TMJ in previous studies. Conventional two-dimensional radiographs, such as tomography or panoramic radiographs, were widely used in the early days. However, these modalities are inadequate for quantitative evaluation because of certain limitations, for example, they cannot reflect the three-dimensional shape accurately and may have image distortion and magnification [1,27]. Magnetic resonance imaging (MRI) can provide visualization in both osseous and soft tissue abnormalities, including the morphology of bone structures, the articular disk, and associated muscles and ligaments, in addition to evaluating the functional relationships between them [28]. It is considered the gold standard imaging diagnostic method for TMDs and is widely used in the qualitative evaluation of TMDs [28]. Unfortunately, it was difficult for us to use MRI for all participants included in the present study due to the limitations of the research conditions. The appearance of helical CT makes it possible to evaluate osseous components in three dimensions without superimposition or distortion. Nowadays, CBCT has already replaced helical CT as a superior method in the stomatological area because of the high spatial resolution, lower radiation dose, shorter scanning time, and greater cost-effectiveness [24,25]. In this study, the CBCT was selected for angular and linear measurements of the TMJ osseous morphology.

The development stage of the articular eminence may influence the quantitative measurements of the TMJ. After reviewing the previous studies, the time to full development time of the articular eminence is still controversial. An autopsy study of Oberg reported that the tubercle and the fossa were well developed at the age of 14–15 years [29]. On the other hand, Katsavrias studied the dry skulls from Asiatic Indian individuals in 2002 and found that the articular eminence was 90–94% complete by the age of 20 years [4]. In order to minimize the influence of the growth on the experimental result, we limited the age of the patients in the sample selection to those that were at least 20 years old. Finally, the age range of the samples included in the present study was 20–49 years and the mean age was 27.91 ± 6.94 years. The sample size for understanding anatomical trends in patients should be as large as possible; however, the present study was just a pilot investigation that demonstrated the possibility of a trend existing. We calculated the sample size using the PASS software based on our preliminary data to increase the scientificity of the study, where the minimum sample size was computed to be 38 joints per group. It should be recognized that the present study aimed to access the association between the osseous morphology of the TMJ and the dental malocclusion. Therefore, the skeletal pattern of the individuals of the current study was strictly limited to skeletal class I with average mandibular angle by ANB, FH–MP, and SN–GnGo. After the statistical analysis of the age and basic measurement of the skeletal pattern, there was no statistical difference between the different malocclusion groups, which indicated that the samples of different malocclusion groups had excellent intergroup consistency for comparison.

The articular eminence is a small bone structure belonging to the cranium. The surface of its posterior slope is exposed to mechanical and functional load arising from biomechanical forces from other structures within the TMJ, where these loads influence the morphological characteristics of it [30]. It is crucial to choose a stable and comparable method for measuring the inclination of the articular eminence. The "best-fit line" method and the "top-roof line" method on the central sagittal slice of the TMJ are the two main methods described in previous studies [13]. The "best-fit line" method is considered as the functional inclination of the articular eminence because it is directly related to the movement direction of the condyle–disk complex and reflects the actual condylar path. In contrast, the "top-roof line" method is more concerned about the localization of the articular eminence in relation to the glenoid fossa and it largely depends on the development of the articular eminence. Therefore, it depicts the anatomical inclination of the articular eminence better. In the current study, the class II division 2 group showed the highest value of AEI-BFL, followed by the class II division 1 group, then the class I group, where the differences between the three groups were significant. For the AEI-TRL, class II division 2 also revealed the highest value. However, the statistical differences were only found between the dental class I and class II malocclusions. These results indicated that there might be some correlation between the AEI-TRL and the molar relationship. However, for the functional AEI, the angle was not only related to the molar relationship but was also affected by the inclination of the anterior teeth.

In previous studies, the fossa shapes were assessed in subjective ways and traditionally classified as triangular, trapezoidal, oval, and round [31]. In this study, the shapes of the fossa were studied quantitatively using their width and depth. Considering that the size of the fossa may have great variability in different individuals, we also introduced the variable of GFW/GFD to describe the relative relationship between the width and depth. The GFD and AEH were both used to analyze the vertical depth of the fossa; however, the GFD is focused more on describing the anatomical height of the glenoid fossa, regardless of the patient's head position. The AEH was highly related to the shape of the articular eminence, which reflected the vertical sliding space of the condyle in the normal head position. Based on the results of this study, the difference in the fossa shapes only appeared in the GFW and its ratio to GFD between the class II division 2 and class I groups. There were no significant differences in the anatomic and functional fossa depths between different malocclusion groups. It indicated that the fossa shapes of class II divisions 1 and 2 were relatively similar, which was consistent with the findings obtained by Katsavrias and Halazonetis [32]. In addition, the height of the articular fossa might not be a specific index to distinguish between different malocclusions according to samples of the study. Moreover, Sümbüllü et al., Cğlayan et al., and Poluha et al. [24,33,34] affirmed that the AEH and GFD were also not specific indicators to discriminate between the normal and TMD patients, though the opposite opinion was expressed by Paknahad et al. [25].

TMJ is the only diarthrodial joint with a bilateral linkage in human bodies. It can move synchronously during the symmetrical movement (open–close, protrusion–retrusion) or with its own movements on each side during the lateral movement. Several published papers only noted TMJ as an individual joint without taking into account the contralateral side [24,25]. In the present study, the left and right joints were measured separately and the differences between both sides were evaluated. Based on the results of the study, all the angular and linear measurements of the glenoid fossa showed no significant differences between the left and right sides. The findings of Shahidi et al. and Wu et al. also mentioned that the inclination of the left and right articular eminences did not display any significant differences, which is in agreement with the current study [1,11]. However, the condylar angle of the left joint in both class II division 1 and division 2 groups was significantly lower than that of the right, which was not seen in the class I group. This may indicate that the mandible of the class II patients revealed more asymmetry than that of the class I patients. The values of CA and IA also showed differences between different malocclusion groups. Compared with other types of malocclusion, the condyles of individuals in the class II division 2 group had a greater tendency to rotate inward.

The morphological discrepancies of TMJ due to differences in sex hormones and metabolic activity between male and female individuals have been reported in previous studies [35]. Beyond that, differences in the functional loading of TMJ according to gender can also cause changes in TMJ morphology [36]. Jasinevicius et al. [37] found a gender difference in AEI, which demonstrated a contrary result to the study of Sümbüllü et al. [24]. Based on our results, it was observed that the diversities of TMJ morphology between the two genders were only revealed in the CA and IA values of the class I group. As for the differences in the TMJ morphology variables between malocclusion groups that were separately analyzed according to gender, the AEI showed similar trends in different genders. However, the differences in other morphological parameters of both the glenoid fossa and condyle in female individuals between the three malocclusion groups mentioned in the current study were higher than those in males, which might be one of the possible reasons why TMJ dysfunctions occur more often in females than in males.

5. Conclusions

On the basis of our study, the following conclusions could be drawn:

1. The inclination of articular eminence displayed a great difference between class I and class II malocclusions in the normal skeletal pattern, and the individuals of class II division 2 showed the highest AEI.

2. The height of the glenoid fossa might not be a specific index to distinguish between different malocclusions.

3. The condyles of individuals in the class II division 2 group had a greater tendency to rotate inward.

4. The shape of the glenoid fossa showed no significant difference between the left and right sides.

5. The differences in morphological parameters of TMJ in female individuals between the three malocclusion groups were higher than those in males.

Author Contributions: Conceptualization, X.-C.F. and X.R.-F.; data curation, X.-C.F. and L.-S.M.; formal analysis, L.C.; funding acquisition, X.-F.H.; investigation, X.-C.F. and L.-S.M.; methodology, X.-C.F. and D.S.; project administration, X.-C.F., X.R.-F., and X.-F.H.; supervision, X.R.-F. and X.-F.H.; writing—original draft, X.-C.F.; writing—review and editing, L.C., X.R.-F., and X.-F.H. All authors have read and agreed to the published version of the manuscript.

Funding: This study was supported by the Natural Science Foundation of Beijing Municipality (grant no. 7202036) and the Capital Health Research and Development of Special Funding (grant no. 2018-2-1102).

Institutional Review Board Statement: The study was conducted according to the guidelines of the Declaration of Helsinki and approved by the Ethical Committee of Beijing Friendship Hospital (approval number 2021-P2-008-01, updated on 1 February 2021).

Informed Consent Statement: Informed consent was obtained from all subjects involved in the study.

Data Availability Statement: The data presented in this study are available on request from the corresponding author.

Conflicts of Interest: The authors declare no conflict of interest.

References

1. Wu, C.-K.; Hsu, J.-T.; Shen, Y.-W.; Chen, J.-H.; Shen, W.-C.; Fuh, L.-J. Assessments of inclinations of the mandibular fossa by computed tomography in an Asian population. *Clin. Oral Investig.* **2012**, *16*, 443–450. [CrossRef]
2. Som, P.-M.; Curtin, H.D. *Head and Neck Imaging*, 5th ed.; Mosby, Inc.: St. Louis, MO, USA, 2011; p. 1547.
3. Schmolke, C. The relationship between the temporomandibular joint capsule, articular disc and jaw muscles. *J. Anat.* **1994**, *184*, 335–345.
4. Katsavrias, E.G. Changes in articular eminence inclination during the craniofacial growth period. *Angle Orthod.* **2002**, *72*, 258–264. [PubMed]
5. Pandis, N.; Karpac, J.; Trevino, R.; Williams, B. A radiographic study of condyle position at various depths of cut in dry skulls with axially corrected lateral tomograms. *Am. J. Orthod. Dentofac. Orthop.* **1991**, *100*, 116–122. [CrossRef]
6. Isberg, A.; Westesson, P.L. Steepness of articular eminence and movement of the condyle and disk in asymptomatic temporomandibular joints. *Oral Surg. Oral Med. Oral Pathol. Oral Radiol. Endodontol.* **1998**, *86*, 152–157. [CrossRef]
7. Sulun, T.; Cemgil, A.T.; Duc, J.-M.P.; Rammelsberg, P.; Jäger, L.; Gernet, W. Morphology of the mandibular fossa and inclination of the articular eminence in patients with internal derangement and in symptom-free volunteers. *Oral Surg. Oral Med. Oral Pathol. Oral Radiol. Endodontol.* **2001**, *92*, 98–107. [CrossRef]
8. Fan, X.-C.; Singh, D.; Ma, L.-S.; Piehslinger, E.; Huang, X.-F.; Rausch-Fan, X. Is There an Association between Temporomandibular Disorders and Articular Eminence Inclination? A Systematic Review. *Diagnostics* **2021**, *11*, 29. [CrossRef]
9. Reicheneder, C.; Gedrange, T.; Baumert, U.; Faltermeier, A.; Proff, P. Variations in the inclination of the condylar path in children and adults. *Angle Orthod.* **2009**, *79*, 958–963. [CrossRef]
10. Imanimoghaddam, M.; Madani, A.S.; Mahdavi, P.; Bagherpour, A.; Darijani, M.; Ebrahimnejad, H. Evaluation of condylar positions in patients with temporomandibular disorders: A cone-beam computed tomographic study. *Imaging Sci. Dent.* **2016**, *46*, 127–131. [CrossRef]
11. Shahidi, S.; Vojdani, M.; Paknahad, M. Correlation between articular eminence steepness measured with cone-beam computed tomography and clinical dysfunction index in patients with temporomandibular joint dysfunction. *Oral Surg. Oral Med. Oral Pathol. Oral Radiol.* **2013**, *116*, 91–97. [CrossRef]
12. Kubein-Meesenburg, D.; Nagerl, H. Basic principles of relation of anterior and posterior guidance in stomatognathic systems. *Anat. Anz.* **1990**, *171*, 1–12.
13. İlgüy, D.; İlgüy, M.; Fişekçioğlu, E.; Dölekoğlu, S.; Ersan, N. Articular eminence inclination, height, and condyle morphology on cone beam computed tomography. *Sci. World J.* **2014**, *2014*, 761714. [CrossRef]
14. Verner, F.S.; Roque-Torres, G.D.; Ramírez-Sotello, L.R.; Devito, K.L.; Almeida, S.M. Analysis of the correlation between dental arch and articular eminence morphology: A cone beam computed tomography study. *Oral Surg. Oral Med. Oral Pathol. Oral Radiol.* **2017**, *124*, 420–431. [CrossRef]
15. Cevidanes, L.H.; Hajati, A.K.; Paniagua, B.; Lim, P.F.; Walker, D.G.; Palconet, G.; Nackley, A.G.; Styner, M.; Ludlow, J.-B.; Zhu, H.; et al. Quantification of condylar resorption in temporomandibular joint osteoarthritis. *Oral Surg. Oral Med. Oral Pathol. Oral Radiol. Endodontol.* **2010**, *110*, 110–117. [CrossRef] [PubMed]
16. Zabarović, D.; Jerolimov, V.; Carek, V.; Vojvodić, D.; Zabarović, K.; Buković, D., Jr. The effect of tooth loss on the TM-joint articular eminence inclination. *Coll. Antropol.* **2000**, *24*, 37–42.
17. Kurita, H.; Ohtsuka, A.; Kobayashi, H.; Kurashina, K. Is the morphology of the articular eminence of the temporomandibular joint a predisposing factor for disc displacement? *Dentomaxillofac. Radiol.* **2000**, *29*, 159–162. [CrossRef]

18. Kurita, H.; Ohtsuka, A.; Kobayashi, H.; Kurashina, K. Flattening of the articular eminence correlates with progressive internal derangement of the temporomandibular joint. *Dentomaxillofac. Radiol.* **2000**, *29*, 277–279. [CrossRef]
19. Mengi, A.; Sharma, V.P.; Tandon, P.; Agarwal, A.; Singh, A. A cephalometric evaluation of the effect of glenoid fossa location on craniofacial morphology. *J. Oral Biol. Craniofac. Res.* **2016**, *6*, 204–212. [CrossRef]
20. Proffit, W.R. *Contemporary Orthodontics*, 3rd ed.; Mosby, Inc.: St. Louis, MO, USA, 2000; pp. 435–439.
21. Iodice, G.; Danzi, G.; Cimino, R.; Paduano, S.; Michelotti, A. Association between posterior crossbite, masticatory muscle pain, and disc displacement: A systematic review. *Eur. J. Orthod.* **2013**, *35*, 737–744. [CrossRef] [PubMed]
22. Fu, M.-K.; Mao, X.-J. Cephalometric study of 144 normal subjects. *Chin. Med. J.* **1975**, *55*, 865–867.
23. Park, I.-Y.; Kim, J.-H.; Park, Y.-H. Three-dimensional cone-beam computed tomography based comparison of condylar position and morphology according to the vertical skeletal pattern. *Korean J. Orthod.* **2015**, *45*, 66–73. [CrossRef]
24. Sümbüllü, M.A.; Çağlayan, F.; Akgül, H.M.; Yilmaz, A.B. Radiological examination of the articular eminence morphology using cone beam CT. *Dentomaxillofac. Radiol.* **2012**, *41*, 234–240. [CrossRef] [PubMed]
25. Paknahad, M.; Shahidi, S.; Akhlaghian, M.; Abolvardi, M. Is Mandibular Fossa Morphology and Articular Eminence Inclination Associated with Temporomandibular Dysfunction? *J. Dent.* **2016**, *17*, 134–141.
26. Shrout, P.E.; Fleiss, J.L. Intraclass correlations: Uses in assessing rater reliability. *Psychol. Bull.* **1979**, *86*, 420–428. [CrossRef] [PubMed]
27. Unal Erzurumlu, Z.; Celenk, P. A radiological evaluation of the effects of edentulousness on the temporomandibular joint. *J. Oral Rehabil.* **2020**, *47*, 319–324. [CrossRef] [PubMed]
28. Larheim, T.A.; Westesson, P.; Sano, T. Temporomandibular joint disk displacement: Comparison in asymptomatic volunteers and patients. *Radiology* **2001**, *218*, 428–432. [CrossRef] [PubMed]
29. Oberg, T.; Carlsson, G.E.; Fajers, C.M. The temporomandibular joint: A morphological study on a human autopsy material. *Acta Odontol. Scand.* **1971**, *29*, 349–383. [CrossRef]
30. O'Ryan, F.; Epker, B.N. Temporomandibular joint function and morphology: Observations on the spectra of normalcy. *Oral Surg. Oral Med. Oral Pathol.* **1984**, *58*, 272–279. [CrossRef]
31. Katsavrias, E.G. Morphology of the temporomandibular joint in subjects with Class II Division 2 malocclusions. *Am. J. Orthod. Dentofac. Orthop.* **2006**, *129*, 470–478. [CrossRef]
32. Katsavrias, E.G.; Halazonetis, D.J. Condyle and fossa shape in Class II and Class III skeletal patterns: A morphometric tomographic study. *Am. J. Orthod. Dentofac. Orthop.* **2005**, *128*, 337–346. [CrossRef]
33. Çağlayan, F.; Sümbüllü, M.A.; Akgül, H.M. Associations between the articular eminence inclination and condylar bone changes, condylar movements, and condyle and fossa shapes. *Oral Radiol.* **2013**, *30*, 84–91. [CrossRef]
34. Poluha, R.L.; Cunha, C.O.; Bonjardim, L.R.; Conti, P.C.R. Temporomandibular joint morphology does not influence the presence of arthralgia in patients with disk displacement with reduction: A magnetic resonance imaging–based study. *Oral Surg. Oral Med. Oral Pathol. Oral Radiol.* **2020**, *129*, 149–157. [CrossRef]
35. Siriwat, P.P.; Jarabak, J.R. Malocclusion and facial morphology is there a relationship? An epidemiologic study. *Angle Orthod.* **1985**, *55*, 127–138. [PubMed]
36. Zivko-Babić, J.; Pandurić, J.; Jerolimov, V.; Mioc, M.; Pizeta, L.; Jakovac, M. Bite force in subjects with complete dentition. *Coll. Antropol.* **2002**, *26*, 293–302. [PubMed]
37. Jasinevicius, T.R.; Pyle, M.A.; Lalumandier, J.A.; Nelson, S.; Kohrs, K.J.; Türp, J.C.; Sawyer, D.R. Asymmetry of the articular eminence in dentate and partially edentulous populations. *Cranio* **2006**, *24*, 85–94. [CrossRef] [PubMed]

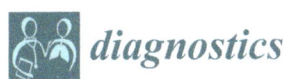

Article

SPECT/CT Correlation in the Diagnosis of Unilateral Condilar Hyperplasia

Diego Fernando López [1,*], Valentina Ríos Borrás [2], Juan Manuel Muñoz [3], Rodrigo Cardenas-Perilla [3] and Luis Eduardo Almeida [4]

1. Orthodontics Department, Universidad del Valle, Cali 760043, Colombia
2. Escuela de Odontología, Universidad del Valle, Cali 760043, Colombia; valentina.rios@correounivalle.edu.co
3. Nuclear Medicine Department, Centro Médico Imbanaco, Cali 760043, Colombia; juan.munoz@imbanaco.com.co (J.M.M.); rodrigo.cardenas@imbanaco.com.co (R.C.-P.)
4. Surgical Clinical Sciences, School of Dentistry, Marquette University, Milwaukee, WI 53206, USA; luis.almeida@marquette.edu
* Correspondence: diego.f.lopez@correounivalle.edu.co

Abstract: Objective: To evaluate the correlation between metabolic bone activity measured by single photon emission computed tomography (SPECT) and the anatomic condylar characteristics acquired by computed tomography (CT), in patients with unilateral condylar hyperplasia (UCH). Method and Materials/Patients: Observational, descriptive study in a group of 71 patients with clinical diagnosis of UCH and indication of SPECT/CT. Bone SPECT images obtained in a gamma-camera GE Infina and processed in a station Xeleris 3 with the program Volumetrix MI Evolution for bone. CT images acquired in a PET/CT Biograph mcT20 equipment (Siemens) processed in a station Osirix V 7.5.1 (Pixmeo, Bomex, Switzerland). Results: The sample included 24 men (33.8%) and 47 women (66.2%). Active state UCH was detected in 40 (56.3%) cases (over 55% uptake in the affected condyle) and 38 (53.5%) presented mandibular deviation to the right side. No significant differences related to sex, age, or mandibular deviation side were found. Mandibular deviation was the only morphologic feature related to active/inactive UCH ($p = 0.003$). The likelihood of active CH was significantly higher in patients with mandibular deviation higher than 6 mm compared with <6 mm (odds ratio (OR): 3.51, confidence interval (CI) 95%: 1.27–9.72). Conclusion: There is a significant correlation between the magnitude of mandibular deviation quantified on CT and metabolic findings obtained by SPECT in patients with UCH. The risk of active UCH is 3.5 times higher in patients with a mandibular deviation ≥6 mm.

Keywords: bone scintigraphy; computed tomography; condylar hyperplasia; SPECT; ^{99m}Tc-MDP

1. Introduction

Condylar hyperplasia (CH) is a progressive and self-limiting pathology affecting the mandibular condyle growth and compromising the temporomandibular joint (TMJ) anatomy [1–3].

The functional, occlusal, and esthetic effects of CH in patients demand a multidisciplinary intervention to confirm a clinically suspected diagnosis and establish the therapeutic approach [4]. Early diagnosis and adequate treatment are important to avoid complicated sequelae [5].

UCH is effectively diagnosed by measurement of bone metabolic hyperactivity in SPECT mandibular TMJ 3D images [1,6,7]. Recent studies show that 3D SPECT images are superior to planar images [8]. Uptake radioactive values equal or higher than 55% for the suspected condyle or a percentage side difference over 10% are commonly accepted as positive results indicating hyperactivity (active disease) of the mandibular condyle [9,10]. However, the functional SPECT images are not adequate to show in detail the anatomic

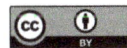

structures in the region of interest (ROI). Therefore, it is recommended to combine SPECT with CT images to characterize the pathology by both its anatomy and metabolism [11,12].

The correlation of metabolic and anatomic findings by a team of experts in the management and interpretation of SPECT/CT techniques allows the establishment of clear-cut parameters of the pathology to precisely indicate the extension of the altered region. This approach is a recent breakthrough in the procedures of diagnosis and treatment of UCH [12,13].

The authors' hypothesis from the existing literature is that the fusion of images and information obtained from SPECT/CT to diagnose UCH improves the precision and specificity of the diagnostic tests and, consequently, allows better therapeutic decisions [11,12,14–16]. Considering that there are few published studies and they provide information from poorly representative populations, the objective of the present study was to correlate the metabolic bone activity of the condyle measured by SPECT with the anatomic information provided by CT images, in patients with active or inactive UCH.

2. Materials and Methods/Patients

This is a retrospective observational study with no intervention or manipulation of variables from the patients. Therefore, it is a no risk investigation and was approved by the Institutional Ethics Committee (Approval number CEI-403) and conducted following all the regulations of the Declaration of Helsinki, last version.

A population of 153 image sets from patients tested by SPECT/CT (Figure 1), performed in the Nuclear Medicine deparment of a High Complexity Center, between January 2015 and January 2020, was evaluated for the study. The patients had been sent to Nuclear Medicine by the clinical specialists owing to facial asymmetry and suspected UCH. Following the classification of Lopez et al. 2019 [17], the patients were classified by types of facial asymmetry, obtaining 71 cases with UCH diagnosis. Taking into account the information from clinical records, patients with antecedents of TMJ trauma or fracture, previous orthognatic surgery, dentofacial syndromes, and arthritis were excluded. When the SPECT/CT information was not complete, the set of images was excluded as well.

The mandibular bone SPECT procedure was carried out 2 h after the endovenous administration of a dose of 15 mCi ^{99m}Tc-MDP for patients over 18 year and normalized according to the EANM Pediatric Dosage Card for patients under 18. The images were obtained using a double head gamma-camera GE Infinia (Chicago, IL, USA), with low energy collimators, and a 128×128 high resolution matrix to obtain 45 images, 18 s of exposure, for each $180°$ of detection.

The data were reconstructed in the processing station Xeleris 3 (General Electric, Chicago, IL, USA) using the program "Volumetrix MI Evolution for Bone", with the ordered subsets expectations maximization (OSEM) algorithm for iterative reconstruction, applying four interactions and eight subsets with a Butterworth 0.45 filter and Power 12, plus correction of resolution recovery. From the reconstruction, five transaxial images for quantification in the condyles were obtained, extracting the total counts for a fixed-size ROI (1.76 cm^2) [18].

The SPECT report provided quantitative information expressed as radionuclide percentage uptake in the condyles. The counts observed within the selected ROI were used to calculate the % uptake using the following equations:

% right condyle uptake = Maximum counts in the right condyle $\times$ 100

Right side counts + left side counts

% left condyle uptake = Maximum counts in the left condyle $\times$ 100.

Right side counts + left side counts

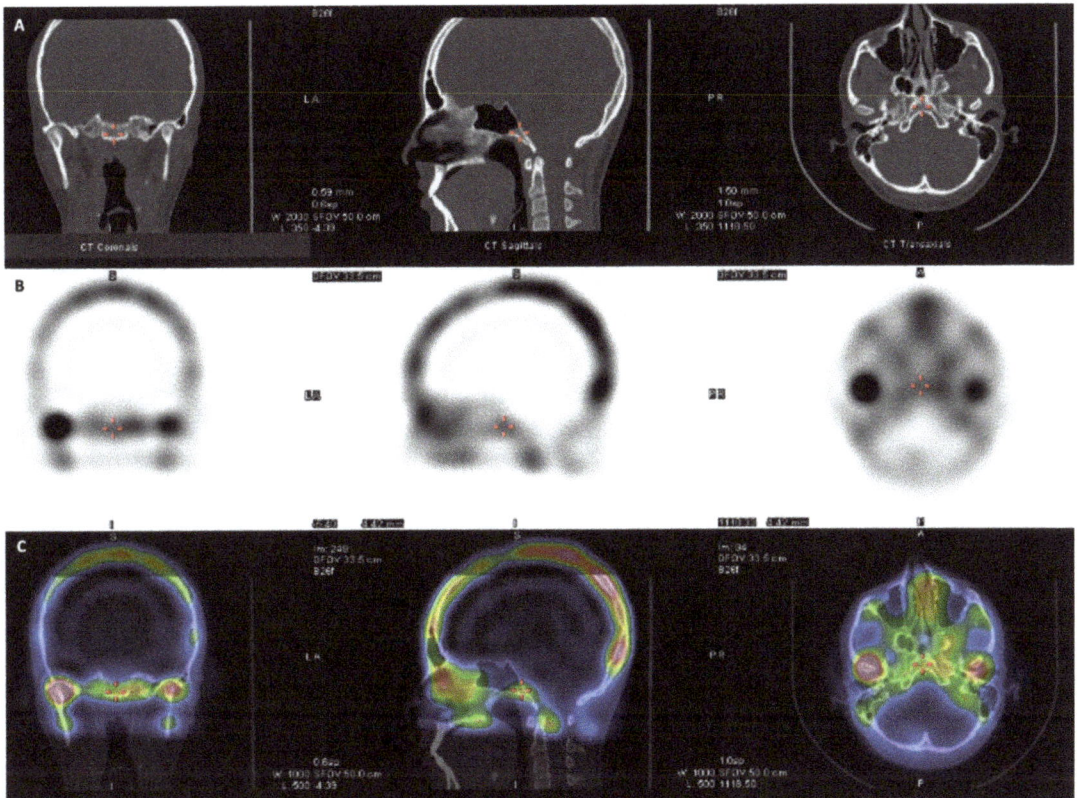

Figure 1. (**A**) Computed tomography (CT) images: coronal, sagittal, and axial sections. (**B**) Single photon emission CT (SPECT) images: coronal, sagittal, and axial sections. (**C**) Fused functional images (SPECT and CT) in a patient with right side active unilateral condylar hyperplasia (UCH).

A difference in percentage uptake between condyles = or >10% was interpreted as a positive result indicating active pathology [3].

CT cranial images were acquired in a PET/CT Biograph mCT20 (Siemens, Erlangen, Germany) equipment without contrast enhanced, from vertex to sternal notch, applying the following parameters: section thickness: 1.0 mm, pitch: 1.0, and a 512 × 512 cubic matrix with isotropic voxel (size 0.75 × 0.75 × 0.75 mm) to avoid image distortion in the different planes. The same parameters were applied to adult and pediatric patients. The CT images were reconstructed using a B26F homogeneous low dose filter for anatomic localization. All the patients were positioned with a head fixing device to avoid artifacts owing to movement and facilitate the image fusion.

The set of DICOM images was processed in a work station Osirix V 7.5.1 (Pixmeo, Bernex, Switzerland) obtaining linear measurements in sagittal and frontal planes. The description of measurements taken in the 3D bone tissue reconstruction is described in Table 1.

Table 1. Description of craniofacial measurements taken in the 3D bone tissue reconstruction, frontal, and sagittal planes.

Measurement (mm)	Description
Condylar length	In the sagittal view, a line parallel to a tangent to the posterior ridge of the mandibular ramus was traced and extended from the most superior point of the condyle to a perpendicular line, passing through the most inferior point of the mandibular notch. This length was obtained in a corrected image of the axial axis of the mandibular ramus (Figure 2A).
Mandibular ramus length	In the sagittal view of 3D reconstruction, a line perpendicular to the Frankfort plane, was traced and extended from the deepest point of the notch to the inferior ridge of mandibular body (Figure 2B).
Anteroposterior condylar length	In the axial view, a line from the most anterior point of condylar cortical bone to the most posterior limit of cortical bone was traced. This image was obtained in an orthogonal plane (Figure 3A).
Midlateral condylar length	In the axial view, a line from the most anterior limit of proximal cortical of the condyle to the most anterior limit of its distal cortical was traced. This image was obtained in an orthogonal plane (Figure 3B).
Deviation Magnitude	In the coronal view of the 3D reconstruction, repositioning the skull in a natural position of the head, the magnitude of the deviation is quantified as follows: the distance in mm from menton to the facial midline projected from the apophysis *crista galli*, perpendicular to the zygomatic plane was measured (Figure 4).
Side of mandibular deviation (laterognathism)	In the coronal view of the bone tissue 3D reconstruction, this qualitative variable was visually detected, indicating the mandibular deviation side (right/left) (Figure 4).

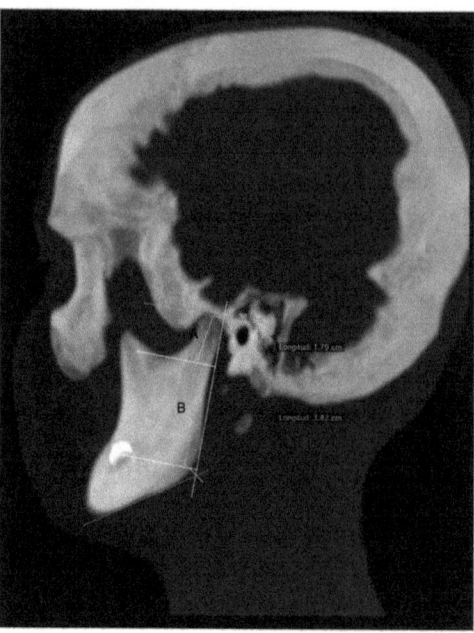

Figure 2. Bone tissue CT, sagittal view. (**A**) Condylar length. (**B**) Mandibular ramus length.

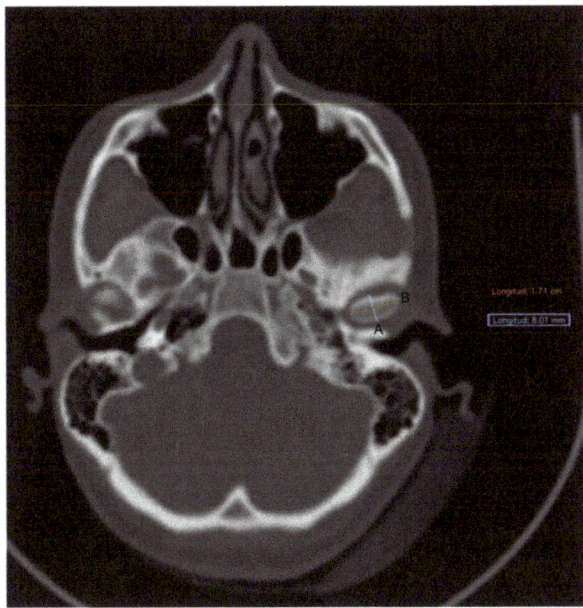

Figure 3. Bone tissue CT, axial view. (**A**) Anteroposterior condylar length. (**B**) Midlateral condylar length.

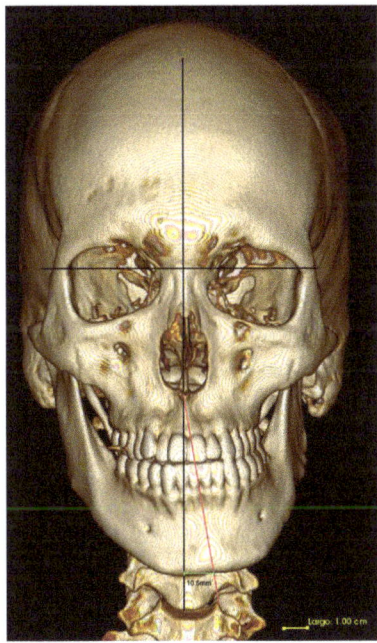

Figure 4. Bone tissue CT, 3D reconstruction. Coronal view. Mandibular deviation magnitude and deviation side.

The tomographic measurements were taken by a trained and calibrated operator. Each data set was simultaneously revised and classified according to the craniofacial characteristics of the asymmetry [17], together by the operator and a specialist with experience in diagnosis and treatment of patients with facial asymmetry.

To assess the reproducibility of the measurements, a duplicate reading was taken by the same observer on a subsample of 20 patients with a four-week interval between the two measurements. The correlation coefficients (Rho) indicate an agreement higher than 0.90 for all of the variables (Table 2).

Table 2. Intraobserver agreement for craniofacial measurements obtained in frontal and sagittal views.

Measurement in mm	Difference * Average ± SD	Rho	p-Value
Right side total condylar length	0.01 ± 0.19	0.99 (0.99–1.00)	0.000
Left side total condylar length	0.10 ± 0.31	0.99 (0.99–1.00)	0.000
Right side ramus length	−0.19 ± 0.33	0.99 (0.99–1.00)	0.000
Left side ramus length	0.10 ± 0.57	0.99 (0.99–1.00)	0.000
Anteroposterior pole of right condyle	0.07 ± 0.19	0.98 (0.96–0.99)	0.000
Anteroposterior pole of left condyle	0.19 ± 0.28	0.95 (0.91–0.99)	0.000
Lateral pole of right condyle	−0.19 ± 0.31	0.99 (0.98–1.00)	0.000
Lateral pole of left condyle	−0.05 ± 0.30	0.99 (−0.99–1.00)	0.000
Mandibular deviation in mm	0.13 ± 0.51	0.99 (0.98–1.00)	0.000
Difference in percentage uptake	0 ± 0	1	0.000

Difference between first and second measurement *. SD: standard deviation. Rho: Spearman correlation coefficient.

Statistical Analysis

The data were processed by one operator expert in the software management. All statistical analyses were carried out in the software Stata13® (StataCorp, College Station, TX, USA). Normality of distribution was tested by the method of Shapiro–Wilk and, according to it and the kind of variable, the results are expressed as average ± standard deviation, median, inter-quartile range, and absolute/relative frequencies. The Chi square test or Fisher test was applied for bivariate analysis of qualitative variables and either Student's t-test or U-test for quantitative variables, according to the distribution normality. Correlations were evaluated by the Spearman coefficient rho. The level of significance was $p < 0.05$.

Intraobserver agreement was evaluated by the intraclass correlation coefficient of Lin.

Receiver operating characteristics (ROC) curves were determined to establish the best cut-off value of mandibular deviation to classify the hyperplasia as active or inactive. ROC curves were obtained from estimated sensitivity, specificity, and positive and negative predictive values calculating their 95% confidence intervals.

3. Results

Data from 71 SPECT/CT files were analyzed. The sample included 47 (66.2%) women and 24 (33.8%) men, with a median age of 19 years. From the total number of patients, 40 (56.3%) presented active UCH (≥55% uptake in the affected condyle) and 38 (53.5%) presented right side deviation. No significant differences in the frequency of active UCH were detected in relation to age, ($p = 0.1$), sex ($p = 0.22$), or side of mandibular deviation ($p = 0.99$) (Table 3).

Table 3. General characteristics of the patients with active/inactive condylar hyperplasia. SPECT, single photon emission computed tomography.

Variable	Active n = 40	Inactive n = 31	Total n = 71	p-Value
Age	19 (16–26.25)	17 (13–21.5)	19 (15–25.5)	0.10
	22.15 (8.54)	19.29 (7.47)	20.90 (8.16)	0.14
Male sex	11 (27.5)	13 (41.93)	24 (33.80)	0.22
Female sex	29 (72.5)	18 (58.06)	47 (66.20)	
Right Laterognathism	21 (52.5)	17 (54.84)	38 (53.52)	0.99
Left Laterognathism	19 (47.5)	14 (45.16)	33 (46.48)	
Difference in percentage uptake in SPECT *	17.2 (7.52)	3.93 (3.16)	11.41 (8.93)	<0.001

Median (P25–P75); n (%); average (standard deviation). * ($\geq$10% active stage).

Morphologic Data and Active Hyperplasia

The measurements obtained in CT images of the patients were related to the active or inactive state of UCH. The results are presented in Table 4 and Figure 5. A statistically significant difference was found only for the amount of mandibular deviation, which was higher in active cases of UCH (6.3 ± 3.4 mm) compared with inactive cases (4.1 ± 2.2) ($p = 0.003$).

Table 4. Comparison of morphologic measurements in active/inactive unilateral condylar hyperplasia (UCH) cases.

Morphologic Measurements in mm	Active	Inactive	p-Value
Right condyle total length	19.75 (3.41)	20.21 (3.07)	0.55
Left condyle total length	19.95 (4.48)	19.53 (4.88)	0.71
Right mandibular ramus length	34.96 (5.0)	37.29 (6.37)	0.09
Left mandibular ramus length	34.48 (5.26)	37.05 (5.30)	0.05
Anteroposterior pole of right condyle	8.15 (1.15)	7.88 (1.1)	0.32
Anteroposterior pole of left condyle	7.72 (1.01)	8.08 (1.2)	0.19
Midlateral pole of left condyle	16.04 (3.41)	15.94 (3.53)	0.90
Midlateral pole of right condyle	15.82 (2.41)	15.57 (3.73)	0.73
Mandibular Deviation (mm)	6.31 (3.46)	4.11 (2.20)	0.003 **

Average (standard deviation); ** $p < 0.005$.

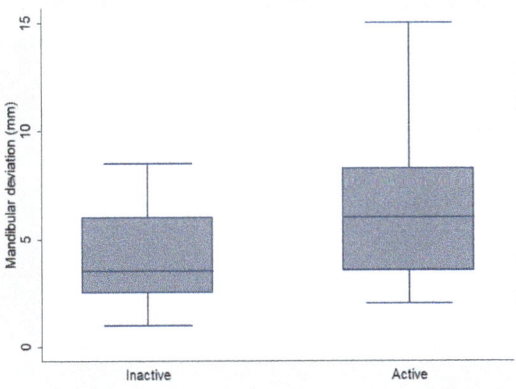

Figure 5. Mandibular deviation 95% confidence intervals (CIs) in active and inactive UCH patients.

The ability of mandibular deviation to classify the state of UCH as active or inactive was studied by ROC analysis. The area under ROC curve (AUC) was 0.695 (CI 95%: 0.57–0.82), indicating acceptable ability to distinguish the states, as the area is >0.5 (Figure 6).

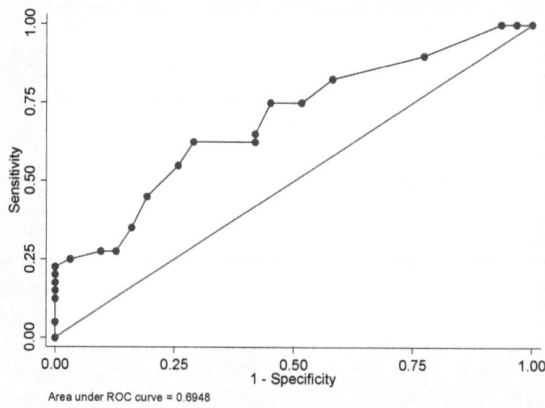

Figure 6. Receiver operating characteristics (ROC) curve (sensitivity vs. 1—specificity) for condylar hyperplasia activity detection by mandibular deviation.

Two cut-off values of mandibular deviation were selected. The first was a 6 mm value because it is more specific, that is, it detects inactive UCH with 55% sensitivity and 74.19% specificity, providing a positive predictive value (PPV) of 73.3% and negative predictive value (NPV) of 56.1%. The other cut-off value was 4 mm, which shows the best sensitivity, that is, it detects more active cases of UCH with a sensitivity of 75% and 54.8% specificity, PPV of 68–18%, and NPV of 63% (Table 5).

Table 5. Diagnostic performance for two criteria (cut-off values: MD = 6 mm and MD = 4) to classify UCH as active/inactive based upon MD.

Diagnostic Performance	Cut-Off Value MD = 6mm	Cut-Off Value MD = 4mm
TP	22	30
TN	23	17
FP	8	14
FN	18	10
Sensitivity	55.00%	75.00%
Specificity	74.19%	54.84%
Correct classification	63.8%	66.2%
PPV	73.33%	68.18%
NPV	56.10%	62.96%
LR (+)	2.13	1.66
LR (−)	0.61	0.46

MD: mandibular deviation; TP (true positive); TN (true negative); FP (false positive); FN (false negative); PPV (positive predictive value); NPV (negative predictive value); LR+ (likelihood ratio positive); LR− (likelihood ratio negative).

The likelihood of having active UCH in patients with mandibular deviation equal or higher than 6 mm was 3.5× higher than the likelihood associated with mandibular deviations <6 mm (OR: 3.51, CI 95%: 1.27–9.72).

When the cut-off value was set to 4 mm, the likelihood of inactive UCH was 73% (OR: 0.27, CI 95%: 0.10–0.75).

4. Discussion

Image fusion for diagnostic purposes, as in the case of SPECT/CT, is known as a co-register or hybrid technique and it is used to improve the diagnostic precision and, therefore, to aid in the development of a better treatment plan positively determined by the prognosis [19]. In nuclear medicine, the use of hybrid tests increases the diagnostic precision by about 30% in skeletal conditions, as well as in tumors and inflammatory processes, owing to a better correction of attenuation, higher specificity, and a more accurate description of the disease location and possible compromise of the adjacent tissues [20,21].

In connection with this, Jacene et al. [11] postulated that the hybrid SPECT/CT image compared with SPECT alone provides additional interpretative information because the CT data indicate the anatomic location of abnormal findings.

The radioactive uptake in bone SPECT depends on the blood circulation and the absorption by the structure of hydroxyapatite crystals. The areas of high uptake of the radioactive tracer are correlated with hyperemia and more metabolic bone activity and, additionally, identify activity at the molecular level. Therefore, nuclear medicine images are highly sensitive for early detection of lesions, very much earlier than X-ray or tomographic images. Bone SPECT is very useful and has been validated for early diagnosis of UCH [1,6,7,22], because this is a condition that could be active during growth and development, but may be self-limited and finally expressed only by sequelae of the pathology [2,23]. Although the diagnosis is strictly clinical, based on intraoral and extraoral findings and tomographic or radiographic images, the evaluation of bone metabolism by SPECT is very useful to differentiate the active/inactive stages [17].

The hybrid SPECT/CT technique for the diagnosis of UCH provides detailed morphologic information about the mandibular condyles and other craniofacial structures that may be compromised in the pathology. This information is associated with the data of bone metabolic activity in the condyles [12], obtained by the comparative lateral uptake of ^{99m}Tc-MPD. In this context, Suh et al. [24] point out the need to have a standardized value for the radiopharmaceutical uptake and the CT data to evaluate temporomandibular disorders.

In the present study, the fusion of data from SPECT/CT to classify UCH conditions as active or inactive detected a significant difference in the magnitude of mandibular deviation (MD) associated with active cases. This finding is concordant with the results of Wang et al. [25], postulating that only MDs exceeding 5 mm are unacceptable according to the patient perception and demand for surgical treatment.

Regarding the diagnostic added value of SPECT/CT compared with SPECT alone to evaluate UCH, Fokoue et al. [26] indicate that this image fusion is superior to detect the hyperplasic area. Agarwal et al. [15] also evaluated, in 21 patients, the diagnostic improvement obtained by the SPECT/TCT fusion compared with SPECT alone, which is more sensitive (80%), but SPECT/CT is more specific (100%) and accurate (85.5%), while planar scintigraphy had the lowest diagnostic performance. However, Theerakulpisut et al. [14], in a study of 61 scintigraphies, concluded that the diagnostic specificity is not improved by fused tests and, as the radiation is increased, did not recommend its use. In the same sense, Verhelst et al. [27] reported that the anatomic changes detected by CT in the hybrid test are evident only in 50% of the patients, adding a minimum benefit, and Liu et al. [16] concluded that ROI delimitation in the drawing of condylar outline was not superior when SPECT/CT was used.

Taking into account these observations, the authors of the present study postulate that the specificity of the SPECT test is improved by the clinical and tomographic pre-diagnostic findings [17], and by the technique applied. The ROI selection; the number of trans-axial sections; and the quantification of radioactive uptake, either by total counts or mean counts, are critical aspects having an influence on the results of the test [18].

International studies indicate that, in different populations, the prevalence of UCH is higher in women than in men [13], as was found in the present study (66.2% women). However, the difference in number of active/inactive cases of the pathology was not significantly sex-dependent. Additionally, in the present study, the difference in laterognathia was not statistically significant, in agreement with previous reports [1,28].

Regarding the age distribution of UCH, the average age in the active UCH group was similar to that of inactive UCH (19 and 17, respectively), both including ranges of residual growth [29]. Although the early detection of UCH reduces the sequelae and invasiveness of the treatment, the fact that that only 10% of changes in bone metabolism appear as positive uptake in SPECT deserves consideration, but the anatomic changes detected by CT are able to indicate the compromise of a higher percentage of bone density [22]. Therefore, in very young patients or in patients that at the moment of examination have initial development of the pathology, the SPECT/CT correlation may not be positive because the pathology is not sufficiently expressed.

The difference between the average DM (6.3 mm) in active states of UCH and the average for inactive conditions (4.1 mm) is statistically significant ($p = 0.003$) and clinically relevant.

Therefore, a significant outcome of the study is the demonstration that a mandibular deviation >6 mm is able to classify the UCH condition as active or inactive, because the AUC in the ROC curve was 0.695. López et al. [30] recently evaluated the ability of mandibular deviation to differentiate the hemi-mandibular elongation (the most common form of condylar hyperplasia [17]) from the asymmetric mandibular prognathism, determining that MDs >5.1 mm are more frequent in hemi-mandibular elongation cases.

The present study provides data from a sample higher than other studies published to study the correlation SPECT/CT in UCH patients. However, a limitation of the study is that hybrid equipment was not used, but rather image fusion. There is no correction for attenuation in this case. Additionally, the use of two separate techniques generates more radiation and is more expensive than the SPECT alone, but the hybrid special scanning system is not yet available in development countries, except in a limited number of research institutions. It is also important to mention that volumetric assessment of the mandible and the articular surfaces provides information on the entire structure under study [31]; although, for this research, what was taken into account were linear measurements, including those of the active condylar surfaces such as the medial–lateral pole and the anterior–posterior pole, which represent the functional area, it is recommended that volumetric assessment of the articular structures be carried out in future studies.

5. Conclusions

The correlation between the magnitude of mandibular deviation measured in CT images and the percentage uptake obtained by SPECT is statistically significant ($p = 0.003$) and ROC analysis established that a mandibular deviation >6 mm is a risk factor for active UCH (OR: 3.51; CI 95%: 1.27–9.72).

Author Contributions: Conceptualization, D.F.L.; Formal analysis, R.C.-P. and J.M.M.; Investigation, D.F.L. and V.R.B.; Methodology, R.C.-P. and J.M.M.; Supervision, D.F.L., R.C.-P. and L.E.A.; Validation, J.M.M.; Visualization, V.R.B.; Writing—original draft, V.R.B., R.C.-P. and J.M.M.; Writing—review & editing, D.F.L. All authors have read and agreed to the published version of the manuscript.

Funding: This research received no external funding.

Institutional Review Board Statement: This is a study with no intervention or manipulation of variables from the patients. Therefore, it is a no risk investigation and was approved by the Institutional Ethics Committee (Approval number CEI-403) and conducted following all the regulations of the Declaration of Helsinki, last version.

Informed Consent Statement: Without patient consent due, this is a study with no intervention or manipulation of variables from the patients, therefore, it is a no risk investigation.

Acknowledgments: The authors wish to express their sincere acknowledge to the Imbanaco Medical Center, Research Institute staff for their support during the development of this study.

Conflicts of Interest: The authors declare no conflict of interest.

References

1. López, B.D.F.; Corral, S.C.M. Comparison of planar bone scintigraphy and single photon emission computed tomography for diagnosis of active condylar hyperplasia. *J. Cranio-Maxillo-Facial Surg. Off. Publ. Eur. Assoc. Cranio-Maxillo-Facial Surg.* **2016**, *44*, 70–74. [CrossRef] [PubMed]
2. Veeranki, S.; Park, J.; Pruzansky, D.; Takagi, M.; Tai, K. A current review of asymmetry. *J. Clin. Orthod.* **2018**, *52*, 325–341. [PubMed]
3. Nolte, J.; Schreurs, R.; Karssemakers, L.; Tuinzing, D.; Becking, A. Demographic features in Unilateral Condylar Hyperplasia: An overview of 309 asymmetric cases and presentation of an algorithm. *J. Cranio Maxillofac. Surg.* **2018**, *46*, 1484–1492. [CrossRef]
4. Almeida, L.E.; Zacharias, J.; Pierce, S. Condylar hyperplasia: An updated review of the literature. *Korean J. Orthod.* **2015**, *45*, 333–340. [CrossRef] [PubMed]
5. Nelke, K.H.; Pawlak, W.; Morawska-Kochman, M.; Łuczak, K. Ten years of observations and demographics of hemimandibular hyperplasia and elongation. *J. Cranio Maxillofac. Surg.* **2018**, *46*, 979–986. [CrossRef]
6. López Buitrago, D.F.; Ruiz Botero, J.; Corral, C.M.; Carmona, A.R.; Sabogal, A. Comparison of (99m)Tc-MDP SPECT qualitative vs. quantitative results in patients with suspected condylar hyperplasia. *Rev. Española Med. Nucl. Imagen Mol.* **2017**, *36*, 207–211. [CrossRef] [PubMed]
7. Saridin, C.P.; Raijmakers, P.G.H.M.; Tuinzing, D.B.; Becking, A.G. Bone scintigraphy as a diagnostic method in unilateral hyperactivity of the mandibular condyles: A review and meta-analysis of the literature. *Int. J. Oral Maxillofac. Surg.* **2011**, *40*, 11–17. [CrossRef]
8. Shintaku, W.H.; Venturin, J.S.; Langlais, R.P.; Clark, G.T. Imaging Modalities to Access Bony Tumors and Hyperplasic Reactions of the Temporomandibular Joint. *J. Oral Maxillofac. Surg.* **2010**, *68*, 1911–1921. [CrossRef] [PubMed]
9. Wen, B.; Shen, Y.; Wang, C.-Y. Clinical Value of 99Tcm-MDP SPECT Bone Scintigraphy in the Diagnosis of Unilateral Condylar Hyperplasia. *Sci. World J.* **2014**, *2014*, 1–6. [CrossRef]
10. Fahey, F.H.; Abramson, Z.R.; Padwa, B.L.; Zimmerman, R.E.; Zurakowski, D.; Nissenbaum, M.; Kaban, L.B.; Treves, S.T. Use of 99mTc-MDP SPECT for assessment of mandibular growth: Development of normal values. *Eur. J. Nucl. Med. Mol. Imaging* **2010**, *37*, 1002–1010. [CrossRef]
11. Jacene, H.A.; Goetze, S.; Patel, H.; Wahl, R.L.; Ziessman, H.A. Advantages of Hybrid SPECT/CT vs. SPECT Alone. *Open Med. Imaging J.* **2008**, *2*, 67–79. [CrossRef]
12. Hamed, M.A.G.; AlAzzazy, M.Z.; Basha, M.A.A. The validity of SPECT/CT in diagnosis of condylar hyperplasia. *Egypt J. Radiol. Nucl. Med.* **2017**, *48*, 451–459. [CrossRef]
13. Raijmakers, P.G.; Karssemakers, L.H.; Tuinzing, D.B. Female Predominance and Effect of Gender on Unilateral Condylar Hyperplasia: A Review and Meta-Analysis. *J. Oral. Maxillofac. Surg.* **2012**, *70*, e72–e76. [CrossRef]
14. Theerakulpisut, D.; Somboonporn, C.; Wongsurawat, N. Single Photon Emission Computed Tomography without and with Hybrid Computed Tomography in Mandibular Condylar Hyperplasia. *J. Med. Assoc. Thail.* **2016**, *99*, S65–S73.
15. Agarwal, K.K.; Mukherjee, A.; St, A.; Tripathi, M.; Bal, C. Incremental value of single-photon emission computed tomography/computed tomography in the diagnosis of active condylar hyperplasia. *Nucl. Med. Commun.* **2017**, *38*, 29–34. [CrossRef] [PubMed]
16. Liu, P.; Shi, J. Is Single-Photon Emission Computed Tomography/Computed Tomography Superior to Single-Photon Emission Computed Tomography in Assessing Unilateral Condylar Hyperplasia? *J. Oral. Maxillofac. Surg.* **2019**, *77*, 1279.e1–1279.e7. [CrossRef]
17. López, D.F.; Botero, J.R.; Muñoz, J.M.; Cárdenas-Perilla, R.; Moreno, M. Are There Mandibular Morphological Differences in the Various Facial Asymmetry Etiologies? A Tomographic Three-Dimensional Reconstruction Study. *J. Oral. Maxillofac. Surg. Off. J. Am. Assoc. Oral. Maxillofac. Surg.* **2019**, *77*, 2324–2338. [CrossRef]
18. López Buitrago, D.F.; Muñoz Acosta, J.M.; Cárdenas-Perilla, R.A. Comparison of four methods for quantitative assessment of (99m)Tc-MDP SPECT in patients with suspected condylar hyperplasia. *Rev. Española Med. Nucl. Imagen Mol.* **2019**, *38*, 72–79. [CrossRef]
19. Konidena, A.; Shekhar, S.; Dixit, A.; Patil, D.J.; Gupta, R. Fusion imaging: A bipartite approach. *Oral. Radiol.* **2017**, *34*, 1–9. [CrossRef]
20. Kuwert, T.; Schillaci, O. SPECT/CT: Yesterday, today, tomorrow. *Clin. Transl. Imaging* **2014**, *2*, 443–444. [CrossRef]
21. Mariani, G.; Bruselli, L.; Kuwert, T.; Kim, E.E.; Flotats, A.; Israel, O.; Dondi, M.; Watanabe, N. A review on the clinical uses of SPECT/CT. *Eur. J. Nucl. Med. Mol. Imaging* **2010**, *37*, 1959–1985. [CrossRef]
22. Wassef, H.R.; Colletti, P.M. Nuclear Medicine Imaging in the Dentomaxillofacial Region. *Dent. Clin. N. Am.* **2018**, *62*, 491–509. [CrossRef]
23. Elbaz, J.; Wiss, A.; Raoul, G.; Leroy, X.; Hossein-Foucher, C.; Ferri, J. Condylar Hyperplasia. *J. Craniofac. Surg.* **2014**, *25*, 1085–1090. [CrossRef]

24. Suh, M.S.; Lee, W.W.; Kim, Y.-K.; Yun, P.-Y.; Kim, S.E. Maximum Standardized Uptake Value of99mTc Hydroxymethylene Diphosphonate SPECT/CT for the Evaluation of Temporomandibular Joint Disorder. *Radiology* **2016**, *280*, 890–896. [CrossRef] [PubMed]
25. Wang, T.T.; Wessels, L.; Hussain, G.; Merten, S. Discriminative Thresholds in Facial Asymmetry: A Review of the Literature. *Aesthetic Surg. J.* **2017**, *37*, 375–385. [CrossRef] [PubMed]
26. Fokoue, F.; El Mselmi, S.; Abaouz, N.; Alaoui, N.I. Added Value of SPECT-CT Imaging in the Diagnosis of Unilateral Active Mandibular Hypercondylia in Adult: A Case Report and Review. *Adv. Mol. Imaging* **2020**, *10*, 1–5. [CrossRef]
27. Verhelst, P.-J.; Shaheen, E.; Vasconcelos, K.D.F.; Van Der Cruyssen, F.; Shujaat, S.; Coudyzer, W.; Salmon, B.; Swennen, G.; Politis, C.; Jacobs, R. Validation of a 3D CBCT-based protocol for the follow-up of mandibular condyle remodeling. *Dentomaxillofac. Radiol.* **2020**, *49*, 20190364. [CrossRef]
28. Nitzan, D.W.; Katsnelson, A.; Bermanis, I.; Brin, I.; Casap, N. The Clinical Characteristics of Condylar Hyperplasia: Experience with 61 Patients. *J. Oral. Maxillofac. Surg.* **2008**, *66*, 312–318. [CrossRef]
29. Aarts, B.; Convens, J.; Bronkhorst, E.; Kuijpers-Jagtman, A.; Fudalej, P. Cessation of facial growth in subjects with short, average, and long facial types—Implications for the timing of implant placement. *J. Cranio Maxillofac. Surg.* **2015**, *43*, 2106–2111. [CrossRef] [PubMed]
30. López Buitrago, D.F. Diferencias en la morfología ósea entre el lado desplazado y contralateral en pacientes con asimetría facial. *Rev. Ces. Odontol.* **2020**, *2*. in press.
31. Farronato, M.; Cavagnetto, D.; Abate, A.; Cressoni, P.; Fama, A.; Maspero, C. Assessment of condylar volume and ramus height in JIA patients with unilateral and bilateral TMJ involvement: Retrospective case-control study. *Clin. Oral Investig.* **2019**, *24*, 2635–2643. [CrossRef]

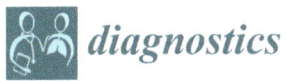

Case Report

Chemical Diagnosis of Calcium Pyrophosphate Deposition Disease of the Temporomandibular Joint: A Case Report

Masahiko Terauchi [1,*], Motohiro Uo [2], Yuki Fukawa [3], Hiroyuki Yoshitake [1], Rina Tajima [1], Tohru Ikeda [3] and Tetsuya Yoda [1]

1. Department of Maxillofacial Surgery, Graduate School of Medical and Dental Sciences, Tokyo Medical and Dental University, 1-5-45 Yushima, Bunkyo, Tokyo 113-8549, Japan; h-yoshitake.mfs@tmd.ac.jp (H.Y.); r_tajima.mfs@tmd.ac.jp (R.T.); yoda.mfs@tmd.ac.jp (T.Y.)
2. Department of Advanced Biomaterials, Graduate School of Medical and Dental Sciences, Tokyo Medical and Dental University, 1-5-45 Yushima, Bunkyo, Tokyo 113-8549, Japan; uo.abm@tmd.ac.jp
3. Department of Oral Pathology, Graduate School of Medical and Dental Sciences, Tokyo Medical and Dental University, 1-5-45 Yushima, Bunkyo, Tokyo 113-8549, Japan; yfkwmpa@tmd.ac.jp (Y.F.); tohrupth.mpa@tmd.ac.jp (T.I.)
* Correspondence: terauchi.org@tmd.ac.jp; Tel.: +81-3-5803-5500

Abstract: Calcium pyrophosphate dihydrate (CPPD) deposition disease is a benign disorder characterized by acute gouty arthritis-like attacks and first reported by McCarty. CPPD deposition disease rarely occurs in the temporomandibular joint (TMJ), and although confirmation of positive birefringence by polarized light microscopy is important for diagnosis, it is not reliable because other crystals also show birefringence. We reported a case of CPPD deposition disease of the TMJ that was diagnosed by chemical analysis. A 47-year-old man with a chief complaint of persistent pain in the right TMJ and trismus was referred to our department in 2020. Radiographic examination revealed destruction of the head of the mandibular condyle and cranial base with a neoplastic lesion involving calcification tissue. We suspected CPPD deposition disease and performed enucleation of the white, chalky masses. Histopathologically, we confirmed crystal deposition with weak birefringence. SEM/EDS revealed that the light emitting parts of Ca and P corresponded with the bright part of the SEM image. Through X-ray diffraction, almost all peaks were confirmed to be CPPD-derived. Inductively coupled plasma atomic emission spectroscopy revealed a Ca/P ratio of nearly 1. These chemical analyses further support the histological diagnosis of CPPD deposition disease.

Keywords: calcium pyrophosphate dihydrate deposition disease; pseudogout; temporomandibular joint; X-ray diffraction; inductively coupled plasma atomic emission spectroscopy

1. Introduction

McCarty was the first to report a case of calcium pyrophosphate dihydrate (CPPD) crystal deposition disease, a rare benign crystalline arthropathy also known as pseudogout [1,2]. This disease is characterized by the accumulation of CPPD crystals in various intra-articular and periarticular tissues [3]. Unfortunately, its etiology is unknown, but the disease has been associated with metabolic disorders such as hyperparathyroidism, hypothyroidism, hypomagnesemia, and hyperphosphatemia [4–6]. Diabetes mellitus is associated with a greater incidence of CPPD deposition disease [1,7]. CPPD deposition disease predominantly involves relatively large joints such as the knee, shoulder, hip, wrist, and pubic symphysis; small joints such as the temporomandibular joint (TMJ) are rarely affected [4,8,9]. Pritzker et al. were the first to describe pseudogout in the TMJ in 1976 [10]. Almost all previously reported cases of CPPD deposition disease of the TMJ were diagnosed using a polarized microscope to find positive birefringence. However, we consider this modality insufficient for diagnosis because, in addition to those in CPPD and gout, many birefringent crystals such as those of calcium oxalate, synthetic steroids, and ethylenediaminetetraacetic acid are present in the joint fluid, joint tissue, and bone [11]. Herein, we describe a case of CPPD deposition disease of the TMJ diagnosed using chemical analyses, scanning electronic microscopy (SEM)/energy-dispersive X-ray spectroscopy (EDS), XRD, and inductively coupled plasma atomic emission spectroscopy (ICP-AES).

2. Case Presentation

2.1. Clinical Summary

A 47-year-old man with a chief complaint of persistent pain in the right TMJ and trismus was referred to our department in 2020. He experienced a traffic accident approximately 25 years ago, which damaged his liver and pancreas and caused wrist and left shoulder bone fractures. His clinical history appeared related to the accident, in which he had also bruised his right TMJ but had not sought treatment for it. Since the accident, the patient experienced discomfort with irregular sudden pain in the right TMJ. This pain resolved after the use of analgesics at every episode. He visited a local hospital when the frequency and intensity of pain increased in 2020. He was then referred to our department when surgical management was anticipated.

Clinical examination revealed bilateral symmetry of the face. His mouth opening was limited, and there was limited lateral excursion to the left. The maximal mouth opening was 28 mm and accompanied by pain in the right TMJ. His uric acid level was normal.

The panoramic radiograph showed an unclear right mandibular condyle with a cloud-like mass (Figure 1). Computed tomography (CT) revealed that the right mandibular condyle was destroyed, and that mottled-like hard tissues had formed around the condyle as viewed on the axial plane (Figure 2A). Similarly, it was confirmed on the coronal plane that the mandibular fossa and cranial base were destroyed. Furthermore, calcified opacity was observed in the bone resorption fossa (Figure 2B). Proton density-weighted imaging showed no disc dislocation in the right TMJ, and the area corresponding to the upper and lower joint space was filled with uneven hypointensity, and the joint space appeared dilated. Additionally, the high signal inside and granular low-signal images were scattered inside the mandibular condyle and fossa (Figure 3). The left TMJ showed no abnormal findings. Based on these findings, we suspected CPPD deposition disease as a clinical diagnosis and excised the lesion under general anesthesia. The right TMJ was exposed using a preauricular approach. During surgery, we confirmed and removed the white chalk-like masses (Figure 4). These masses were present in the articular capsule, articular eminence, mandibular condyle, the upper and lower joint cavities, and articular disc. The maximum size of the masses was $16 \times 5 \times 5$ mm, although various sizes were extracted. CT images were obtained after surgery, and we confirmed that the masses were extracted from the right temporomandibular joint (Figure 5). The postoperative healing was uneventful. This was six months post-surgery, and although the pain in the right TMJ was persistent when opening the mouth, the maximal mouth opening had improved to 42 mm.

2.2. Pathological Findings

Histologically, the masses consisted of chondroid tissue with island-like or nodular deposition of basophilic crystals (Figure 6A). A foreign body granulomatous reaction was observed in some areas around the crystal deposition (Figure 6B). The crystals appeared rhombus or needle shaped and showed weak birefringence under the polarized light microscopy (Figure 6C,D).

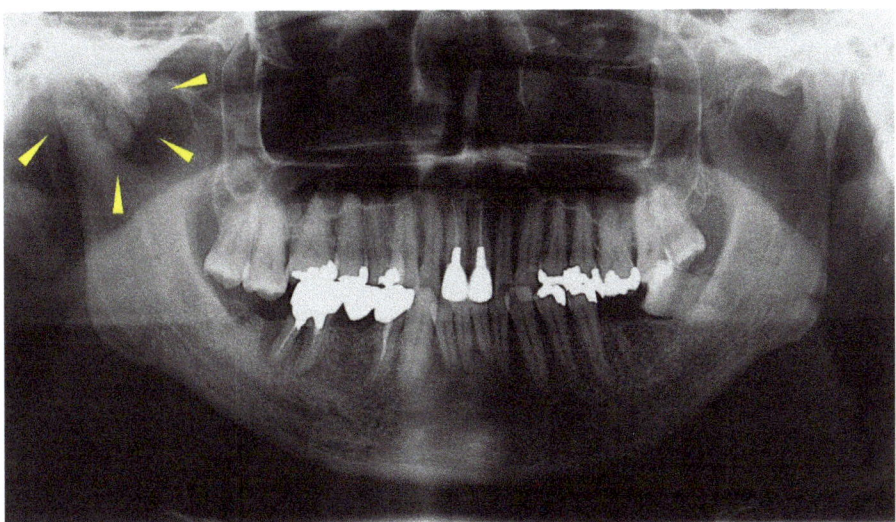

Figure 1. Panoramic radiograph from the first visit. The ill-defined calcification around the mandibular condyle is shown (yellow arrows).

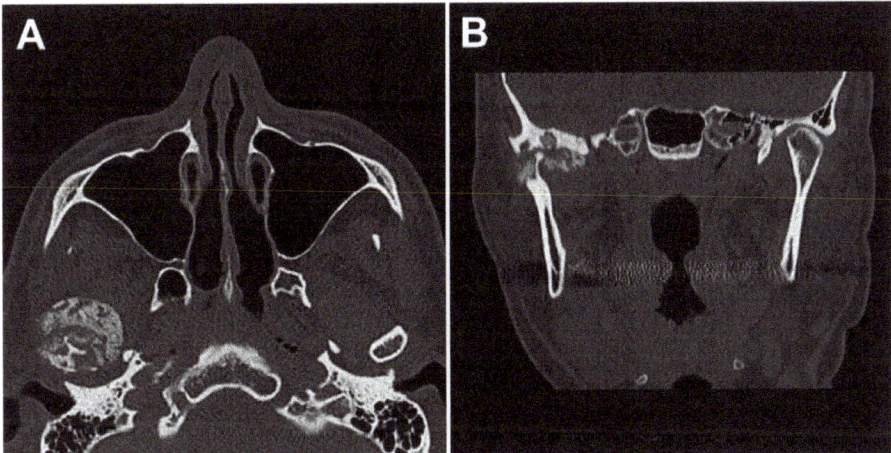

Figure 2. Preoperative computed tomography (CT) images. (**A**) Axial CT images showing the intra-articular localized, non-corticated, and ill-marginated calcified lesion that abuts the articular surface of the glenoid fossa around the right mandibular condyle. (**B**) Coronal CT images of the right temporomandibular joint revealed resorption of part of the mandibular condyle and cranial base.

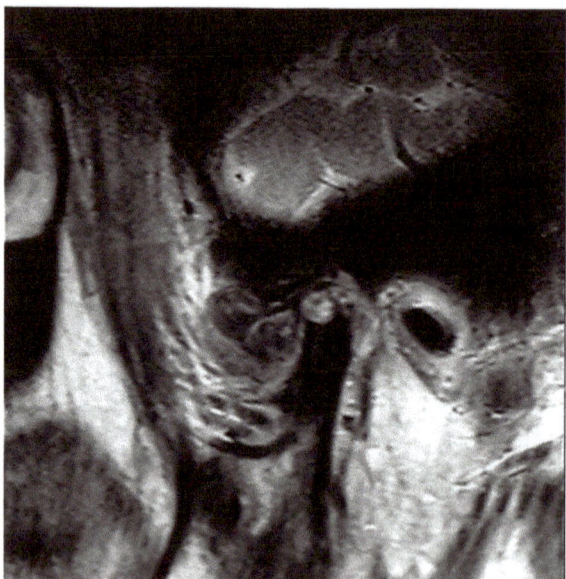

Figure 3. Magnetic resonance image. Proton density-weighted image of the sagittal plane.

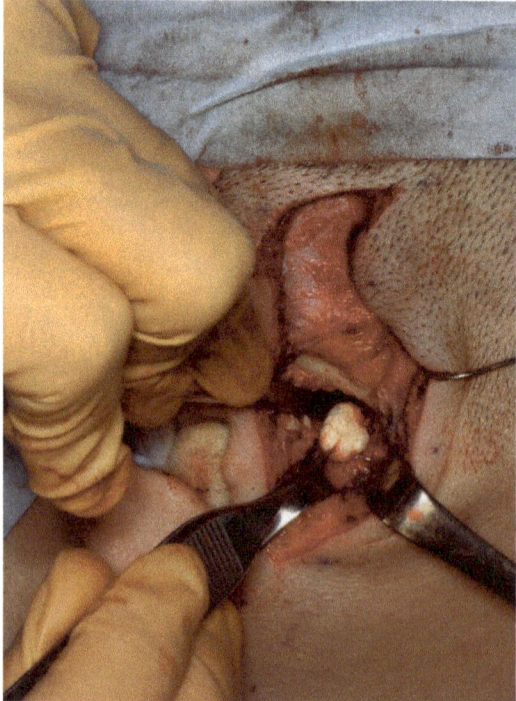

Figure 4. Intraoperative photograph. The whitish calcified tumorous mass was enucleated from the right infratemporal fossa.

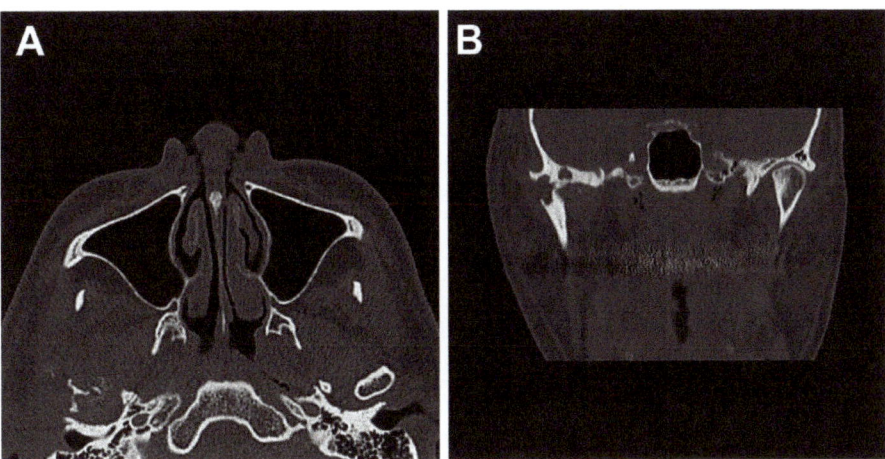

Figure 5. Postoperative computed tomography (CT) images. (**A**) Axial CT images and (**B**) Coronal CT images revealed that the masses were extracted from the right temporomandibular joint.

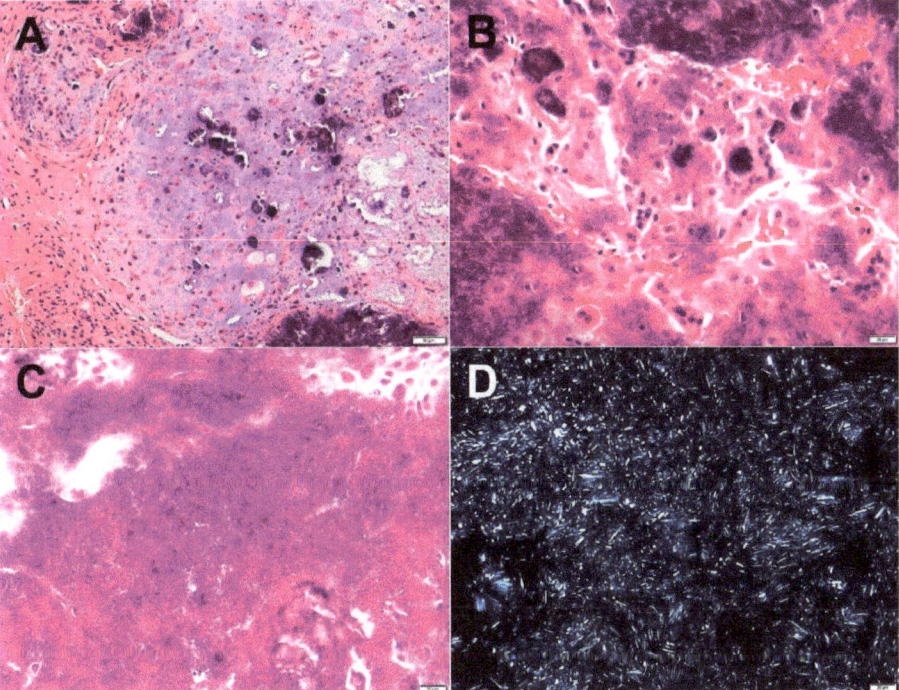

Figure 6. Histopathological examination. Representative specimen from the upper joint cavity showed the histopathological features of calcium pyrophosphate dihydrate deposition disease. (**A**) Chondroid metaplasia forms around basophilic islands of crystalline deposits. (**B**) A foreign body granulomatous reaction with multinucleated giant cells phagocytosing the crystals. (**C**) Deposited crystals appeared rhombus or needle shaped. (**D**) Under polarized light, these crystals demonstrated weak birefringence.

2.3. Elemental Analysis Using SEM/EDS

The two large deposits extracted from the upper and lower joint cavities were chosen as representative specimens for the chemical analysis. SEM/EDS microanalysis was performed to evaluate the calcified mass. Each deposit was fixed with 10% paraformaldehyde solution and washed with distilled water. Thereafter, it was dehydrated in a series of alcohol baths of increasing concentration and dried using vacuum drying. SEM was performed to observe the fine structure around the deposit surface. A carbon coat was formed on these surfaces and observed using SEM (TM4000Plus, Hitachi High-Tech Corporation, Tokyo, Japan) at an acceleration voltage of 15 kV. The elemental distribution around the interface was estimated using EDS (Quantax75 (Oxford Instruments, Oxford, England). The elemental distribution images of the interface were acquired with a resolution of 256 × 200 pixels with an integration time of 200 µs per point. The results are shown in Figure 7. The calcified mass from the upper joint cavity consisted of needle-like crystals, rhomboid masses, and soft tissue that lacked the crystal. However, the specimens from the lower joint cavity consisted of needle-like crystals. Both crystals were the same size with no more than 1 µm thickness and a length of approximately 10 µm. The elemental distribution images and spectrum are shown in Figure 8. The same specimen used in Figure 6A (upper joint cavity) was analyzed. The light emitting parts of Ca and P corresponded with each other. Figure 8C shows the elemental distribution diagram: Ca, P, O, and C were detected. The specimen in Figure 7B (lower joint cavity) was also analyzed, and the same results were obtained (data not shown).

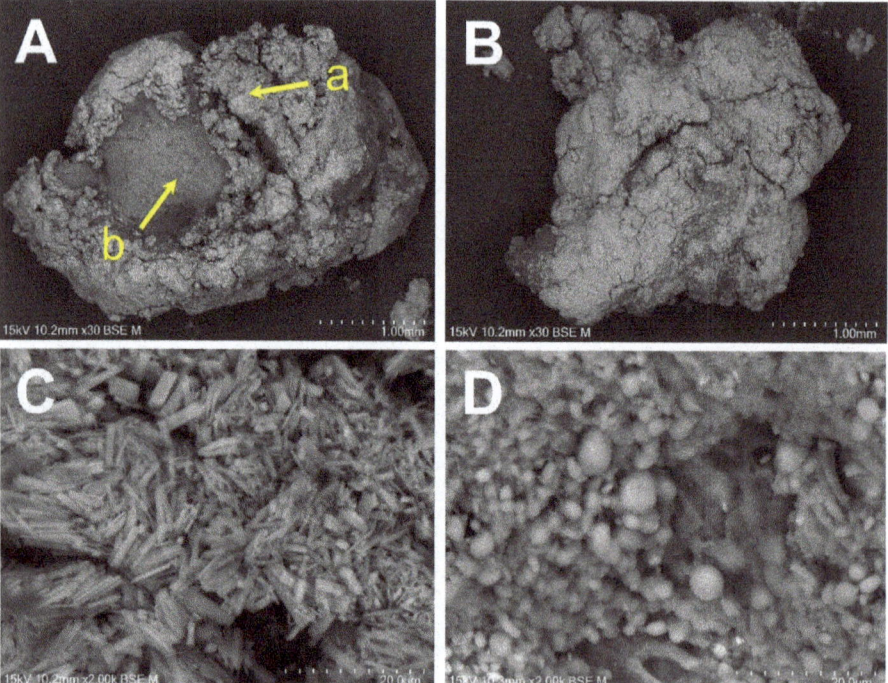

Figure 7. Scanning electronic microscopic images of the masses from the joint cavities. Masses were extracted from the (**A**) upper and (**B**) lower joint cavities (30×). (**C,D**) present the 2000× high power fields of (**A-a**) and (**A-b**), respectively.

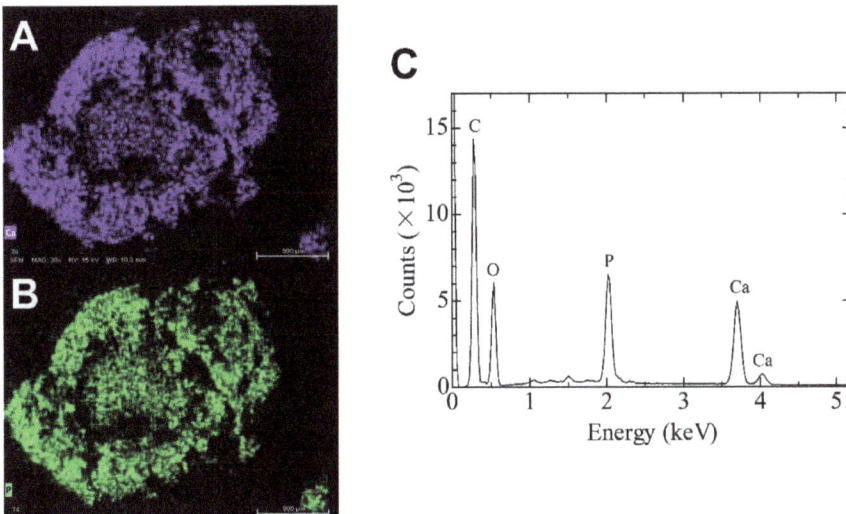

Figure 8. Elemental distribution images of (**A**) Ca and (**B**) P. (**C**) The EDS spectrum for the entire specimen (from Figure 6A) obtained by SEM/EDS.

2.4. Crystal Phase Analysis Using XRD

The calcified specimens extracted from the upper and lower joint cavities (Figure 6A,B) were washed several times with distilled water, dried at 180 °C for 1 h, and ground into powder using an agate mortar. The crystal phases of the powder specimens were analyzed using XRD (Miniflex, Rigaku Cooporation, Tokyo, Japan) under the following conditions: 40 kV, 15 mA, and 2°/min.

Most diffraction peaks of both crystals were assigned to those of CPPD, and a few small peaks were assigned to those of hydroxyapatite (HAp). Therefore, the main crystal was CPPD (Figure 9).

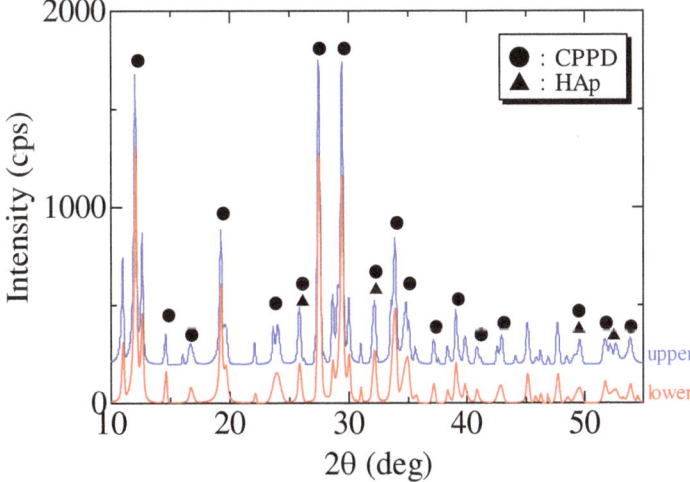

Figure 9. X-ray diffraction. The blue and red wavelengths represent the specimens extracted from the upper and lower joint cavities, respectively. The circles and triangles indicate the intrinsic peaks of calcium pyrophosphate dihydrate (CPPD) and hydroxyapatite (HAp), respectively.

2.5. Quantitative Elemental Analysis for ICP-AES

The tissue concentrations of Ca and P were quantitatively evaluated using ICP-AES. The specimens of the deposits were washed several times with distilled water and weighed while wet (upper: 0.0322 g, lower: 0.0582 g). The specimens were then dissolved in concentrated nitric acid (HNO_3; 38 w/v%, UltraPur100, Kanto Chemical Co. Ltd., Tokyo, Japan) overnight at 90 °C. The trace element concentrations in the solutions were quantitated using ICP-AES (Spectro Arcos, Hitachi High-technologies, Tokyo, Japan). Multi-element (100 ppm, XSTC-22, Seishin Trading Co. Ltd., Kobe, Japan) and Sr standard solutions (1000 ppm, Nacalai Tesque, Kyoto, Japan) were used for ICP-AES analyses. The measurement results are presented in Table 1. In the upper cavity specimen, 11.20 wt% Ca and 9.20 wt% P were detected. In the lower cavity specimen, 9.12 wt% Ca and 6.75 wt% P were found (Table 1). Fe, K, Mg, Na, Zn, and Sr were also detected as the trace elements present in the specimens, while the other elements could not be detected or the detection limit or less by this method. In other words, it was clearly composed of elements of biological origin. Accordingly, a Ca/P molar ratio of 0.94 and 1.04 was obtained in the upper and lower cavity specimens, respectively. CPPD is a calcium phosphate that has a Ca/P molar ratio of 1.0. Therefore, the elemental analyses with ICP-AES further supported the histological diagnosis of CPPD deposition disease.

Table 1. ICP-AES for quantitative analysis of elements.

Element	Quantity		Unit
	Upper	Lower	
Ca	11.2	9.12	wt%
P	9.2	6.75	
Fe	24	22	µg/g (ppm)
K	153	102	
Mg	274	267	
Na	1920	2140	
Zn	7	16	
Sr	16	12	

3. Discussion

McCarty's diagnostic criteria for CPPD deposition disease are based on the following: (1) the validation of the specimen by reliable methods such as XRD or chemical analysis or (2) the presence of typical calcific deposition and the detection of crystals suggestive of calcium pyrophosphate deposition through a polarized microscope [1]. The crystal deposits in CPPD deposition disease had a rhomboid structure and were positively birefringent under polarized light, whereas those in gout exhibited negative birefringence. Therefore, birefringence is an important differential diagnostic criterion for gout and CPPD [3,12]. In our case, these crystals clearly demonstrated a rhomboid and rod-shaped appearance, and they exhibited birefringence under a polarized microscope (Figure 6D). Based on these findings, CPPD deposition disease was suspected. However, definitive diagnosis of CPPD can be difficult because not only are these crystals small and often show weak birefringence, but there are also many other birefringent crystals such as those of calcium oxalate, synthetic steroids, and ethylenediaminetetraacetic acid, present in the joint fluid, joint tissue, and bone [11,13]. Therefore, because other quantitative and chemical analyses are required for definitive diagnosis of CPPD deposition disease, we performed SEM/EDS, XRD, and ICP-AES.

Asghar et al. described how crystals demonstrate peaks corresponding to Ca and P in SEM/EDS; therefore SEM/EDS is a rapid and effective method for diagnosing CPPD [3]. In elemental analysis using EDS, only Ca, P, and O derived from CPPD and C and O derived from soft tissue were observed, and the distribution of Ca and P was the same as the bright part of the SEM image (Figures 7A and 8). These results suggest that the specimens contained CPPD. Most previous reports of CPPD deposition disease describe the detection of Ca and P using SEM/EDS or the diagnosis of CPPD based on a Ca/P ratio of approximately 1 on a rough composition analysis using EDS [3–5]. However, these diagnostic methods are considered inappropriate for the following reasons: (1) Since there are innumerable calcium phosphate compounds such as HAp, tricalcium phosphate (TCP), octacalcium phosphate, and dibasic calcium phosphate anhydrous, it is not possible to determine the exact calcium phosphate compound present despite the detection of Ca and P (Table 2), so accurate Ca and P concentrations should be determined to distinguish calcium phosphate compounds; and (2) most EDS composition analyses have a "standardless method," and their accuracy is lower than that of other analyses calibrated with the concentration standard specimens. Therefore, additional analyses are required to definitively diagnose the precipitation as CPPD.

Table 2. A list of the major calcium phosphate compounds.

Composition Formula	Ca/P Ratio	Name	Abbreviation (Mineral Name)
$Ca(H_2PO_4)_2 \cdot H_2O$	0.5	Calcium bis(dihydrogenphosphate) monohydrate	MCPM
$CaHPO_4$	1	Calcium monohydrogen phosphate	DCPA (monetite)
$CaHPO_4 \cdot 2H_2O$	1	Calcium hydrogen phosphate dihydrate	DCPD (brushite)
$Ca_2P_2O_7$	1	Calcium pyrophosphate	
$Ca_2P_2O_7 \cdot 2H_2O$	1	Calcium pyrophosphate dihydrate	CPPD
$Ca_8(PO_4)_4(HPO_4)_2(OH)_2$	1.33	Octacalcium phosphate	OCP
$Ca_3(PO_4)_2$	1.5	Tricalcium phosphate	TCP
$Ca_{10}(PO_4)_6(OH)_2$	1.66	Hydroxyapatite	HAp
$Ca_4(PO_4)_2O$	2	Tetracalcium phosphate	TTCP

XRD is a powerful method for the crystal phase and structure analyses of inorganic compounds. The basic method for the crystal identification of inorganic compounds through a database is XRD, and if the results are combined with the identification of major elements using EDS elemental analysis, the elements can be identified with high reliability [14]. XRD revealed that all diffraction peaks were consistent with those of CPPD. Even small peaks were thought to be derived from hydroxyapatite, and the main crystals were strongly considered to be derived from CPPD (Figure 9). XRD can help distinguish crystal phase identification and form, but cannot correctly quantify the chemical composition. This method uses a "standardless method," but SEM/EDS can be used for pseudo-analysis. Thus, the accuracy of the numerical value is questionable.

In this study, we focused on ICP-AES analysis to further accumulate evidence. Bones and teeth are not purely composed of calcium phosphate and often contain divalent cations of Mg, Sr, and Zn instead of Ca (for example, Sr exists at a concentration of one hundred to several hundred parts per million) [15]. Additionally, ICP-AES can help reliably quantify the Ca/P ratio and confirm CPPD based on the chemical composition of the specimen. In CPPD, the Ca/P ratio was 1, which was lower than that of HAp and TCP (Table 1). In our results, the Ca/P ratio in the upper and lower joint cavities was 0.94 and 1.04, respectively. The analysis value retention Ca/P ratio obtained through ICP-AES was approximately 1. These results indicate that there is no possibility that other calcium phosphate compounds are present, which supports the diagnosis of CPPD deposition from the perspective of the chemical composition. In addition, only cations contained in the human organism were detected in our case. In other words, heavy metals and other substances are unlikely to accumulate or be the cause of the problem. Assuming that all the aforementioned Ca values were associated with CPPD deposits, the weight ratio of CPPD in the tissue was estimated to be 40.6 wt% on the upper side and 33.0 wt% on the lower side. Considering this number as wet weight, most of the tissue was CPPD, which corresponds reasonably well with the SEM observations. Thus, we diagnosed CPPD deposition disease of the right TMJ. The diagnosis of CPPD deposition disease by chemical analysis is not simple considering the special equipment and the number of specimens required for analysis. For this reason, in this study, we preoperatively suspected CPPD, consulted with pathologists and engineers, and used chemical analysis for postoperative diagnosis. Collaborating with pathologists and engineers on preoperatively suspected CPPD deposition disease was effective in obtaining a more reliable diagnosis.

4. Conclusions

In summary, the diagnosis of CPPD deposition disease of the TMJ is based on the presence of rhomboid positively birefringent crystals; however, because it is considered as a weak diagnostic criterion, performing chemical analyses such as SEM/EDS, XRD, and ICP-AES offers a reliable method for the diagnosis of CPPD deposition disease.

Author Contributions: Conceptualization, M.T. and M.U.; Surgeon, H.Y.; Data curation, M.T., R.T., Y.F. and M.U.; Funding acquisition: M.T.; Writing—original draft, M.T.; Writing—editing: M.U., H.Y., T.I. and T.Y. All authors have read and agreed to the published version of the manuscript.

Funding: This research received no external funding.

Institutional Review Board Statement: Not applicable.

Informed Consent Statement: Informed consent was obtained from the patient to publish this paper.

Data Availability Statement: Not applicable.

Acknowledgments: We are grateful to Kaoru Kobayashi (Tsurumi University, Kanagawa, Japan) for his advice on the image readings.

Conflicts of Interest: The authors declare no conflict of interest.

References

1. McCarty, D.J. Calcium pyrophosphate dihydrate crystal deposition disease: Pseudogout: Articular chondrocalcinosis. In *Arthritis and Allied Conditions*, 9th ed.; McCarty, D.J., Ed.; Lea & Febiger: Philadelphia, PA, USA, 1979; pp. 1276–1299.
2. Kohn, N.N.; Hughes, R.E.; McCarty, D.R., Jr.; Faires, J.S. The significance of calcium phosphate crystals in the synovial fluid of arthritic patients: The "pseudogout syndrome": II. Identification of crystals. *Ann. Intern. Med.* **1962**, *56*, 738–745. [CrossRef] [PubMed]
3. Naqvi, A.H.; Abraham, J.L.; Kellman, R.M.; Khurana, K.K. Calcium pyrophosphate dihydrate deposition disease (CPPD)/pseudogout of the temporomandibular joint–FNA findings and microanalysis. *Cytojournal* **2008**, *5*, 8. [CrossRef] [PubMed]
4. Meng, J.; Guo, C.; Luo, H.; Chen, S.; Ma, X. A case of destructive calcium pyrophosphate dihydrate crystal deposition disease of the temporomandibular joint: A diagnostic challenge. *Int. J. Oral Maxillofac. Surg.* **2011**, *40*, 1431–1437. [CrossRef] [PubMed]
5. Kwon, K.J.; Seok, H.; Lee, J.H.; Kim, M.K.; Kim, S.G.; Park, H.K.; Choi, H.M. Calcium Pyrophosphate Dihydrate Deposition Disease in the Temporomandibular Joint: Diagnosis and Treatment. *Maxillofac. Plast. Reconstr. Surg.* **2018**, *40*, 19. [CrossRef] [PubMed]
6. Nakagawa, Y.; Ishibashi, K.; Kobayashi, K.; Westesson, P.L. Calcium pyrophosphate deposition disease in the temporomandibular joint: Report of two cases. *J. Oral Maxillofac. Surg.* **1999**, *57*, 1357–1363. [CrossRef]
7. Abdelsayed, R.A.; Said-Al-Naief, N.; Salguerio, M.; Holmes, J.; El-Mofty, S.K. Tophaceous pseudogout of the temporomandibular joint: A series of 3 cases. *Oral Surg. Oral Med. Oral Pathol. Oral Radiol.* **2014**, *117*, 369–375. [CrossRef] [PubMed]
8. Scott, J.T. *Copeman's Textbook of the Rheumatic Diseases*, 5th ed.; Churchill Livinstone: Edinburgh, UK, 1978.
9. Resnick, D. Calcium pyrophosphate dihydrate (CPPD) crystal deposition disease. In *Diagnosis of Bone and Joint Disorders*, 4th ed.; Hotokezaka, Y., Ed.; W B Saunders: Philadelphia, PA, USA, 2002.
10. Pritzker, K.P.; Phillips, H.; Luk, S.C.; Koven, I.H.; Kiss, A.; Houpt, J.B. Pseudotumor of temporomandibular joint: Destructive calcium pyrophosphate dihydrate arthropathy. *J. Rheumatol.* **1976**, *3*, 70–81. [PubMed]
11. Aoyama, S.; Kino, K.; Amagasa, T.; Kayano, T.; Ichinose, S.; Kimijima, Y. Differential diagnosis of calcium pyrophosphate dihydrate deposition of the temporomandibular joint. *Br. J. Oral Maxillofac. Surg.* **2000**, *38*, 550–553. [CrossRef] [PubMed]
12. Shidham, V.; Chivukula, M.; Basir, Z.; Shidham, G. Evaluation of crystals in formalin-fixed, paraffin-embedded tissue sections for the differential diagnosis of pseudogout, gout, and tumoral calcinosis. *Mod. Pathol.* **2001**, *14*, 806–810. [CrossRef] [PubMed]
13. Ann, K.; Rosenthal, A.K.; Ryan, L.M. Calcium pyrophosphate deposition disease. *N. Engl. J. Med.* **2016**, *374*, 2575–2584. [CrossRef]
14. Kudoh, K.; Kudoh, T.; Tsuru, K.; Miyamoto, Y. A case of tophaceous pseudogout of the temporomandibular joint extending to the base of the skull. *Int. J. Oral Maxillofac. Surg.* **2017**, *46*, 355–359. [CrossRef] [PubMed]
15. Dedhiya, M.G.; Young, F.; Higuchi, W.I. Mechanism for the retardation of the acid dissolution rate of hydroxyapatite by strontium. *J. Dent. Res.* **1973**, *52*, 1097–1109. [CrossRef] [PubMed]

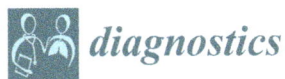

Article

Synovial Tissue Proteins and Patient-Specific Variables as Predictive Factors for Temporomandibular Joint Surgery

Mattias Ulmner [1,2,*], Rachael Sugars [2], Aron Naimi-Akbar [2,3], Nikolce Tudzarovski [2], Carina Kruger-Weiner [2,4] and Bodil Lund [2,5,6]

1 Unit of Cranio- and Maxillofacial Surgery, Karolinska University Hospital, 171 76 Stockholm, Sweden
2 Department of Dental Medicine, Karolinska Institutet, 141 04 Huddinge, Sweden; rachael.sugars@ki.se (R.S.); aron.naimi-akbar@mau.se (A.N.-A.); nikolce.tudzarovski@ki.se (N.T.); carina.kruger-weiner@sll.se (C.K.-W.); Bodil.Lund@uib.no (B.L.)
3 Health Technology Assessment-Odontology, Malmö University, 205 06 Malmö, Sweden
4 Department of Oral and Maxillofacial Surgery, Folktandvården Stockholm, Eastmaninstitutet, 113 24 Stockholm, Sweden
5 Department of Clinical Dentistry, Faculty of Medicine, University of Bergen, 5020 Bergen, Norway
6 Department of Oral and Maxillofacial Surgery, Haukeland University Hospital, 5021 Bergen, Norway
* Correspondence: mattias.ulmner@sll.se; Tel.: +46-851-772-633

Citation: Ulmner, M.; Sugars, R.; Naimi-Akbar, A.; Tudzarovski, N.; Kruger-Weiner, C.; Lund, B. Synovial Tissue Proteins and Patient-Specific Variables as Predictive Factors for Temporomandibular Joint Surgery. *Diagnostics* **2021**, *11*, 46. https://doi.org/10.3390/diagnostics11010046

Received: 12 December 2020
Accepted: 28 December 2020
Published: 30 December 2020

Publisher's Note: MDPI stays neutral with regard to jurisdictional claims in published maps and institutional affiliations.

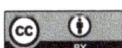

Copyright: © 2020 by the authors. Licensee MDPI, Basel, Switzerland. This article is an open access article distributed under the terms and conditions of the Creative Commons Attribution (CC BY) license (https://creativecommons.org/licenses/by/4.0/).

Abstract: Our knowledge of synovial tissues in patients that are scheduled for surgery as a result of temporomandibular joint (TMJ) disorders is limited. Characterising the protein profile, as well as mapping clinical preoperative variables, might increase our understanding of pathogenesis and forecast surgical outcome. A cohort of 100 patients with either disc displacement, osteoarthritis, or chronic inflammatory arthritis (CIA) was prospectively investigated for a set of preoperative clinical variables. During surgery, a synovial tissue biopsy was sampled and analysed via multi-analytic profiling. The surgical outcome was classified according to a predefined set of outcome criteria six months postoperatively. Higher concentrations of interleukin 8 ($p = 0.049$), matrix metalloproteinase 7 ($p = 0.038$), lumican ($p = 0.037$), and tissue inhibitor of metalloproteinase 2 ($p = 0.015$) were significantly related to an inferior surgical outcome. Several other proteins, which were not described earlier in the TMJ synovia, were detected but not related to surgical outcome. Bilateral masticatory muscle palpation pain had strong association to a poor outcome that was related to the diagnoses disc displacement and osteoarthritis. CIA and the patient-reported variable TMJ disability might be related to an unfavourable outcome according to the multivariate model. These findings of surgical predictors show potential in aiding clinical decision-making and they might enhance the understanding of aetiopathogenesis in TMJ disorders.

Keywords: temporomandibular joint; surgery; synovial tissue; synovitis; interleukin; lumican; matrix metalloproteinases; tissue inhibitor of metalloproteinases; cytokine; biomarker

1. Introduction

Temporomandibular joint (TMJ) diseases might be painful and restrictive by nature, hampering dietary intake and with a negative impact on psychosocial well-being [1]. Surgery is often not considered before a substantial period of failing non invasive treatments has been tried. From this perspective, the demands on surgery from the affected patients are higher, which accounts for the long duration of symptoms and it is regarded as chronic at this timepoint. Arthroscopy is a minimally invasive surgical alternative that is often used in cases of disc displacement (DD), osteoarthritis (OA), and chronic inflammatory arthritis (CIA) [2–4]. Discectomy is an open surgical procedure that is mainly used for DD [5,6]. The outcome of arthroscopy or discectomy, when applied to patients with DD, OA, and CIA, has been reported to be 60 to 88%, where open joint surgery seems to be slightly superior when compared to arthroscopy in a meta-analysis [2–7]. Inferior surgical outcome can be prevented by examining the patient in an organised fashion and applying strict diagnostic criteria in search of the correct diagnosis [8,9]. This is the foundation for the surgical decision, but, since TMJ DD, as well as TMJ OA, still lack formal explanatory grounds, a better understanding of the aetio-pathogenesis might shed new light on both diagnostic criteria and best-practice treatment. Characterising the synovial tissue profile and identifying patient-specific predictive factors is a possible approach for enhancing the surgical outcome. This will benefit the patient, as well as regulatory authorities, since a good surgical outcome often prevents further treatment, reduces medication, and minimises sick leave.

Potential predictive factors for TMJ surgery, such as age, TMJ pain, maximal interincisal opening (MIO), psychiatric co-morbidity, and masticatory muscle palpation pain, have been investigated [2,10–13]. In addition, cytokines have been identified in the TMJ synovial fluid, and high concentrations of interleukin (IL) 10 have been proposed for predicting a successful surgical outcome [14]. Studies have already highlighted cytokine localisation in synovial tissue as a valuable biomarker and predictor for treatment in rheumatoid arthritis [15,16]. However, this has not been assessed for the TMJ and diagnoses that are associated with TMJ disease or disorder.

The primary aim of the present study was to investigate synovial tissue protein concentrations and relate them to surgical outcome. The hypothesis was that the concentrations of pro-inflammatory cytokines were higher in patients with inferior outcome, whilst the anti-inflammatory cytokines were higher in patients with superior surgical outcomes. The secondary aim was to control for recorded objective and subjective patient variables, and their relation to surgical outcome. Identifying clinical variables or synovial tissue proteins that might influence surgical outcome could be a valuable contribution to oral- and maxillofacial surgeons decision-making. To our knowledge, this is the first attempt to investigate TMJ synovial tissue proteins in relation to surgical outcome.

2. Materials and Methods

2.1. Study Design

A prospective cohort study was performed at the Unit of Cranio- and Maxillofacial Surgery, Karolinska University Hospital, Stockholm, Sweden. The Regional Ethics Review Board approved the study (registration number 2014/622-31/1, approved on 23 April 2014. The patients referred due to DD with reduction (DDwR), DD without reduction (DDwoR), OA together with arthralgia, and CIA were eligible for inclusion. The patients were enrolled from December 2014 to January 2017 and written informed consent was mandatory before inclusion. The study was designed, and the article written, in accordance with the STROBE statement.

2.2. Study Population

TMJ diagnoses were set according to the Diagnostic Criteria for Temporomandibular Disorders (DC/TMD), except for CIA diagnosis, where the requirement was rheumatic diagnosis that was set by a rheumatologist [8]. Criterions for surgery and inclusion were that the patient had one of the diagnoses DDwR, DDwoR, OA, or CIA, had tried non-invasive therapy for at least 3–6 months, visual analogue scale (VAS) value of ≥ 4 for TMJ functional pain or TMJ disability, and that DDwoR patients had a MIO of ≤ 35 mm. The patients were excluded if they had prior open TMJ surgery, were unable to give informed consent, or were younger than 18 years.

2.3. Clinical Examination

Patient-specific data were registered preoperatively, one and six months postoperatively, while using a standardised case record form. Patient inclusion and data gathering were performed by M.U., A.N.-A., C.K.-W, and B.L., who were calibrated for patient classification and clinical examination. The anamnestic variables collected included present illnesses, medication, prior jaw trauma, ongoing tinnitus/ear fullness affected side, duration of present TMJ symptoms, and subjective grading on a 0–10 graded VAS of TMJ pain, TMJ disability, psychosocial impact of TMJ problems, and global pain [17]. Joint mobility was measured with the Beighton scoring system, and a value of ≥ 4 was regarded to be indicative of general joint hypermobility [18]. Positive findings of palpation pain of the masticatory muscles and the TMJ's, and measurements of MIO, lateral excursion, and protrusion were registered in accordance with DC/TMD [8]. A calibration exercise preceded Wilks classification and two of the researchers (M.U. and B.L.) subsequently individually performed the grading [19]. Divergent conclusions were discussed, and consensus was reached.

Surgical outcome was based on four parameters: MIO, TMJ pain, TMJ disability, and TMJ psychosocial impact registered at the last planned visit six months after surgery, and classified as either successful, good, intermediate, or deteriorated. The criteria for successful treatment were objective measurement of MIO ≥ 35 mm, and all subjective VAS scoring of TMJ pain, TMJ disability, and TMJ psychosocial impact of ≤ 3 or $\geq 40\%$ improvement. A good surgical outcome was defined as MIO ≥ 35 mm and whether one or two of the VAS values of pain, functional disabilities, and psycho-social impact showed $\geq 40\%$ improvement or a VAS value of ≤ 3. If the above-mentioned criteria got obviously worse, then the outcome was deemed to be deteriorated. With minor or no improvements, the result was classified as intermediate.

2.4. Surgical Procedure and Collection of Tissue Samples

According to the departments' research-based guidelines, patients with DDwR were scheduled for discectomy, and patients with DDwoR, OA, or CIA had arthroscopic lysis and lavage generally. One surgeon performed all of the operations (M.U.). Two synovial tissue biopsies were taken from the posterior bilaminar zone in the superior joint compartment. The triangulation technique was used in order to collect biopsies under direct visualisation during arthroscopy (Figure 1) [20]. Biopsy forceps (Karl Storz SE & Co, Tuttlingen, Germany) were used, resulting in approximately 4 mm^2 tissue samples. Synovial tissue samples that were destined for protein extraction were placed in RNAlater (ThermoFisher Scientific, Waltham, MA, USA) and then refrigerated for 24 h. RNAlater was then removed and the samples stored at -80 °C.

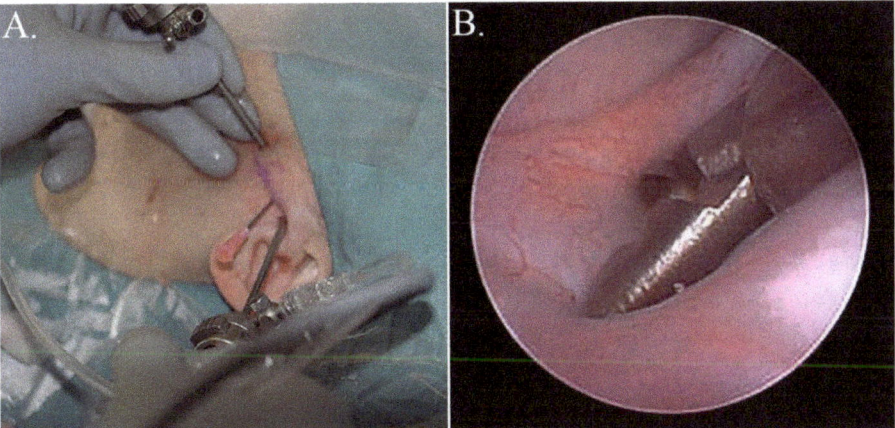

Figure 1. Photographs showing the synovial sample procedure. (**A**) In the triangulation technique, the instrument canal closest to the patient's ear contained the optic and the second instrument canal the biopsy forceps. (**B**) A synovial tissue sample from the posterior bilaminar zone in the superior temporomandibular joint (TMJ) compartment was taken with the biopsy forceps.

2.5. Analysis of Synovial Tissues

Synovial tissue was ground in liquid nitrogen in order to disrupt the tissue piece. The proteins were extracted in ice-cold cell lysis buffer NP40, prepared according to the manufacturer's instructions (ThermoFisher Scientific) [21]. 50 µL cell lysis buffer per 10 mg of tissue was used. The mixtures were centrifuged at $20,000 \times g$ at 4 °C for 10 min., and the supernatant stored at −80 °C until analysis.

The total protein concentration in each tissue sample was determined while using the Qubit Protein Assay Kit (ThermoFisher Scientific) and the Qubit Fluorometer (ThermoFisher Scientific). Magnetic bead panels HTMP2MAG-54K, HMMP2MAG-55K, and HCYTOMAG-60K (Merck Millipore, Burlington, MA, USA), and LXSAHM-20 (R&D Systems, Bio-Techne Corp., Minneapolis, MN, USA), were used in order to determine the levels of synovial tissue proteins with multi-analytic profiling while using a Luminex 200 system (Luminex, Austin, TX, USA) and xMAP technology. Attained data were analysed by xPONENT 3.1 software (Luminex). HCYTOMAG-60K and LXSAHM-20 were customised and contained the following proteins: a disintegrin and metalloproteinase with a thrombospondin type 1 motif member 13 (ADAMTS13), aggrecan, bone morphogenetic protein (BMP) 2, 4, and 9, collagen 1-α1, collagen 4-α1, epidermal growth factor (EGF), eotaxin, fibroblast activation protein (FAP), fibroblast growth factor 2 (FGF-2), fibronectin, granulocyte-colony stimulating factor (G-CSF), granulocyte-macrophage (GM) CSF, hepatocyte growth factor receptor (HGFR), intercellular adhesion molecule 1 (ICAM-1), IL-1β, IL-1ra, IL-6, IL-7, IL-8, IL-10, IL-17, interferon gamma-induced protein 10 (IP-10), lumican, monocyte chemoattractant protein 1 (MCP-1), macrophage inflammatory protein 1α (MIP-1α), MIP-1β, neural cell adhesion molecule (NCAM), osteoprotegerin (OPG), osteonectin, platelet-derived growth factor (PDGF) AA, PDGF-AB/BB, regulated on activation normal T-cell expressed and secreted (RANTES), syndecan-1, syndecan-4, tenascin C, transforming growth factor α (TGF-α), tumour necrosis factor α (TNF-α), TNF-β, triggering receptor expressed on myeloid cells 1 (TREM-1), and vascular endothelial growth factor (VEGF). In addition, HTMP2MAG-54K and HMMP2MAG-55K contained matrix metalloproteinase 1 (MMP-1), MMP-2, MMP-7, MMP-9, MMP-10, tissue inhibitor of metalloproteinase 1 (TIMP-1), TIMP-2, TIMP-3, and TIMP-4. Fifty-one proteins were analysed in total.

2.6. Statistical Analyses

Stata version 15 (StataCorp, Collage Station, TX, USA) and IBM SPSS version 25.0 (IBM Corp, Armonk, NY, USA) were used to analyse the data. The descriptive statistics were calculated as mean ± SD for all continuous data and as a number and percentage for bivariate data. Data on patient characteristics were analysed with Student's T-test for continuous data and Fisher's exact test for categorical data. For the statistical analyses of synovial tissue proteins, the surgical outcome groups intermediate and deteriorated were merged into one group, since there was only one patient in the deteriorated group. The concentration of specified proteins (pg/mL) was used in the statistical analyses. The surgical outcome was the dependent variable and ordered logistic regression were used for both univariate and multivariate computations. The multivariate regression model was tested with Akaike's information criterion (AIC) in order to estimate the performance of the model. The best performance was reached by including the specific protein and the potential confounders CIA, TMJ disability, masticatory muscle palpation, and the interaction of CIA and positive finding of masticatory muscle palpation pain. Masticatory muscle palpation was dichotomised, and no finding of palpation pain was merged with unilateral positive sign, since it made the model perform better according to AIC. A p-value of ≤0.05 was regarded as significant.

3. Results

3.1. Patient Demographics and Patient-Specific Clinical Variables

One-hundred patients had followed the protocol at study closure (Figure 2). The 27 patients who were excluded or did not participate had a mean age of 40.4 years (SD 15.3) and 81% were women. No differences were found when comparing participating patients to the non-participating with regards to sex and age. In six patients out of the hundred included, it was not possible to harvest any synovial tissue; therefore, their data were only included in the clinical parameter analyses. Table 1 compiles demographic data and preoperative patient-specific symptoms and signs. The outcome of surgery, as well as measured mean differences before and after surgery are displayed in Table 2. Patients in the diagnosis-group OA were significantly older when compared to the other groups ($p = 0.022$) and they had more co-morbidities, classified as "other diseases" ($p = 0.041$). Both OA ($p = 0.003$) and DDwR patients ($p < 0.001$) had larger MIO as compared to the rest of the cohort. The group with DDwR had significantly lower TMJ pain VAS-value ($p = 0.008$) and fewer patients with both palpation pain of the masticatory muscles ($p < 0.001$) and the TMJ ($p < 0.001$). On the other hand, the CIA-group had significantly more patients with palpation pain on muscles ($p = 0.006$) and TMJ ($p < 0.001$). Patients with DDwoR had significantly lower TMJ psychosocial impact ($p = 0.003$), as well as lower global pain ($p = 0.050$), when compared to the other three diagnoses.

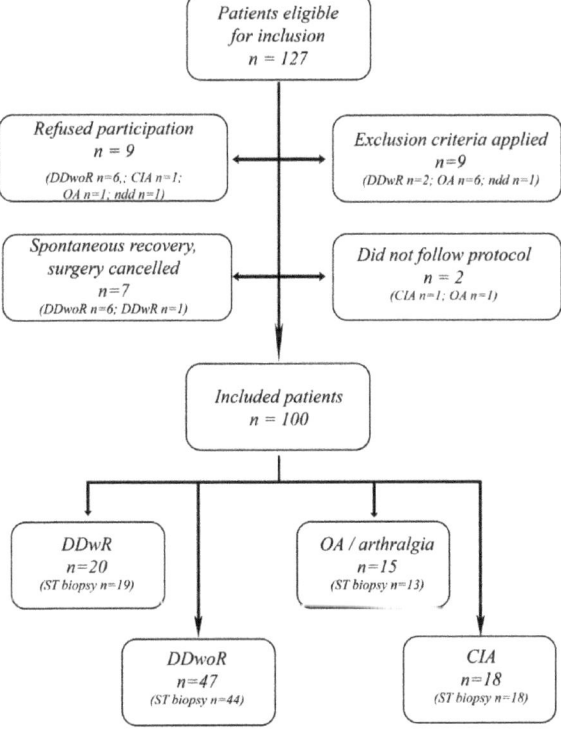

Figure 2. Flow chart illustrating patients´ eligibility for inclusion into the study, reasons for not participating, and TMJ diagnoses. CIA, chronic inflammatory arthritis; DDwoR, disc displacement without reduction; DDwR, disc displacement with reduction; OA, osteoarthritis; *n*, number; ndd, no diagnosis defined; ST, synovial tissue.

Table 1. Preoperative registration of demographic data, anamnestic information, objective and subjective measurements of included patients.

Classification	DDwR	DDwoR	OA	CIA	Total
Demographic data					
Number of patients	20	47	15	18	100
Sex, W/M	15/5	40/7	15/0	17/1	87/13
Age (years), mean (SD)	37.5 (11.7)	43.1 (15.8)	50.7 (20.3)	38.1 (13.0)	42.2 (15.8)
Patient history					
Duration (mos.) mean (SD)	43.3 (40.4)	20.7 (24.0)	29.3 (44.1)	43.5 (42.7)	30.4 (35.7)
Tinnitus/ear fullness, n (%)	5 (25)	14 (30)	5 (33)	5 (28)	29 (29)
TMJ trauma, n (%)	8 (40)	10 (21)	3 (20)	3 (17)	24 (24)
Medical history, n (%)					
Healthy	10 (50)	19 (40)	2 (13)	0 (0)	31 (31)
Psychiatric disorder	4 (20)	15 (32)	1 (7)	3 (17)	23 (23)
Neuropsychiatric disorder	1 (5)	1 (2)	0 (0)	1 (6)	3 (3)
Autoimmune disease	0 (0)	0 (0)	1 (7)	18 (100)	19 (19)
Metabolic disease	2 (10)	6 (13)	3 (20)	0 (0)	11 (11)
Other disease	6 (30)	22 (47)	11 (73)	10 (56)	49 (49)
Objective measures					
MIO, mm (SD)	43.8 (9.7)	29.2 (4.7)	40.4 (5.7)	31.2 (7.0)	34.1 (8.9)
Wilks classification, mean (SD)	2.6 (0.9)	3.9 (0.6)	na	na	3.6 (1.0)
TMJ palp pain, n (bilat/lat/no)	0/6/14	4/28/15	2/10/3	7/10/1	13/54/33
Muscle palp pain, n (bilat/lat/no)	2/4/14	7/10/28	6/3/6	9/3/5	24/20/53
Subjective measures (VAS 0–10), mean (SD)					
TMJ pain	4.3 (2.5)	5.6 (2.4)	6.3 (2.2)	6.2 (1.9)	5.6 (2.4)
TMJ disability	6.1 (2.0)	6.3 (1.7)	5.7 (2.2)	5.8 (1.8)	6.1 (1.8)
TMJ psychosocial impact	5.1 (3.3)	3.7 (2.8)	5.7 (3.6)	5.7 (2.4)	4.6 (3.0)
Global pain	3.1 (3.2)	3.0 (3.0)	4.9 (2.5)	4.8 (2.9)	3.6 (3.0)

Bilat, bilateral; CIA, chronic inflammatory arthritis; DDwoR, disc displacement without reduction; DDwR, disc displacement with reduction; lat, lateral; M, men; MIO, maximum interincisal opening; mos., months; n, number; na, not applicable; OA, osteoarthritis; palp, palpation; SD, standard deviation; TMJ, temporomandibular joint; VAS, visual analogue scale; W, women.

All of the registered diagnoses and patient-specific factors were tabulated and those showing signs of association to outcome were further analysed in a univariate fashion. TMJ palpation pain (coef., 0.89; $p = 0.044$) and masticatory muscle palpation pain (coef., 1.97; $p < 0.001$) were both positively associated to a worse outcome (Figure 3). The four subjective VAS variables all had a linear association with surgical outcome, which was significant for TMJ disability (coef., 0.29; $p = 0.011$), TMJ psychosocial impact (coef., 0.15; $p = 0.032$), and global pain (coef., 0.13; $p = 0.043$), but not for TMJ pain (coef., 0.16; $p = 0.073$) (Figure 4). Tinnitus, sex, age, MIO, psychiatric disorder, TMJ pain, and the TMJ diagnoses showed no significant correlation to outcome.

Table 2. Outcome of surgery for the total cohort and for the different TMJ diagnoses, comparing mean differences of preoperative and postoperative values using paired samples t-test.

Outcome	Successful	Good	Intermediate	Deteriorated [a]
Number of patients (%)				
Total	56 (56)	22 (22)	21 (21)	1 (1)
DDwR	14 (70)	3 (15)	3 (15)	0 (0)
DDwoR	24 (51)	14 (30)	9 (19)	0 (0)
OA	9 (60)	4 (27)	2 (13)	0 (0)
CIA	9 (50)	1 (6)	7 (39)	1 (6)
Preoperative measurements sorted according to outcome				
Sex, W/M	48/8	18/4	20/1	
Age (years), mean (SD)	44.5 (16.0)	39.1 (16.2)	39.4 (14.6)	
Patient history				
Duration (mos.) mean (SD)	30.9 (39.5)	30.0 (31.1)	30.5 (31.8)	
Tinnitus/ear fullness, n (%)	13 (23)	7 (32)	9 (43)	
TMJ trauma, n (%)	15 (27)	7 (32)	2 (10)	
GJH, n (%)	12 (21)	7 (32)	5 (23)	
Medical history, n (%)				
Healthy	19 (34)	6 (27)	6 (29)	
Psychiatric disorder	12 (21)	5 (23)	6 (29)	
Neuropsychiatric disorder	0 (0)	2 (9)	1 (5)	
Autoimmune disease	1 (2)	1 (5)	1 (5)	
Metabolic disease	7 (13)	3 (14)	1 (5)	
Other disease	26 (46)	13 (59)	10 (48)	
Objective measures, mean (SD)				
MIO (mm)	34.4 (7.6)	33.9 (11.8)	33.5 (9.3)	
Wilks classification	3.5 (1.0)	3.6 (0.9)	4.0 (0.9)	
Mean differences of pre- and postoperative measurements in relation to outcome				
Objective measures (mm), mean (SD)				
MIO	8.4 (7.2) **	7.1 (8.0) **	0.5 (7.2)	
LTR left	0.3 (2.2)	1.9 (2.8) *	−0.7 (3.0)	
LTR right	0.8 (3.1) *	0.3 (2.8)	0.7 (2.1)	
PTR	1.5 (2.9) **	1.7 (2.6) *	0.6 (2.0)	
Subjective measures (VAS 0-10), mean (SD)				
TMJ pain	−4.1 (2.4) **	−1.6 (2.4) **	−0.7 (1.7)	
TMJ disability	−4.2 (1.8) **	−2.5 (2.2) **	−0.5 (1.9)	
TMJ psychosocial	−3.5 (2.6) **	−0.8 (3.2)	−0.1 (2.6)	
Global pain	−1.2 (2.8) **	−0.3 (2.0)	0.5 (3.3)	

CIA, chronic inflammatory arthritis; DDwoR, disc displacement without reduction; DDwR, disc displacement with reduction; GJH, general joint hypermobility; LTR, lateral excursion; M, men; MIO, maximum interincisal opening; mm, millimetre; mos., months; n, number; OA, osteoarthritis; PTR, protrusion; SD, standard deviation; TMJ, temporomandibular joint; VAS, visual analogue scale; W, women. [a] The patient with deteriorated outcome was transferred to the intermediate group for statistical analyses. * $p \leq 0.05$, ** $p \leq 0.005$.

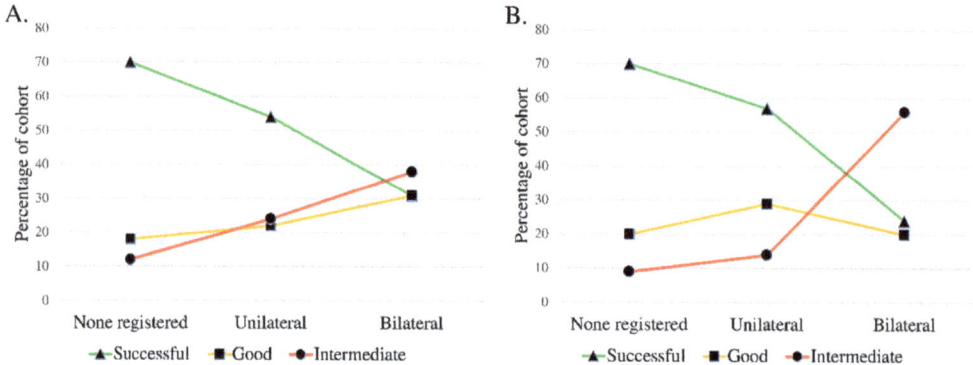

Figure 3. Line charts illustrating the preoperative TMJ and muscle palpation variables related to surgical outcome groups. The intermediate outcome group also contains the single deteriorated patient. Palpation of the lateral aspect of the TMJ and palpation of the masseter and temporal muscle was performed in accordance with the Diagnostic Criteria for Temporomandibular Disorders (DC/TMD). Positive palpation findings were recorded as being unilateral or bilateral. Negative palpation findings were recorded as none registered. (**A**) The line chart shows the significant linear association of increased positive findings of TMJ palpation pain related to a worse outcome ($p \leq 0.05$). (**B**) Masticatory muscle palpation pain had a strong association to surgical outcome in a similar manner as TMJ palpation pain ($p \leq 0.005$). DC/TMD, diagnostic criteria for temporomandibular disorders; TMJ, temporomandibular joint.

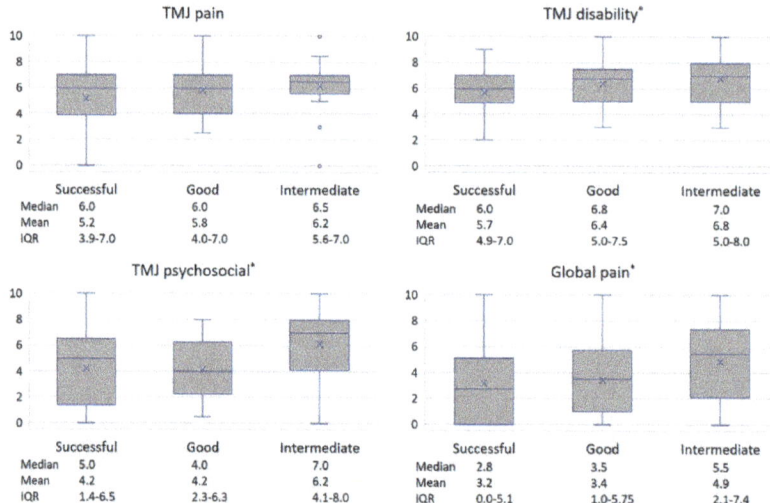

Figure 4. Box plot showing the relation between preoperative patient-reported 0–10 VAS values of TMJ pain, TMJ disability, TMJ psychosocial, and global pain according to surgical outcome groups. The top of the box indicates the 75th percentile, and the bottom the 25th percentile. The line within the box shows the median and the cross indicates the mean. The whiskers show the 10th and 90th percentile and points outside the 10th and 90th percentile shows outliers. All four preoperative VAS values were higher in relation to a worsened outcome, but only TMJ pain were not significant. TMJ, temporomandibular joint; VAS, visual analogue scale. * $p < 0.05$.

3.2. Synovial Tissue Analysis, Univariate Analysis

When examining the proteins in the multi-analytic profiling system, some of the proteins were identified as being below or above the standard limits, as defined by the manufacturers. Those samples that were below the lowest standard were set at the lowest standard value and those above the highest standard were set at the highest standard value. The processed tissue samples with protein measurements out of the assay's precision and recovery were treated as the missing values.

ADAMTS13, BMP-9, HGFR, IL-7, MMP-10, NCAM, osteonectin, syndecan-1 and 4, TIMP-4, and TREM-1 were found with detectable concentrations in most patients. These proteins have not been previously described in the human TMJ.

All of the analysed proteins were related to outcome in a univariate ordered logistic regression model. Higher concentrations of both eotaxin (coef., 2.89×10^{-3}; $p = 0.038$) and syndecan-1 (coef., 1.11×10^{-4}; $p = 0.024$) significantly changed the outcome in a negative direction. None of the other proteins had any significant correlation to outcome.

3.3. Multivariate Analysis of Synovial Tissue and Potential Confounders

The significant results from univariate analyses with respect to patient-specific variables were tested in a multivariate model. The tested variables were TMJ disability (coef., 0.23; $p = 0.054$), TMJ psychosocial impact (coef., 0.06, $p = 0.424$), global pain (coef., 0.07, $p = 0.352$), and masticatory muscle palpation pain (coef., 1.69; $p = 0.001$). Table 3 presents multivariate ordered logistic regression analyses of association between the outcome of TMJ surgery and the specific proteins, including potential confounders and the interaction between CIA and positive bilateral masticatory muscle palpation pain. Higher concentrations of IL-8, lumican, MMP-7, and TIMP-2 were all associated to an inferior outcome in a significant way. ADAMTS13, BMP-4, eotaxin, NCAM-1, and TIMP-1 were close to significant, with p-values of ≤ 0.075. Patients with the interaction CIA and bilateral masticatory muscle palpation pain showed a significant association to a positive surgical outcome in the analysis of ADAMTS13, IL-1β, and TNF-β (Table 3). All of the analyses of the interaction variable showed a negative coefficient, indicating that positive bilateral muscle palpation pain does not predict a poor surgical outcome in patients that are suffering from CIA.

Table 3. Ordered logistic regression relating the dependent variable surgical outcome (successful, good, intermediate/deteriorated) to analysed proteins, potential confounders and the interaction of CIA and positive jaw muscle palpation tenderness.

Protein	No. obs.	Specified Protein [a] Coef.	CIA [b] Coef.	Masticatorymuscle Palpation [b] Coef.	TMJ Disability [b] Coef.	Interaction CIA/Palp.[c] Coef.
ADAMTS13	87	7.29×10^{-7}	3.78 **	2.15 **	0.27 *	−4.19 *
Aggrecan	94	-8.25×10^{-6}	1.77	1.93 **	0.22	−2.07
BMP-2	94	-9.06×10^{-5}	1.24	1.87 **	0.23	−1.69
BMP-4	94	8.05×10^{-4}	1.34	1.95 **	0.22	−1.62
BMP-9	44	1.45×10^{-3}	1.00	1.73	0.24	−1.54
Collagen-1 α1	94	4.28×10^{-6}	1.31	1.90 **	0.21	−1.66
Collagen-4 α1	94	-2.38×10^{-6}	1.15	1.86 **	0.23	−1.64
EGF	94	4.33×10^{-4}	1.16	1.86 **	0.22	−1.64
Eotaxin	93	2.69×10^{-3}	1.19	1.92 **	0.22	−1.61
FAP	94	1.05×10^{-5}	1.37	1.95 **	0.18	−1.72
FGF-2	94	4.03×10^{-5}	1.22	1.99 **	0.23	−1.77
Fibronectin	94	5.12×10^{-8}	1.26	1.83 *	0.20	−1.66

Table 3. Cont.

Protein	No. obs.	Specified Protein [a] Coef.	CIA [b] Coef.	Masticatory muscle Palpation [b] Coef.	TMJ Disability [b] Coef.	Interaction CIA/Palp. [c] Coef.
G-CSF	94	-2.32×10^{-4}	1.82	2.01 **	0.22	-2.37
HGFR	94	6.68×10^{-5}	1.34	1.92 **	0.21	-1.68
ICAM-1	94	1.54×10^{-8}	1.17	1.86 **	0.22	-1.65
IL-1β	85	-2.57×10^{-2}	1.98 *	2.01 **	0.20	-3.27 *
IL-1ra	94	2.51×10^{-3}	1.24	1.90 **	0.21	-1.64
IL-6	46	8.66×10^{-3}	1.33	0.91	0.04	-0.55
IL-7	94	-6.60×10^{-4}	1.54	1.91 **	0.22	-2.01
IL-8	93	2.17×10^{-2} *	1.11	2.11 **	0.20	-1.33
IL-10	92	5.66×10^{-3}	1.56	1.88 *	0.25 *	-2.00
IP-10	94	6.99×10^{-5}	1.13	1.68 *	0.23	-1.40
Lumican	94	9.99×10^{-8} *	1.48	2.02 **	0.17	-1.82
MCP-1	94	-2.43×10^{-4}	1.09	1.91 **	0.23	-1.53
MIP-1α	49	1.70×10^{-3}	1.71	1.97	-0.09	-2.80
MIP-1β	60	3.61×10^{-3}	1.73 *	1.63 *	0.16	-1.70
MMP-1	66	9.72×10^{-4}	17.74	2.56 **	0.26	$-$ [d]
MMP-2	93	1.92×10^{-7}	1.55	1.86 **	0.24	-2.04
MMP-7	62	3.06×10^{-5} *	$-$ [e]	3.22 **	0.23	$-$ [e]
MMP-9	93	1.92×10^{-6}	1.61 *	1.90 **	0.24	-2.07
MMP-10	89	-5.65×10^{-5}	1.57	1.80 *	0.26 *	-2.02
NCAM-1	94	1.74×10^{-5}	1.33	1.90 **	0.22	-1.58
OPG	94	1.73×10^{-5}	1.31	1.80 *	0.20	-1.61
Osteonectin	94	2.98×10^{-8}	1.17	1.86 **	0.22	-1.66
PDGF-AA	94	1.28×10^{-4}	1.16	1.84 *	0.22	-1.61
PDGF-AB/BB	94	-4.84×10^{-5}	1.27	1.88 **	0.21	-1.84
RANTES	94	-4.13×10^{-5}	1.22	1.80 *	0.22	-1.92
Syndecan-1	94	7.62×10^{-5}	0.60	1.72 *	0.19	-0.98
Syndecan-4	90	9.74×10^{-5}	1.20	1.89 **	0.19	-1.66
Tenascin C	94	4.13×10^{-6}	1.23	1.89 **	0.20	-1.70
TIMP-1	93	3.91×10^{-5}	2.01 *	1.89 **	0.20	-2.04
TIMP-2	93	3.11×10^{-5} *	2.12 *	2.18 **	0.21	-2.25
TIMP-3	93	5.68×10^{-5}	1.87 *	2.02 **	0.25 *	-2.22
TIMP-4	93	4.30×10^{-4}	1.57	1.86 **	0.23	-2.08
TNF-α	91	-2.89×10^{-2}	2.57 *	1.91 **	0.27 *	-2.47
TNF-β	65	-1.53×10^{-2}	3.36 *	3.03 **	0.11	-4.48 *
TREM-1	85	9.48×10^{-5}	1.18	1.60 *	0.22	-1.39
VEGF	93	6.03×10^{-4}	1.49	1.79 *	0.23	-1.94
GM-CSF [f]	41	$-$	$-$	$-$	$-$	$-$
IL-17 [f]	13	$-$	$-$	$-$	$-$	$-$
TGF-α [f]	32	$-$	$-$	$-$	$-$	$-$

ADAMTS13, a disintegrin and metalloproteinase with a thrombospondin type 1 motif member 13; BMP, bone morphogenetic protein; CIA, chronic inflammatory arthritis; Coef., coefficient; EGF, epidermal growth factor; FAP, fibroblast activation protein; FGF, fibroblast growth factor; G-CSF, granulocyte-colony stimulating factor; GM, granulocyte-macrophage; HGFR, hepatocyte growth factor receptor; ICAM, intercellular adhesion molecule; IL, interleukin; IP, interferon gamma-induced protein; MCP, monocyte chemoattractant protein; MIP, macrophage inflammatory protein; MMP, matrix metalloproteinase; NCAM, neural cell adhesion molecule; No., number; obs., observations; OPG, osteoprotegerin; palp., palpation; PDGF, platelet-derived growth factor; TIMP, tissue inhibitors of metalloproteinases; TGF, transforming growth factor; TNF, tumour necrosis factor; TREM, triggering receptor expressed on myeloid cells; VEGF, vascular endothelial growth factor. [a] The ordered logistic regression was modelled from successful outcome in three steps down to intermediate/deteriorated outcome as the worst outcome. A positive coefficient thereby indicating that the higher the specific protein concentration, the worse the outcome. [b] A positive coefficient shows that the diagnosis or variable affects the outcome in a negative way. [c] Describes the interaction between CIA and positive jaw muscle palpation related to outcome. A negative coefficient indicates a positive correlation to outcome. [d] No observations in the sample. [e] Omitted because of collinearity. [f] Too few observations why calculations could not be done. * $p \leq 0.05$, ** $p \leq 0.005$.

4. Discussion

The success rates in TMJ surgery have been reported as variable and they often not better than 80%. Identifying patient-specific predictors might be a valuable tool for surgeons, patients, and health-care providers to improve outcome.

The investigation of TMJ synovial fluid proteins potentially reflecting surgical outcome has to our knowledge been done twice before, where higher concentrations of IL-10 were significantly associated with a positive outcome of arthrocentesis, and TMJ pain was associated with higher concentrations of IL-6 and IL-8 indicating a negative outcome [14,22]. The TMJ synovial tissue proteins have not been investigated in relation to outcome earlier. In this study, four proteins—IL-8, lumican, MMP-7, and TIMP-2—were found to be associated with an impaired surgical outcome in a concentration dependent matter in multivariate analyses. The chemokine IL-8 exerts effects on cells, such as fibroblasts, neutrophils, and synovial cells during normal function and with an inflammatory state [23]. Higher levels of IL-8 have been associated with a higher severity of disease in rheumatoid arthritis and when comparing DDwR to DDwoR [23,24]. In oral squamous cell carcinoma, IL-8 was reported to up-regulate the production of MMP-7 via the IL-8 receptor β [25]. MMP´s are a group of proteases with the ability to degrade components of extracellular matrix (ECM) [26,27]. MMP-7 has been found to act on several collagens and proteoglycans directing to its role in joint degradation [26–28]. The main endogenous inhibitors of MMPs are TIMPs that bind MMPs in a 1:1 ratio [29]. TIMP-2 has been proposed to serve as a continuous ECM protector. Some of the studies have suggested that its mRNA expression does not respond to different stimuli during basal or inflammatory activity in joints, whereas other studies have detected mRNA in response to osteopontin or relaxin levels [30–32]. The small, leucine-rich, proteoglycan lumican has been associated with wound healing and found to be increased in degenerated TMJ discs when compared to normal discs [33,34]. All four proteins with a negative correlation to outcome are related to tissue turnover and remodeling, where lumican and TIMP-2 are suggested to promote TMJ healing, whilst IL-8 and MMP-7 possibly have degenerative properties. Therefore, they may potentially be useful as individual markers for a negative outcome and, if they are also demonstrated to relate to each other, they might provide a protein pattern that is indicative of biomarker quality.

In the univariate statistical analyses, higher concentrations of eotaxin and syndecan-1 showed a correlation to a suboptimal surgical outcome. Eotaxin is a chemokine that has been shown to increase osteoclast activity in bone inflammation, while syndecan-1 might be associated with attempted cartilage repair [35,36]. Fibrocartilage stem-cells (FCSC) with chondrogenic differentiation abilities have been identified in the human TMJ cartilage [37]. The association between the transmembrane proteoglycan syndecan-1 and FCSC reparative traits is unknown, but it deserves attention.

The age of the patient and preoperative MIO have previously been described as predictive factors for TMJ surgical outcome [2,13,38,39]. In the current study, this could not be confirmed for MIO and age. Univariate analysis revealed that TMJ disability, TMJ psychosocial impact, global pain, masticatory muscle, and TMJ palpation pain were significantly related to outcome. In the multivariate analysis, only masticatory muscle palpation pain remained significant. TMJ disability and CIA were included in the multivariate model, because they, according to AIC, strengthened the model. CIA showed a significant negative correlation to outcome in 10 of the 51 multivariate analyses of specified proteins, and TMJ disability in six of 51. This might imply that the diagnosis CIA and the variable TMJ disability individually can be valid predictors for a negative outcome of TMJ surgery.

The association between masticatory muscle palpation pain and negative outcome has earlier been presented by our group in two different patient cohorts [2,13]. Considering that the variable was significant in all but four multivariate calculations advocates its potential as a predictive factor. In contrast, CIA patients with the presence of bilateral muscle palpation pain did not seem to have any additional negative impact on outcome. The result strongly suggests that bilateral masticatory muscle palpation pain is an important predictive factor, which is why DDwR-, DDwoR-, and OA-patients with these findings should alert the clinician to consider a new round of non-invasive therapy.

A shortcoming of the study was the loss of 27 eligible patients, who did not participate for different reasons. Potential bias might be considered because the only variables possible to analyse for the non-participant group were sex, age, and TMJ diagnosis. A relatively short follow-up period was used, which might also implicate a bias in some of the diagnostic groups. Because only four out of 51 proteins correlated with outcome, there was a risk that these associations are by chance. This suggests that further investigations should be made to verify these findings.

To conclude, preoperative bilateral palpation pain of the masticatory muscles was found to be a predictor for negative surgical outcome, and it might alert the surgeon to consider non-invasive interventions that have not yet been tried before scheduling surgery. However, in patients diagnosed with CIA, bilateral masticatory muscle pain did not indicate a negative surgical outcome when compared to the other included TMJ diagnoses. TMJ disability was the only outcome measure that showed potential as predicting factor. IL-8, lumican, MMP-7, and TIMP-2 were individually shown to have a positive correlation to worse outcome. Altogether, the results demonstrate that the clinical variable bilateral masticatory muscle palpation pain seems to be a more robust predictor for surgical outcome when compared to any of the investigated proteins. Description of protein alterations due to diagnosis, severity, and progress of TMJ disease, but also in relation to different treatment modalities, has to continue. Further mapping will possibly reveal more of the potential multi-factorial pathogenesis.

Author Contributions: Conceptualization, M.U., R.S., C.K.-W., B.L.; Methodology, M.U., R.S., C.K.-W., B.L.; Validation, M.U., R.S., B.L.; Formal Analysis, M.U., R.S., A.N.-A., B.L.; Investigation, M.U., R.S., N.T., B.L.; Resources, M.U., R.S., A.N.-A., N.T., B.L.; Data Curation, M.U., R.S.; Writing—Original Draft Preparation, M.U., B.L.; Writing—Review & Editing, M.U., R.S., A.N.-A., N.T., C.K.-W., B.L.; Visualization, M.U., R.S., A.N.-A., B.L.; Supervision, R.S., B.L.; Project Administration, M.U., R.S., B.L.; Funding Acquisition, M.U., B.L. All authors have read and agreed to the published version of the manuscript.

Funding: This study was supported by grants from the Swedish Dental Society, Karolinska Institutet funding, University of Bergen and HelseVest funding, Haukeland University Hospital, Bergen, Norway.

Institutional Review Board Statement: The study was conducted according to the guidelines of the Declaration of Helsinki, and approved by the Regional Ethics Review Board in Stockholm (registration number 2014/622-31/1, approved on 23 April 2014).

Informed Consent Statement: Informed consent was obtained from all subjects involved in the study.

Data Availability Statement: The data presented in this study are available on request from the corresponding author.

Acknowledgments: The authors wish to thank the technical support of Janne Elin Reseland, Safiyye Suslu, and Aina Mari Lian at Oral Research Laboratory, Institute of Clinical Dentistry, University of Oslo.

Conflicts of Interest: The authors declare no conflict of interest.

References

1. Fillingim, R.B.; Slade, G.D.; Greenspan, J.D.; Dubner, R.; Maixner, W.; Bair, E.; Ohrbach, R. Long-term changes in biopsychosocial characteristics related to temporomandibular disorder: Findings from the OPPERA study. *Pain* **2018**, *159*, 2403–2413. [CrossRef] [PubMed]
2. Ulmner, M.; Weiner, C.K.; Lund, B. Predictive factors in temporomandibular joint arthroscopy: A prospective cohort short-term outcome study. *Int. J. Oral Maxillofac. Surg.* **2020**, *49*, 614–620. [CrossRef]
3. Gynther, G.W.; Holmlund, A.B. Efficacy of arthroscopic lysis and lavage in patients with temporomandibular joint symptoms associated with generalized osteoarthritis or rheumatoid arthritis. *J. Oral Maxillofac. Surg.* **1998**, *56*, 147–151. [CrossRef]
4. Machoň, V.; Šedý, J.; Klíma, K.; Hirjak, D.; Foltán, R. Arthroscopic lysis and lavage in patients with temporomandibular anterior disc displacement without reduction. *Int. J. Oral Maxillofac. Surg.* **2012**, *41*, 109–113. [CrossRef] [PubMed]
5. Miloro, M.; McKnight, M.; Han, M.D.; Markiewicz, M.R. Discectomy without replacement improves function in patients with internal derangement of the temporomandibular joint. *J. Cranio-Maxillofacial Surg.* **2017**, *45*, 1425–1431. [CrossRef] [PubMed]

6. Holmlund, A.; Lund, B.; Weiner, C.K. Discectomy without replacement for the treatment of painful reciprocal clicking or catching and chronic closed lock of the temporomandibular joint: A clinical follow-up audit. *Br. J. Oral Maxillofac. Surg.* **2013**, *51*, 211–214. [CrossRef]
7. Al-Moraissi, E. Open versus arthroscopic surgery for the management of internal derangement of the temporomandibular joint: A meta-analysis of the literature. *Int. J. Oral Maxillofac. Surg.* **2015**, *44*, 763–770. [CrossRef]
8. Schiffman, E.; Ohrbach, R.; Truelove, E.; Look, J.; Anderson, G.; Goulet, J.P.; List, T.; Svensson, P.; Gonzalez, Y.; Lobbezoo, F.; et al. Diagnostic criteria for temporomandibular disorders (DC/TMD) for clinical and research applications: Recommendations of the international RDC/TMD consortium network* and orofacial pain special interest groupdagger. *J Oral Facial Pain Headache* **2014**, *28*, 6–27. [CrossRef]
9. Lund, B.; Ulmner, M.; Bjørnland, T.; Berge, T.; Olsen-Bergem, H.; Rosèn, A. A disease-focused view on the temporomandibular joint using a Delphi-guided process. *J. Oral Sci.* **2020**, *62*, 1–8. [CrossRef]
10. Haeffs, T.H.; D'Amato, L.N.; Khawaja, S.N.; Keith, D.A.; Scrivani, S.J. What variables are associated with the outcome of arthroscopic lysis and lavage surgery for internal derangement of the temporomandibular joint? *J. Oral Maxillofac. Surg.* **2018**, *76*, 2081–2088. [CrossRef]
11. Bouloux, G.F.; Zerweck, A.G.; Celano, M.; Dai, T.; Easley, K.A. Can preoperative psychological assessment predict outcomes after temporomandibular joint arthroscopy? *J. Oral Maxillofac. Surg.* **2015**, *73*, 2094–2102. [CrossRef] [PubMed]
12. Cho, J.; Israel, H. Does the age of a patient affect the outcome of temporomandibular joint arthroscopic surgery? *J. Oral Maxillofac. Surg.* **2017**, *75*, 1144–1150. [CrossRef] [PubMed]
13. Ulmner, M.; Kruger-Weiner, C.; Lund, B. Patient-specific factors predicting outcome of temporomandibular joint arthroscopy: A 6-year retrospective study. *J. Oral Maxillofac. Surg.* **2017**, *75*, 1643. [CrossRef] [PubMed]
14. Hamada, Y.; Kondoh, T.; Holmlund, A.B.; Sakota, K.; Nomura, Y.; Seto, K. Cytokine and clinical predictors for treatment outcome of visually guided temporomandibular joint irrigation in patients with chronic closed lock. *J. Oral Maxillofac. Surg.* **2008**, *66*, 29–34. [CrossRef] [PubMed]
15. Orr, C.; Vieira-Sousa, E.; Boyle, D.L.; Buch, M.H.; Buckley, C.D.; Cañete, J.D.; Catrina, A.I.; Choy, E.H.S.; Emery, P.; Fearon, U.; et al. Synovial tissue research: A state-of-the-art review. *Nat. Rev. Rheumatol.* **2017**, *13*, 463–475. [CrossRef]
16. Veale, D.J. Synovial tissue biopsy research. *Front. Med.* **2019**, *6*, 72. [CrossRef]
17. Holmlund, A. Disc derangements of the temporomandibular joint: A tissue-based characterization and implications for surgical treatment. *Int. J. Oral Maxillofac. Surg.* **2007**, *36*, 571–576. [CrossRef]
18. Beighton, P.; Horan, F. Orthopaedic aspects of the Ehlers-Danlos syndrome. *J. Bone Jt. Surgery. Br.* **1969**, *51*, 444–453. [CrossRef]
19. Wilkes, C.H. Internal derangements of the temporomandibular joint: Pathological variations. *Arch. Otolaryngol. Head Neck Surg.* **1989**, *115*, 469–477. [CrossRef]
20. McCain, J.P. *Principles and Practice of Temporomandibular Joint Arthroscopy*; Mosby: Maryland Heights, MO, USA, 1996.
21. Rosengren, S.; Firestein, G.S.; Boyle, D.L. Measurement of inflammatory biomarkers in synovial tissue extracts by enzyme-linked immunosorbent assay. *Clin. Diagn. Lab. Immunol.* **2003**, *10*, 1002–1010. [CrossRef]
22. Hamada, Y.; Kondoh, T.; Holmlund, A.B.; Yamamoto, M.; Horie, A.; Saito, T.; Ito, K.; Seto, K.; Sekiya, H. Inflammatory cytokines correlated with clinical outcome of temporomandibular joint irrigation in patients with chronic closed lock. *Oral Surg. Oral Med. Oral Pathol. Oral Radiol. Endodontol.* **2006**, *102*, 596–601. [CrossRef] [PubMed]
23. Russo, R.C.; Garcia, C.C.; Teixeira, M.M.; Amaral, F.A. The CXCL8/IL-8 chemokine family and its receptors in inflammatory diseases. *Expert Rev. Clin. Immunol.* **2014**, *10*, 593–619. [CrossRef] [PubMed]
24. Ulmner, M.; Sugars, R.; Naimi-Akbar, A.; Suslu, S.; Reseland, J.E.; Kruger-Weiner, C.; Lund, B. Synovial tissue cytokine profile in disc displacement of the temporomandibular joint. *J. Oral Rehabilitation* **2020**, *47*, 1202–1211. [CrossRef] [PubMed]
25. Khurram, S.A.; Bingle, L.; McCabe, B.M.; Farthing, P.M.; Whawell, S.A. The chemokine receptors CXCR1 and CXCR2 regulate oral cancer cell behaviour. *J. Oral Pathol. Med.* **2014**, *43*, 667–674. [CrossRef]
26. Ferreira, L.M.; Moura, Á.F.B.; Barbosa, G.A.S.; Pereira, H.S.G.; Calderon, P.D.S. Do matrix metalloproteinases play a role in degenerative disease of temporomandibular joint? a systematic review. *CRANIO* **2016**, *34*, 112–117. [CrossRef]
27. Itoh, Y. Metalloproteinases in rheumatoid arthritis: Potential therapeutic targets to improve current therapies. *Prog. Mol. Biol. Transl. Sci.* **2017**, *148*, 327–338. [CrossRef]
28. Edman, K.; Furber, M.; Hemsley, P.; Johansson, C.; Pairaudeau, G.; Petersen, J.; Stocks, M.; Tervo, A.; Ward, A.; Wells, E.; et al. The discovery of MMP7 inhibitors exploiting a novel selectivity trigger. *ChemMedChem* **2011**, *6*, 769–773. [CrossRef]
29. Liu, J.; Khalil, R.A. Matrix metalloproteinase inhibitors as investigational and therapeutic tools in unrestrained tissue remodeling and pathological disorders. *Prog. Mol. Biol. Transl. Sci.* **2017**, *148*, 355–420. [CrossRef]
30. Zafarullah, M.; Su, S.; Martel-Pelletier, J.; Dibattista, J.A.; Costello, B.G.; Stetler-Stevenson, W.G.; Pelletier, J.-P. Tissue inhibitor of metalloproteinase-2 (TIMP-2) mRNA is constitutively expressed in bovine, human normal, and osteoarthritic articular chondrocytes. *J. Cell. Biochem.* **1996**, *60*, 211–217. [CrossRef]
31. Ko, J.H.; Kang, Y.M.; Yang, J.H.; Kim, J.S.; Lee, W.J.; Kim, S.H.; Yang, I.H.; Moon, S.-H. Regulation of MMP and TIMP expression in synovial fibroblasts from knee osteoarthritis with flexion contracture using adenovirus-mediated relaxin gene therapy. *Knee* **2019**, *26*, 317–329. [CrossRef]
32. Zhang, F.-J.; Yu, W.-B.; Luo, W.; Gao, S.-G.; Li, Y.-S.; Lei, G.-H. Effect of osteopontin on TIMP-1 and TIMP-2 mRNA in chondrocytes of human knee osteoarthritis in vitro. *Exp. Ther. Med.* **2014**, *8*, 391–394. [CrossRef] [PubMed]

33. Karamanou, K.; Perrot, G.; Maquart, F.-X.; Brézillon, S. Lumican as a multivalent effector in wound healing. *Adv. Drug Deliv. Rev.* **2018**, *129*, 344–351. [CrossRef] [PubMed]
34. Kiga, N.; Tojyo, I.; Matsumoto, T.; Hiraishi, Y.; Shinohara, Y.; Fujita, S. Expression of lumican in the articular disc of the human temporomandibular joint. *Eur. J. Histochem.: EJH* **2010**, *54*, 148–153. [CrossRef] [PubMed]
35. Kindstedt, E.; Holm, C.K.; Sulniute, R.; Martinez-Carrasco, I.; Lundmark, R.; Lundberg, P. CCL11, a novel mediator of inflammatory bone resorption. *Sci. Rep.* **2017**, *7*, 1–10. [CrossRef]
36. Pap, T.; Bertrand, J. Syndecans in cartilage breakdown and synovial inflammation. *Nat. Rev. Rheumatol.* **2012**, *9*, 43–55. [CrossRef]
37. Bi, R.; Yin, Q.; Mei, J.; Chen, K.; Luo, X.; Fan, Y.; Zhu, S. Identification of human temporomandibular joint fibrocartilage stem cells with distinct chondrogenic capacity. *Osteoarthr. Cartil.* **2020**, *28*, 842–852. [CrossRef]
38. Kurita, K.; Goss, A.N.; Ogi, N.; Toyama, M. Correlation between preoperative mouth opening and surgical outcome after arthroscopic lysis and lavage in patients with disc displacement without reduction. *J. Oral Maxillofac. Surg.* **1998**, *56*, 1394–1397. [CrossRef]
39. Breik, O.; Devrukhkar, V.; Dimitroulis, G. Temporomandibular joint (TMJ) arthroscopic lysis and lavage: Outcomes and rate of progression to open surgery. *J. Cranio-Maxillofacial Surg.* **2016**, *44*, 1988–1995. [CrossRef]

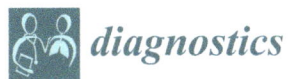

Article

Proteomic Expression Profile in Human Temporomandibular Joint Dysfunction

Andrea Duarte Doetzer [1,*], Roberto Hirochi Herai [1], Marília Afonso Rabelo Buzalaf [2] and Paula Cristina Trevilatto [1]

[1] Graduate Program in Health Sciences, School of Medicine, Pontifícia Universidade Católica do Paraná (PUCPR), Curitiba 80215-901, Brazil; rherai@gmail.com (R.H.H.); paula.trevilatto@pucpr.br (P.C.T.)
[2] Department of Biological Sciences, Bauru School of Dentistry, University of São Paulo, Bauru 17012-901, Brazil; mbuzalaf@fob.usp.br
* Correspondence: duarte.andrea@pucpr.br; Tel.: +55-41-991-864-747

Abstract: Temporomandibular joint dysfunction (TMD) is a multifactorial condition that impairs human's health and quality of life. Its etiology is still a challenge due to its complex development and the great number of different conditions it comprises. One of the most common forms of TMD is anterior disc displacement without reduction (DDWoR) and other TMDs with distinct origins are condylar hyperplasia (CH) and mandibular dislocation (MD). Thus, the aim of this study is to identify the protein expression profile of synovial fluid and the temporomandibular joint disc of patients diagnosed with DDWoR, CH and MD. Synovial fluid and a fraction of the temporomandibular joint disc were collected from nine patients diagnosed with DDWoR ($n = 3$), CH ($n = 4$) and MD ($n = 2$). Samples were subjected to label-free nLC-MS/MS for proteomic data extraction, and then bioinformatics analysis were conducted for protein identification and functional annotation. The three TMD conditions showed different protein expression profiles, and novel proteins were identified in both synovial fluid and disc sample. TMD is a complex condition and the identification of the proteins expressed in the three different types of TMD may contribute to a better comprehension of how each pathology develops and evolutes, benefitting the patient with a focus–target treatment.

Keywords: temporomandibular joint; protein expression; temporomandibular joint dysfunction

Citation: Doetzer, A.D.; Herai, R.H.; Buzalaf, M.A.R.; Trevilatto, P.C. Proteomic Expression Profile in Human Temporomandibular Joint Dysfunction. *Diagnostics* **2021**, *11*, 601. https://doi.org/10.3390/diagnostics11040601

Academic Editor: Gustavo Baldassarre

Received: 28 February 2021
Accepted: 24 March 2021
Published: 28 March 2021

Publisher's Note: MDPI stays neutral with regard to jurisdictional claims in published maps and institutional affiliations.

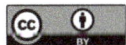

Copyright: © 2021 by the authors. Licensee MDPI, Basel, Switzerland. This article is an open access article distributed under the terms and conditions of the Creative Commons Attribution (CC BY) license (https:// creativecommons.org/licenses/by/ 4.0/).

1. Introduction

Temporomandibular dysfunction (TMD) is a disorder of the masticatory system and it is characterized by pain, loss of function of one or both articulations, and impairment of the masticatory system. TMD impacts not only jaw function, but the life quality of affected patients, increasing their treatment costs and work absence [1]. According to the National Institute of Health [2], TMD management in the USA costs approximately 4 billion dollars per year. A diagnostic protocol developed for research named Research Diagnostic Criteria for TMD (RDC/TMD), classifies TMD as myalgia, arthralgia, condylar pathologies, disc displacement, osteoarthrosis, osteoarthritis, degenerative joint disease and subluxation [3]. TMD has a multifactorial etiology, the most common being trauma, psychological alterations, hormone, inflammatory diseases, parafunction, and genetics [1,4]. TMD usually requires a panorex, and depending on the TMD type, magnetic resonance imaging, scintigraphy and tomography, besides a thorough clinical evaluation [5,6].

Depending on the TMD type, it can be classified as condylar hyperplasia (CH), disc displacement without reduction (DDWoR) and mandibular dislocation (MD). DDWoR is the most common TMD disorder [7], and along with CH, its etiology's understanding is still unclear. MD is a condition that is probably caused by physical alterations [8], and since it is less likely to have hormone contribution, it is a good TMD condition to compare the results with the other pathologies. DDWoR is caused by an abnormal positional association between the disc and the condyle, where the disc is permanently anteriorly displaced in relation to the condyle, causing limited range of mouth opening, pain and may lead to temporomandibular joint (TMJ) degeneration [9]. Disc displacement corresponds to 41% of TMD intra-articular disorders [7], and it is considered a multifactorial disease, with overlapping conditions contributing to its modulation including stress, parafunction, behavioral pattern, emotional status, and genetic background [3]. Among its different types of treatment, clinical handling is firstly employed (splint therapy, medication, physiotherapy) and when unsuccessful, surgery is indicated [6,10]. MD is an involuntary forward movement of the condyle beyond the articular eminence, mostly associated with trauma or excessive mouth opening, impairing its essential functions (speaking, chewing), and it accounts for 3% of all documented dislocations [11]. It usually needs mechanical manipulation to return to its normal position, and recurrent dislocations require surgical treatment [8]. Between these TMD types, CH is the rarest pathology that manifests a head condyle overgrowth, causing facial asymmetry, deformity, malocclusion and sometimes pain and dysfunction [12]. It is a self-limiting condition, more prevalent in female teenagers, but it usually requires surgical treatment to limit facial asymmetry progression and condyle continuous elongation [13]. Studies suggest it has a genetic involvement on its development, but its main etiology is still poorly understood [14].

Despite the etiological differences between CH, DDWoR and MD, current studies have limited understanding of the molecular variations that differentiates these TMD diseases. Condylar hyperplasia, mandibular dislocation and disc displacement have been the aim of many studies, due to their difficulty in targeting the proper treatment to each disease [9]. The employment of specific treatment, which may be improved with the unveiling of its specific etiology factors, will allow us to diminish treatment time and costs.

At the proteomic level, current studies focus only on individual mandibular dysfunctions, without comparing different TMD types to show the proteomic variability that could drive novel biomarkers as targets for disease diagnostic and treatment [15,16]. Proteomic analysis is a gold standard approach to analyze all identifiable proteins in a certain tissue, investigating its abundance, variety of proteoforms, and their stable or transient protein-protein interactions. This approach is especially beneficial in the clinical setting when studying proteins involved in different pathologies [17]. To date, there are very few studies investigating human TMD samples through proteomic output, and these studies analyzed only synovial fluid, focusing on specific target proteins [15,16]. Therefore, analyzing all proteins present in the synovial fluid and disc sample of different types of TMD may potentially lead TMD treatments towards a new reality.

In this research, a high throughput proteomic investigation of the three TMD pathologies CH, DDWoR and MD, was performed. Using state-of-the-art sample extraction procedures, biological samples of synovial fluid and TMJ discs were collected from distinct patients diagnosed with these conditions. The samples were processed, subjected to protein extraction and mass spectrometry proteomic identification. Generated proteomic data were analyzed using bioinformatics methods, and a per-sample protein identification and annotation were performed. The clinical phenotypes were then used to correlate the proteomic profile of each TMD condition.

2. Materials and Methods

2.1. Sample Selection

The sample was composed of 9 disc and synovial fluid specimens from female patients, with a mean age of 31.22 years (18–52). The patients presented different TMJ conditions, with three samples being composed of TMJ displaced disc without reduction ($n = 3$), two mandibular dislocation ($n = 2$) and four patients with condylar hyperplasia ($n = 4$) (Table 1). The specimens were collected from patients treated at the Evangelic University Hospital of Curitiba, Brazil. The study was approved by the Ethical Committee on Research at Pontifical Catholic University of Paraná, Brazil, according to Resolution 196/96 of the National Health Council and approved on 6 May of 2016 under registration number 1.863.521.

Table 1. Baseline characteristics of the sample, showing age and pathology of each female patient.

Number	Age	Diagnostic
1	18	Condylar Hyperplasia
2	20	Condylar Hyperplasia
3	38	Mandibular Dislocation
4	38	Mandibular Dislocation
5	36	Condylar Hyperplasia
6	29	Condylar Hyperplasia
7	25	Disc Displacement Without Reduction
8	25	Disc Displacement Without Reduction
9	52	Disc Displacement Without Reduction

Subjects did not present any of the following criteria: use of orthodontic appliances; chronic usage of anti-inflammatory drugs; history of diabetes, hepatitis, HIV infection; immunosuppressive chemotherapy; history of any disease known to compromise immune function; pregnancy or lactation; major jaw trauma; previous TMJ surgery; and previous steroid injection in the TMJ.

Subjects answered a personal medical history questionnaire and signed a consent form after being advised of the nature of the study. All patients were clinically examined by one experienced oral and maxillofacial surgeon. The clinical examination consisted of palpating the TMJ region, analyzing the occurrence of painful or limitation/excessiveness of mouth opening/closing, and the observation of facial asymmetry. Regarding complementary exams, all patients had a panorex and patients with disc displacement were submitted to a magnetic resonance image. The patients who were considered to be affected with disc displacement were treated surgically when they presented painful clinical signs of disc displacement after unsuccessful non-surgical treatment for at least 6 months [18]. Patients presenting pain related only to muscular spasms were not included in this research. Patients with condylar hyperplasia were diagnosed through clinical evaluation, panorex and when presenting a positive condylar growth in scintilography, a high condylectomy was indicated and performed [19]. Patients with recidivist mandibular dislocation (more than four episodes in six months) were treated with eminectomy [8].

2.2. Sample Acquisition

During access to the TMJ to perform the needed surgery [20], a 21-gauge needle was inserted into the upper TMJ space, then 1 mL of saline was injected into the joint space, which was aspirated thereafter by a second adapted syringe. This procedure was repeated five times to obtain a synovial fluid sample as described previously by Alstergren [21]. For each type of surgery performed, TMJ disc recontouring and repositioning was needed [16], therefore, first the displaced disc was freed, repositioned and sutured to the latero-posterior side of the condyle with a Mitek bone-cleat. The suture was then placed between the posterior and intermediate bands, and recontouring the thickened disk with a scalpel was necessary (this posterior debrided cartilage constituted the disc sample). Synovial fluid was spun down at $300 \times g$ to remove debris, and stored at $-80°C$ until use or analysis, and the disc samples rinsed in phosphate-buffered saline (PBS), and either snap frozen in liquid nitrogen and stored at $-80°C$.

2.3. Proteomic Analysis

The microcentrifuge tubes containing the synovial fluid and TMJ discs were removed from the $-80°C$ freezer, and after defrosting, the discs were cut into small pieces with the aid of sterile scissors, centrifuged, and the supernatants were collected and pooled according to each pathology group. The preparation of the samples for proteomic analysis was carried out as previously reported [22]. The analysis of the tryptic peptides was performed in the nanoACQUITY UPLC system (Waters, Milliford, CT, USA) coupled to the Xevo Q-TOF G2 mass spectrometer (MS) (Waters, Milliford, CT, USA). For this purpose, the UPLC nanoACQUITY system was equipped with a column of type HSS T3 (Acquity UPLC HSS T3 column 75 mm × 150 mm; 1.8 µm, Waters), previously balanced with 7% of the mobile phase B (100% ACN + 0.1% formic acid). The peptides were separated through a linear gradient of 7%–85% of the mobile phase B over 70 min with a flow of 0.35 µL/min and the column temperature maintained at 45 °C. The MS was operated in positive ion mode, with a 75 min data acquisition time. The obtained data were processed using ProteinLynx GlobalServer (PLGS) version 3.03 (Waters, Milliford, CT, USA). Protein identification was obtained using the ion counting algorithm incorporated into the software. The collected data were searched in the database of the species *Homo sapiens* downloaded from the catalog of the UniProt [23] in September of 2020. The identified proteins for the groups DDWoR, MD, and CH of synovial fluid and TMJ disc were classified and attributed by biological function, origin, and molecular interaction with the program Genemania [24]. The overlapping proteins between the groups were clustered by using an automatic Venn diagram generator.

3. Results

In this qualitative study, our aim was to explore, for the first time, a comparative analysis of the proteomic profile of three distinct TMD diseases. Although a statistical analysis was not performed, we were able to identify and describe the function of the proteins, including overlapping proteins between the investigated samples (DDWoR, MD and CH, and between both synovial fluid and disc samples).

In the synovial fluid samples, a total of 225 proteins (351 counting the repeated proteins in all groups) were successfully identified: 190 in the group DDWoR, 154 in the group MD and seven in the group CH. We also compared these three groups to identify shared or condition-specific proteins. We found 114 shared proteins between groups DDWoR and MD, and six proteins were shared by all groups (Table 2).

In the disc sample, 379 proteins were identified (697 counting the repeated proteins in all groups), with 235 proteins in group DDWoR, 196 in group MD and 266 in group CH. These three groups were also compared to identify shared or condition-specific proteins. There were nine shared proteins between groups DDWoR and MD, 28 shared proteins between groups DDWoR and CH, 17 shared proteins between groups MD and CH, and 132 shared proteins by all groups (Table 3).

Regarding the proteins in common in both synovial fluid and disc in the same sample groups, DDWoR presented two common proteins, MD presented three proteins, group CH had no protein in common, and the three groups together had six proteins in common (Table 4).

All synovial fluid and disc samples presented proteins involved in DNA repair, muscle and neural regeneration.

A selective pool of proteins was chosen to be studied according to the pathology group and protein function for synovial fluid and disc sample (Tables 5 and 6).

The synovial fluid sample presented the following proteins functions for each group (Table 5): the DDWoR group presented proteins involved in inflammatory process, apoptosis, hearing, interleukine-6 cascade, and protection against oxidative stress; the MD group showed proteins involved in inflammatory process, apoptosis, hearing, interleukine-6 cascade, protection against oxidative stress, and immune response; in the CH group, the expression of alcohol degradation protein (ADH1) was identified. The group comprising the pathologies DDWoR and MD were mainly involved in inflammatory process inhibition, bone resorption, chondrogenesis, bone and cartilage formation, osteoarthrosis, and neuropathic pain. No proteins were observed in the groups DDWoR and CH, and MD and CH. The proteins expressed in all three groups (DDWoR, MD and CH) were mainly implicated with muscle regeneration.

Table 2. Gene code and name of the proteins expressed in synovial fluid of all groups (disc displacement without reduction (DDWoR), mandibular dislocation (MD), condylar hyperplasia (CH) and between the groups DDWoR and MD, DDWoR and CH, MD and CH and DDWoR, MD and CH.

Protein Expressed in Each Group of TMJ Synovial Fluid Sample (n = 225)												
DDWoR (n = 70)		MD (n = 34)		CH (n = 1)		DDWoR and MD (n = 114)		DDWoR and CH (n = 0)	MD and CH (n = 0)	DDWoR, MD and CH (n = 6)		
Code	Name	Code	Name	Code	Name	Code	Name			Code	Name	
A2M	Alpha-2-Macroglobulin	ACTR3B	Actin Related Protein 3B	ADH1	Alcohol Dehydrogenase Subunit Alpha	ABI3BP	ABI Family Member 3 Binding Protein	X	X	ENO1	Enolase 1	
ANXA5	Annexin A5	ACTR3C	Actin Related Protein 3C			ACTA1	Actin Alpha 1, Skeletal Muscle			ENO2	Enolase 2	
APCS	Amyloid P Component	AKNA	AT-Hook Transcription Factor			ACTA2	Actin Alpha 2, Smooth Muscle			ENO3	Enolase 3	
APOH	Apolipoprotein H	ALDH1L1	Aldehyde Dehydrogenase 1 Family Member L1			ACTB	Actin Beta			MYH16	Myosin Heavy Chain 16 Pseudogene	
ARHGAP21	Rho GTPase Activating Protein 21	C4A	Complement C4A (Rodgers Blood Group)			ACTBL2	Actin Beta Like 2			RPL7L1	Ribosomal Protein L7 Like 1	
CFH	Complement Factor H	C4B_2	Complement Component 4B			ACTC1	Actin Alpha Cardiac Muscle 1			SHLD3	Shieldin Complex Subunit 3	
CHD8	Chromodomain Helicase DNA Binding Protein 8	C7orf57	Complement C7			ACTG1	Actin Gamma 1					
CILP2	Cartilage Intermediate Layer Protein	CAGE1	Cancer Antigen 1			ACTG2	Actin Gamma 2, Smooth Muscle					
CNOT6L	CCR4-NOT Transcription Complex Subunit 6 Like	CPSF2	Cleavage And Polyadenylation Specific Factor 2			ALB	Albumin					
DAGLA	Diacylglycerol Lipase Alpha	DCAF4L2	DDB1 And CUL4 Associated Factor 4 Like 2			ANXA1	Annexin A1					

Table 2. Cont.

Protein Expressed in Each Group of TMJ Synovial Fluid Sample (n = 225)												
DDWoR (n = 70)		MD (n = 34)		CH (n = 1)		DDWoR and MD (n = 114)		DDWoR and CH (n = 0)	MD and CH (n = 0)	DDWoR, MD and CH (n = 6)		
Code	Name	Code	Name	Code	Name	Code	Name			Code	Name	
DPYSL2	Dihydropyrimidinase Like 2	DHRS11	Dehydrogenase/Reductase 11			ANXA2	Annexin A2	X				
DPYSL3	Dihydropyrimidinase Like 3	DMD	Dystrophin			ANXA2P2	Annexin A2 Pseudogene 2					
DYM	Dymeclin	FLNA	Filamin A			APOA1	Apolipoprotein A1					
DYNC1H1	Dynein Cytoplasmic 1 Heavy Chain	HPR	Haptoglobin-Related Protein			ASPN	Asporin					
ENPP3	Ectonucleotide Pyrophosphatase/Phosphodiesterase 3	HPX	Hemopexin			ATP5F1B	ATP Synthase F1 Subunit Beta					
FGFR2	Fibroblast Growth Factor Receptor 2	IFT122	Intraflagellar Transport 122			BGN	Biglycan					
GPSM2	G Protein Signaling Modulator 2	LMO7	LIM Domain 7			C3	Complement C3					
GPX3	Glutathione Peroxidase 3	MYO6	Myosin VI			CILP	Cartilage Intermediate Layer Protein					
GSTP1	Glutathione S-Transferase Pi 1	PDIA3	Protein Disulfide Isomerase Family A Member 3			CLU	Clusterin					
H2BC1	H2B Clustered Histone 1	PPFIA1	PTPRF Interacting Protein Alpha 1			COL12A1	Collagen Type XII Alpha 1 Chain					
H2BE1	H2B.E Variant Histone 1	PPFIA2	PTPRF Interacting Protein Alpha 2			COL14A1	Collagen Type XIV Alpha 1 Chain					
HSPA1A	Heat Shock Protein Family A (Hsp70) Member 1A	PRDX1	Peroxiredoxin 1			COL1A1	Collagen Type I Alpha 1 Chain					

Table 2. Cont.

Protein Expressed in Each Group of TMJ Synovial Fluid Sample (n = 225)											
DDWoR (n = 70)		MD (n = 34)		CH (n = 1)		DDWoR and MD (n = 114)		DDWoR and CH (n = 0)	MD and CH (n = 0)	DDWoR, MD and CH (n = 6)	
Code	Name	Code	Name	Code	Name	Code	Name			Code	Name
HSPA1B	Heat Shock Protein Family A (Hsp70) Member 1B	PRDX2	Peroxiredoxin 2			COL6A1	Collagen Type VI Alpha 1 Chain	X	X		
HSPA1L	Heat Shock Protein Family A (Hsp70) Member 1 Like	RGMB	Repulsive Guidance Molecule BMP Co-Receptor B			COL6A2	Collagen Type VI Alpha 2 Chain				
HSPA2	Heat Shock Protein Family A (Hsp70) Member 2	SACM1L	SAC1 Like Phosphatidylinositide Phosphatase			COL6A3	Collagen Type VI Alpha 3 Chain				
HSPA8	Heat Shock Protein Family A (Hsp70) Member 8	SERPINA9	Serpin Family A Member 9			COMP	Thrombospondin-5				
IGLC1	Immunoglobulin Lambda Constant 1	SERPINH1	Serpin Family H Member 1			DCN	Decorin				
IGLC2	Immunoglobulin Lambda Constant	SLC4A1	Solute Carrier Family 4 Member 1			DES	Desmin				
IGLC3	Immunoglobulin Lambda Constant 3	SMPD3	Sphingomyelin Phosphodiesterase 3			DPT	Dermatopontin				
	Immunoglobulin Lambda Constant 6		Teneurin Transmembrane Protein 4				Fibrillin 1				
IGLC6	Immunoglobulin Lambda Constant 7	TENM4	Transmembrane O-Mannosyltransferase Targeting Cadherins 3			FBN1	Fibrinogen Alpha Chain				
IGLC7	Immunoglobulin Lambda Like Polypeptide 1	TMTC3	Testis Specific 10			FGA	Fibrinogen Beta Chain				
IGLL1	Immunoglobulin Lambda Like Polypeptide 5	TSGA10	Transthyretin			FGB	Fibrinogen Gamma Chain				
IGLL5	Interferon Regulatory Factor 7	TTR	Ubiquitin Specific Peptidase 10			FGG	Fibromodulin				

Table 2. Cont.

Protein Expressed in Each Group of TMJ Synovial Fluid Sample (n = 225)											
DDWoR (n = 70)		MD (n = 34)		CH (n = 1)		DDWoR and MD (n = 114)		DDWoR and CH (n = 0)	MD and CH (n = 0)	DDWoR, MD and CH (n = 6)	
Code	Name	Code	Name	Code	Name	Code	Name			Code	Name
IRF7	Kalirin RhoGEF Kinase	USP10	Actin Related Protein 3B			FMOD	Fibronectin 1	X			
KALRN	Kelch Repeat And BTB Domain Containing 11					FN1	Glyceraldehyde-3-Phosphate Dehydrogenase				
KBTBD11	Keratocan					GAPDH	Gelsolin				
KERA	Keratin 18					GSN	H2B Clustered Histone 11				
KRT18	Keratin 7					H2BC11	H2B Clustered Histone 12				
KRT7	Keratin 8					H2BC12	H2B Clustered Histone 13				
KRT8	Keratin 84					H2BC13	H2B Clustered Histone 14				
KRT84	Putative Uncharacterized Protein					H2BC14	H2B Clustered Histone 15		X		
LOC400499	Leucine Rich Repeat Containing 9					H2BC15	H2B Clustered Histone 17				
LRRC9	Mitogen-Activated Protein Kinase Kinase 7					H2BC17	H2B Clustered Histone 18				
MAP3K7	Microfibril Associated Protein 5					H2BC18	H2B Clustered Histone 21				
MFAP5	Myosin Light Chain 6B					H2BC21	H2B Clustered Histone 3				
MYL6B	NCK Associated Protein 5					H2BC3	H2B Clustered Histone 5				
NCKAP5	Nik Related Kinase					H2BC5	H2B Clustered Histone 9				

Table 2. *Cont.*

Protein Expressed in Each Group of TMJ Synovial Fluid Sample (n = 225)											
DDWoR (n = 70)		MD (n = 34)		CH (n = 1)		DDWoR and MD (n = 114)		DDWoR and CH (n = 0)	MD and CH (n = 0)	DDWoR, MD and CH (n = 6)	
Code	Name	Code	Name	Code	Name	Code	Name			Code	Name
NRK	Pericentriolar Material 1					H2BC9	H2B.S Histone 1	X	X		
PCM1	Procollagen C-Endopeptidase Enhancer					H2BS1	H2B.U Histone 1				
PCOLCE	RAD54 Like					H2BU1	Hemoglobin Subunit Alpha 1				
RAD54L	Retinol Dehydrogenase 5					HBA1	Hemoglobin Subunit Alpha 2				
RDH5	Ret Proto-Oncogene					HBA2	Hemoglobin Subunit Beta				
RET	Regulatory Factor X1					HBB	Hemoglobin Subunit Delta				
RFX1	RPTOR Independent Companion Of MTOR Complex 2					HBD	Hemoglobin Subunit Epsilon 1				
RICTOR	RIMS Binding Protein 3					HBE1	Hemoglobin Subunit Gamma 1				
RIMBP3	RUN And FYVE Domain Containing 2					HBG1	Hemoglobin Subunit Gamma 2				
RUFY2	Serpin Family C Member 1					HBG2	Haptoglobin				
SERPINC1	Serpin Family F Member 1					HP	Heat Shock Protein Family B (Small) Member 1				

Table 2. Cont.

Protein Expressed in Each Group of TMJ Synovial Fluid Sample (n = 225)											
DDWoR (n = 70)		MD (n = 34)		CH (n = 1)		DDWoR and MD (n = 114)		DDWoR and CH (n = 0)	MD and CH (n = 0)	DDWoR, MD and CH (n = 6)	
Code	Name	Code	Name	Code	Name	Code	Name			Code	Name
SERPINF1	SEC14 And Spectrin Domain Containing 1					HSPB1	Immunoglobulin Heavy Constant Alpha 1	X			
SESTD1	Small Nuclear Ribonucleoprotein U5 Subunit 200					IGHA1	Immunoglobulin Heavy Constant Alpha 2 (A2m Marker)				
SNRNP200	SVOP Like					IGHA2	Immunoglobulin Heavy Constant Gamma 1 (G1m Marker				
SVOPL	Transcription Elongation Factor, Mitochondrial					IGHG1	Immunoglobulin Heavy Constant Gamma 2				
TEFM	Thrombospondin 3					IGHG2	Immunoglobulin Heavy Constant Gamma 3				
THBS3	Tenascin C					IGHG3	Immunoglobulin Heavy Constant Gamma 4				
TNC	Trio Rho Guanine Nucleotide Exchange Factor					IGHG4	Immunoglobulin Kappa Constant				
TRIO	Tubulin Beta 1 Class VI					IGKC	Internexin Neuronal Intermediate Filament Protein Alpha				

Table 2. Cont.

	Protein Expressed in Each Group of TMJ Synovial Fluid Sample (n = 225)						
	DDWoR (n = 70)	MD (n = 34)	CH (n = 1)	DDWoR and MD (n = 114)	DDWoR and CH (n = 0)	MD and CH (n = 0)	DDWoR, MD and CH (n = 6)
TUBB1	Ubiquitin Specific Peptidase 42						
USP42	WW Domain Binding Protein 1 Like						
WBP1L	Zinc Finger ZZ-Type And EF-Hand Domain Containing 1						
ZZEF1	H2B Clustered Histone 1						
INA				Galectin 1			
LGALS1				Lamin			
LMNA				Lumican			
LUM				Microfibril Associated Protein 4			
MFAP4				Myosin Light Chain 6			
MYL6				Myocilin			
MYOC				Neurofilament Heavy			
NEFH				Neurofilament Light			
NEFL				Neurofilament Medium			
NEFM				Osteoglycin			
OGN				Pellino E3 Ubiquitin Protein Ligase Family Member 3			
PELI3				Pyruvate Kinase M1/2			
PKM				POTE Ankyrin Domain Family Member E			

Table 2. Cont.

	Protein Expressed in Each Group of TMJ Synovial Fluid Sample (n = 225)				
DDWoR (n = 70)	MD (n = 34)	CH (n = 1)	DDWoR and MD (n = 114)	DDWoR and CH (n = 0)	MD and CH (n = 0)	DDWoR, MD and CH (n = 6)
			POTEE	POTE Ankyrin Domain Family Member F		
			POTEF	POTE Ankyrin Domain Family Member I		
			POTEI	POTE Ankyrin Domain Family Member J		
			POTEJ	POTE Ankyrin Domain Family Member K, Pseudogene		
			POTEKP	Peptidylprolyl Isomerase A		
			PPIA	Proline And Arginine Rich End Leucine Rich Repeat Protein		
			PRELP	Peripherin		
			PRPH	S100 Calcium Binding Protein A10		
			S100A10	Serpin Family A Member 1		
			SERPINA1	Superoxide Dismutase 3		
			SOD3	Transferrin		

Table 2. *Cont.*

		Protein Expressed in Each Group of TMJ Synovial Fluid Sample (n = 225)				
DDWoR (n = 70)	MD (n = 34)	CH (n = 1)	DDWoR and MD (n = 114)	DDWoR and CH (n = 0)	MD and CH (n = 0)	DDWoR, MD and CH (n = 6)
			TF	Transforming Growth Factor Beta Induced		
			TGFBI	Thrombospondin 4		
			THBS4	Tenascin XA		
			TNXA	Tenascin XB		
			TNXB	Tubulin Alpha 1a		
			TUBA1A	Tubulin Alpha 1b		
			TUBA1B	Tubulin Alpha 1c		
			TUBA1C	Tubulin Alpha 3c		
			TUBA3C	Tubulin Alpha 3d		
			TUBA3D	Tubulin Alpha 3e		
			TUBA3E	Tubulin Alpha 4a		
			TUBA4A	Tubulin Alpha 8		
			TUBA8	Tubulin Beta Class I		
			TUBB	Tubulin Beta 2A Class IIa		
			TUBB2A	Tubulin Beta 2B Class IIb		
			TUBB2B	Tubulin Beta 3 Class III		
			TUBB3	Tubulin Beta 4A Class IVa		

Table 2. Cont.

Protein Expressed in Each Group of TMJ Synovial Fluid Sample (n = 225)							
DDWoR (n = 70)		MD (n = 34)		CH (n = 1)	DDWoR and MD (n = 114)	DDWoR and CH (n = 0)	MD and CH (n = 0)	DDWoR, MD and CH (n = 6)
					Tubulin Beta 4B Class IVb			
					Tubulin Beta 6 Class V			
					Tubulin Beta 8 Class VIII			
					Tubulin Beta 8B			
					Versican			
					VIM			
					ABI Family Member 3 Binding Protein			

Table 3. Gene code and name of the proteins expressed in temporomandibular joint (TMJ) discs of all groups (DDWoR, MD, CH) and between the groups DDWoR and MD, DDWoR and CH, MD and CH and DDWoR, MD and CH.

Protein Expressed in Each Group of TMJ Disc Sample (n = 379)														
DDWoR (n = 66)		MD (n = 38)		CH (n = 89)		DDWoR and MD (n = 9)		DDWoR and CH (n = 28)		MD and CH (n = 17)		DDWoR, MD and CH (n = 132)	
Code	Name	Code	Name	Code	Name	Code	Name	Code	Name	Code	Name	Code	Name
ABCC9	ATP Binding Cassette Subfamily C Member 9	AFTPH	Aftiphilin	ACTN1	Actinin Alpha 1	ATP7B	ATPase Copper Transporting Beta	ACAN	Aggrecan	ATP5F1B	ATP Synthase F1 Subunit Beta	A2M	Alpha-2-Macroglobulin
ACSS3	Acyl-CoA Synthetase Short Chain Family Member 3	AKAP13	A-kinase anchor protein 13	ACTN4	Actinin Alpha 4	AXIN2	Axin 2	APOH	Apolipoprotein H	GFAP	Glial Fibrillary Acidic Protein	ABI3BP	ABI Family Member 3 Binding Protein
AGO4	Argonaute RISC Component 4	ALDH3A2	Aldehyde dehydrogenase family 3 member A2	ACTR3	Actin Related Protein 3	C4A	Complement C4A	BRD3	Bromodomain Containing 3	KRT3	Keratin 3	ACTA1	Actin Alpha 1, Skeletal Muscle

Table 3. Cont.

Protein Expressed in Each Group of TMJ Disc Sample (n = 379)												
DDWoR (n = 66)		MD (n = 38)		CH (n = 89)		DDWoR and MD (n = 9)		DDWoR and CH (n = 28)		MD and CH (n = 17)		DDWoR, MD and CH (n = 132)	
Code	Name	Code	Name	Code	Name	Code	Name	Code	Name	Code	Name	Code	Name
AMBP	Alpha-1-Microglobulin/Bikunin Precursor	ANKRD44	Serine/threonine-protein phosphatase 6 regulatory ankyrin repeat subunit B	ADAM10	ADAM Metallopeptidase Domain 10	C4B	Complement C4B	CLTC	Clathrin Heavy Chain	KRT5	Keratin 5	ACTA2	Actin Alpha 2, Smooth Muscle
ANKRD17	Ankyrin Repeat Domain 17	ANKRD52	Serine/threonine-protein phosphatase 6 regulatory ankyrin repeat subunit C	ADSL	Adenylosuccinate Lyase	C4B_2	Complement Component 4B	COL1A1	Collagen Type I Alpha 1 Chain	KRT6A	Keratin 6A	ACTB	Actin Beta
ARHGAP35	Rho GTPase Activating Protein 35	ARMH3	Armadillo-like helical domain-containing protein 3	ALDOA	Aldolase, Fructose-Bisphosphate A	KERA	Keratocan	COL4A6	Collagen Type IV Alpha 6 Chain	KRT6B	Keratin 6B	ACTBL2	Actin Beta Like 2
ARHGEF10	Rho Guanine Nucleotide Exchange Factor 10	CCDC88A	Girdin	ALDOC	Aldolase, Fructose-Bisphosphate C	KIAA0556	Katanin Interacting Protein	DNAH8	Dynein Axonemal Heavy Chain 8	KRT6C	Keratin 6C	ACTC1	Actin Alpha Cardiac Muscle 1
ATAD2B	ATPase Family AAA Domain Containing 2B	CLUH	Clustered mitochondria protein homolog	ANKMY1	Ankyrin Repeat And MYND Domain Containing 1	MAP4	Microtubule Associated Protein 4	EEF1A1	Eukaryotic Translation Elongation Factor 1 Alpha 1	KRT75	Keratin 75	ACTG1	Actin Gamma 1
BCAS2	BCAS2 Pre-MRNA Processing Factor	COL4A1	Collagen alpha-1(IV) chain	ANXA5	Annexin A5	SEMA4F	Semaphorin 4F	EEF1A1P5	Eukaryotic Translation Elongation Factor 1 Alpha 1 Pseudogene 5	KRT76	Keratin 76	ACTG2	Actin Gamma 2
CARNS1	Carnosine Synthase 1	DOCK10	Dedicator of cytokinesis protein 10	ANXA6	Annexin A6			EEF1A2		KRT78	Keratin 78	ALB	Albumin
CCDC187	Coiled-Coil Domain Containing 187	DTHD1	Death domain-containing protein 1	ASXL1	ASXL Transcriptional Regulator 1			HMCN2	Eukaryotic Translation Elongation Factor 1 Alpha 2	KRT79	Keratin 79	ANXA1	Annexin A1

Table 3. Cont.

					Protein Expressed in Each Group of TMJ Disc Sample (n = 379)							
DDWoR (n = 66)		MD (n = 38)		CH (n = 89)		DDWoR and MD (n = 9)		DDWoR and CH (n = 28)		MD and CH (n = 17)		DDWoR, MD and CH (n = 132)	
Code	Name	Code	Name	Code	Name	Code	Name	Code	Name	Code	Name	Code	Name
CDCP1	CUB Domain Containing Protein 1	ERAS	GTPase ERas	ATP2C1	ATPase Secretory Pathway Ca2+ Transporting 1			HSPA2	Hemicentin 2	KRT81	Keratin 81	ANXA2	Annexin A2
CDH3	Cadherin 3	ERBIN	Erbin	BLOC1S1	Biogenesis Of Lysosomal Organelles Complex 1 Subunit 1			HSPA8	Heat Shock Protein Family A (Hsp70) Member 2	KRT83	Keratin 83	ANXA2P2	Annexin A2 Pseudogene 2
CHD7	Chromodomain Helicase DNA Binding Protein 7	FLNA	Filamin-A	BRCA2	BRCA2 DNA Repair Associated			HYDIN	Heat Shock Protein Family A (Hsp70) Member 8	KRT85	Keratin 85	APCS	Amyloid P Component
CHD8	Chromodomain Helicase DNA Binding Protein 8	GOT1L1	Putative aspartate aminotransferase, cytoplasmic 2	CABP5	Calcium Binding Protein 5			IGLC1	HYDIN Axonemal Central Pair Apparatus Protein	KRT86	Keratin 86	APOA1	Apolipoprotein A1
CHD9	Chromodomain Helicase DNA Binding Protein 9	HHLA1	HERV-H LTR-associating protein 1	CACNA2D3	Calcium Voltage-Gated Channel Auxiliary Subunit Alpha2delta 3			IGLC2	Immunoglobulin Lambda Constant 1	PKM	Pyruvate Kinase M1/2	ASPN	Asporin
CSTF2T	Cleavage Stimulation Factor Subunit 2 Tau Variant	IGHV3OR16-9	Immunoglobulin heavy variable 3/OR16-9 (non-functional)	CCDC18	Coiled-Coil Domain Containing 18			IGLC3	Immunoglobulin Lambda Constant 2	TTBK2	Tau Tubulin Kinase 2	BGN	Biglycan
ECH1	Enoyl-CoA Hydratase 1	KDF1	Keratinocyte differentiation factor 1	CDC20	Cell Division Cycle 20			IGLC6	Immunoglobulin Lambda Constant 3			C3	Complement C3
ELAVL3	ELAV Like RNA Binding Protein 3	L1CAM	Neural cell adhesion molecule L1	CENPF	Centromere Protein F			IGLC7	Immunoglobulin Lambda Constant 6			CILP	Cartilage Intermediate Layer Protein
EML4	EMAP Like 4	MARK1	Serine/threonine-protein kinase MARK1	CFAP20DC	CFAP20 Domain Containing			IGLL1	Immunoglobulin Lambda Constant 7			CILP2	Cartilage Intermediate Layer Protein 2
FARP2	FERM, ARH/RhoGEF And Pleckstrin Domain Protein 2	NEIL3	Endonuclease 8-like 3	CNTN1	Contactin 1			IGLL5	Immunoglobulin Lambda Like Polypeptide 1			CLU	Clusterin

Table 3. Cont.

				Protein Expressed in Each Group of TMJ Disc Sample (n = 379)							
DDWoR (n = 66)		MD (n = 38)		CH (n = 89)		DDWoR and MD (n = 9)		DDWoR and CH (n = 28)		MD and CH (n = 17)		DDWoR, MD and CH (n = 132)	
Code	Name	Code	Name	Code	Name	Code	Name	Code	Name	Code	Name	Code	Name
FBN1	Fibrillin 1	NOL8	Nucleolar protein 8	COQ8B	Coenzyme Q8B			LOC441081	Immunoglobulin Lambda Like Polypeptide 5			COL12A1	Collagen Type XII Alpha 1 Chain
GALK2	Galactokinase 2	NUFIP1	Nuclear fragile X mental retardation-interacting protein 1	CTNNA3	Catenin Alpha 3			MIS18BP1	POM121 Membrane Glycoprotein (Rat) Pseudogene			COL14A1	Collagen Type XIV Alpha 1 Chain
GPR162	G Protein-Coupled Receptor 162	NUMA1	Nuclear mitotic apparatus protein	DPYSL2	Dihydropyrimidinase Like 2			MYO15B	MIS18 Binding Protein 1			COL6A1	Collagen Type VI Alpha 1 Chain
GPRASP1	G Protein-Coupled Receptor Associated Sorting Protein 1	PARP10	Protein mono-ADP-ribosyltransferase PARP10	EHD2	EH Domain Containing 2			POSTN	Myosin XVB			COL6A2	Collagen Type VI Alpha 2 Chain
IKBKE	Inhibitor Of Nuclear Factor Kappa B Kinase Subunit Epsilon	PCDHA4	Protocadherin alpha-4	EYS	Eyes Shut Homolog			SERPINA9	Periostin			COL6A3	Collagen Type VI Alpha 3 Chain
INS	Insulin	POLD1	DNA polymerase delta catalytic subunit	F13A1	Coagulation Factor XIII A Chain			VTN	Serpin Family A Member 9			COMP	Cartilage Oligomeric Matrix Protein
IRF2BPL	Interferon Regulatory Factor 2 Binding Protein Like	POM121L2	POM121-like protein 2	GOLGA4	Golgin A4							DCN	Decorin
ITGA6	Integrin Subunit Alpha 6	PPFIA1	Liprin-alpha-1	GSTP1	Glutathione S-Transferase Pi 1							DES	Desmin
KRT26	Keratin 26	PPFIA2	Liprin-alpha-2	GVINP1	GTPase, Very Large Interferon Inducible Pseudogene 1							DMD	Dystrophin
LEMD2	LEM Domain Nuclear Envelope Protein 2	PRR14L	Protein PER14L	H3-2	H3.2 Histone (Putative)							DPT	Dermatopontin
MAP3K21	Mitogen-Activated Protein Kinase Kinase Kinase 21	PTPN7	Tyrosine-protein phosphatase non-receptor type 7	H3-3A	H3.3 Histone A							ENO1	Enolase 1

Table 3. Cont.

					Protein Expressed in Each Group of TMJ Disc Sample (n = 379)							
DDWoR (n = 66)		MD (n = 38)		CH (n = 89)		DDWoR and MD (n = 9)		DDWoR and CH (n = 28)		MD and CH (n = 17)		DDWoR, MD and CH (n = 132)
Code	Name	Code	Name	Code	Name	Code	Name	Code	Name	Code	Name	Code	Name
MDGA1	MAM Domain Containing Glycosylphos-phatidylinositol Anchor 1	RASSF10	Ras association domain-containing protein 10	H3-3B	H3.3 Histone B							ENO2	Enolase 2
MMP10	Matrix Metallopeptidase 10	RPS6KA6	Ribosomal protein S6 kinase alpha-6	H3-4	H3.4 Histone							ENO3	Enolase 3
MMP27	Matrix Metallopeptidase 27	TRIO	TRIO and F-actin-binding protein	H3-5	H3.5 Histone							FBLN1	Fibulin 1
MMP3	Matrix Metallopeptidase 3	TSC1	Hamartin	HEATR6	HEAT Repeat Containing 6							FGA	Fibrinogen Alpha Chain
MOS	MOS Proto-Oncogene, Serine/Threonine Kinas	UPK3A	Uroplakin-3a	HPX	Hemopexin							FGB	Fibrinogen Beta Chain
MYL6	Myosin Light Chain 6	UROD	Uroporphyrinogen decarboxylase	HSP90B1	Heat Shock Protein 90 Beta Family Member 1							FGG	Fibrinogen Gamma Chain
MYO7B	Myosin VIIB			HSPA1A	Heat Shock Protein Family A (Hsp70) Member 1A							FLNB	Filamin B
NT5E	5'-Nucleotidase Ecto			HSPA1B	Heat Shock Protein Family A (Hsp70) Member 1B							FMOD	Fibromodulin
OLFML1	Olfactomedin Like 1			HSPA1L	Heat Shock Protein Family A (Hsp70) Member 1 Like							FN1	Fibronectin 1
PGM5	Phosphoglucomutase 5			HSPA5	Heat Shock Protein Family A (Hsp70) Member 5							GAPDH	Glyceraldehyde-3-Phosphate Dehydrogenase

Table 3. Cont.

				Protein Expressed in Each Group of TMJ Disc Sample (n = 379)							
DDWoR (n = 66)		MD (n = 38)		CH (n = 89)		DDWoR and MD (n = 9)		DDWoR and CH (n = 28)		MD and CH (n = 17)		DDWoR, MD and CH (n = 132)	
Code	Name	Code	Name	Code	Name	Code	Name	Code	Name	Code	Name	Code	Name
PHKA2	Phosphorylase Kinase Regulatory Subunit Alpha 2			IGFN1	Immunoglobulin Like And Fibronectin Type III Domain Containing 1							GPX3	Glutathione Peroxidase 3
PLA2G7	Phospholipase A2 Group VII			INF2	Inverted Formin 2							GSN	Angiotensin 1 Converting Enzyme 2
POR	Cytochrome P450 Oxidoreductase			L3MBTL4	L3MBTL Histone Methyl-Lysine Binding Protein 4							H2BC1	H2B Clustered Histone 1
RANBP17	RAN Binding Protein 17			LMNB1	Lamin B1							H2BC11	H2B Clustered Histone 11
RGS22	Regulator Of G Protein Signaling 22			LMNB2	Lamin B2							H2BC12	H2B Clustered Histone 12
RIF1	Replication Timing Regulatory Factor 1			MFAP5	Microfibril Associated Protein 5							H2BC13	H2B Clustered Histone 13
RTN4	Reticulon 4			MRPL50	Mitochondrial Ribosomal Protein L50							H2BC14	H2B Clustered Histone 14
SARS2	Seryl-TRNA Synthetase 2, Mitochondrial			MS4A6A	Membrane Spanning 4-Domains A6A							H2BC15	H2B Clustered Histone 15
SEPHS2	Selenophosphate Synthetase 2			MUC4	Mucin 4, Cell Surface Associated							H2BC17	H2B Clustered Histone 17
SLFN13	Schlafen Family Member 13			MYH14	Myosin Heavy Chain 14							H2BC18	H2B Clustered Histone 18
SLK	STE20 Like Kinase			MYL6B	Myosin Light Chain 6B							H2BC21	H2B Clustered Histone 21
SPATA20	Spermatogenesis Associated 20			NEK10	NIMA Related Kinase 10							H2BC3	H2B Clustered Histone 3
SPATA5	Spermatogenesis Associated 5			PAK3	P21 (RAC1) Activated Kinase 3							H2BC5	H2B Clustered Histone 5

Table 3. Cont.

Protein Expressed in Each Group of TMJ Disc Sample (n = 379)											
DDWoR (n = 66)		MD (n = 38)		CH (n = 89)		DDWoR and MD (n = 9)		DDWoR and CH (n = 28)		MD and CH (n = 17)		DDWoR, MD and CH (n = 132)	
Code	Name	Code	Name	Code	Name	Code	Name	Code	Name	Code	Name	Code	Name
SPTA1	Spectrin Alpha, Erythrocytic 1			PAPOLA	Poly(A) Polymerase Alpha							H2BC9	H2B Clustered Histone 9
SQLE	Squalene Epoxidase			PAPOLG	Poly(A) Polymerase Gamma							H2BS1	H2B.S Histone 1
ST20-AS1	ST20 Antisense RNA 1			PDIA3	Protein Disulfide Isomerase Family A Member 3							H2BU1	H2B.U Histone 1
STIL	STIL Centriolar Assembly Protein			PDLIM4	PDZ And LIM Domain 4							HBA1	Hemoglobin Subunit Alpha 1
TACC2	Transforming Acidic Coiled-Coil Containing Protein 2			RALBP1	RalA Binding Protein 1							HBA2	Hemoglobin Subunit Alpha 2
TAP1	Transporter 1, ATP Binding Cassette Subfamily B Member			RNF213	Ring Finger Protein 213							HBB	Hemoglobin Subunit Beta
THADA	THADA Armadillo Repeat Containing			SBF2	SET Binding Factor 2							HBD	Hemoglobin Subunit Delta
THBS3	Thrombospondin 3			SERPINF1	Serpin Family F Member 1							HBE1	Hemoglobin Subunit Epsilon 1
UQCRC1	Ubiquinol-Cytochrome C Reductase Core Protein 1			SERPINH1	Serpin Family H Member 1							HBG1	Hemoglobin Subunit Gamma 1
VWA3A	Von Willebrand Factor A Domain Containing 3A			SLC4A5	Solute Carrier Family 4 Member 5							HBG2	Hemoglobin Subunit Gamma 2
ZNF333	Zinc Finger Protein 333			SLIT2	Slit Guidance Ligand 2							HBZ	Hemoglobin Subunit Zeta
				SMPD3	Sphingomyelin Phosphodiesterase 3							HP	Haptoglobin
				TAPT1	Transmembrane Anterior Posterior Transformation 1							HPR	Haptoglobin-Related Protein

Table 3. *Cont.*

Protein Expressed in Each Group of TMJ Disc Sample (n = 379)

DDWoR (n = 66)		MD (n = 38)		CH (n = 89)		DDWoR and MD (n = 9)		DDWoR and CH (n = 28)		MD and CH (n = 17)		DDWoR, MD and CH (n = 132)	
Code	Name	Code	Name	Code	Name	Code	Name	Code	Name	Code	Name	Code	Name
				TBX22	T-Box Transcription Factor 22							HSPB1	Heat Shock Protein Family B (Small) Member 1
				TDRD1	Tudor Domain Containing 1							IGHA1	Immunoglobulin Heavy Constant Alpha 1
				TENM4	Teneurin Transmembrane Protein 4							IGHA2	Immunoglobulin Heavy Constant Alpha 2 (A2m Marker)
				THBS1	Thrombospondin 1							IGHG1	Immunoglobulin Heavy Constant Gamma 1 (G1m Marker)
				TJP2	Tight Junction Protein 2							IGHG2	Immunoglobulin Heavy Constant Gamma 2 (G2m Marker)
				TTR	Transthyretin							IGHG3	Immunoglobulin Heavy Constant Gamma 3 (G3m Marker)
				UBP1	Upstream Binding Protein 1							IGHG4	Immunoglobulin Heavy Constant Gamma 4 (G4m Marker)
				WHRN	Whirlin							IGKC	Immunoglobulin Kappa Constant
				ZNF155	Zinc Finger Protein 155							INA	Internexin Neuronal Intermediate Filament Protein Alpha
				ZNF221	Zinc Finger Protein 221							KRT7	Keratin 7
												KRT8	Keratin 8
												KRT84	Keratin 84
												LGALS1	Galectin 1

Table 3. Cont.

Protein Expressed in Each Group of TMJ Disc Sample (n = 379)												
DDWoR (n = 66)		MD (n = 38)		CH (n = 89)		DDWoR and MD (n = 9)		DDWoR and CH (n = 28)		MD and CH (n = 17)		DDWoR, MD and CH (n = 132)
Code	Name	Code	Name	Code	Name	Code	Name	Code	Name	Code	Name	Code	Name
												LMNA	Lamin A/C
												LUM	Lumican
												MFAP4	Microfibril Associated Protein 4
												MFGE8	Milk Fat Globule EGF And Factor V/VIII Domain Containing
												MYH16	Myosin Heavy Chain 16 Pseudogene
												MYOC	Myocilin
												NEFH	Neurofilament Heavy
												NEFL	Neurofilament Light
												NEFM	Neurofilament Medium
												OGN	Osteoglycin
												POTEE	POTE Ankyrin Domain Family Member E
												POTEF	POTE Ankyrin Domain Family Member F
												POTEI	POTE Ankyrin Domain Family Member I
												POTEJ	POTE Ankyrin Domain Family Member J
												POTEKP	POTE Ankyrin Domain Family Member K, Pseudogene
												PPIA	Peptidylprolyl Isomerase A

Table 3. Cont.

Protein Expressed in Each Group of TMJ Disc Sample (n = 379)												
DDWoR (n = 66)		MD (n = 38)		CH (n = 89)		DDWoR and MD (n = 9)		DDWoR and CH (n = 28)		MD and CH (n = 17)		DDWoR, MD and CH (n = 132)	
Code	Name	Code	Name	Code	Name	Code	Name	Code	Name	Code	Name	Code	Name
												PRDX1	Peroxiredoxin 1
												PRDX2	Peroxiredoxin 2
												PRELP	Proline And Arginine Rich End Leucine Rich Repeat Protein
												PRPH	Peripherin
												RPL7L1	Ribosomal Protein L7 Like 1
												S100A10	S100 Calcium Binding Protein A10
												SALL3	Spalt Like Transcription Factor 3
												SERPINA1	Serpin Family A Member
												SHLD3	Shieldin Complex Subunit 3
												SLC4A1	Solute Carrier Family 4 Member 1
												SOD3	Superoxide Dismutase 3
												TF	Transferrin
												TGFBI	Transforming Growth Factor Beta Induced
												THBS4	Thrombospondin 4
												TNC	Tenascin C
												TNXA	Tenascin XA (Pseudogene)
												TNXB	Tenascin XB
												TUBA1A	Tubulin Alpha 1a

Table 3. *Cont.*

										Protein Expressed in Each Group of TMJ Disc Sample (n = 379)	
DDWoR (n = 66)		MD (n = 38)		CH (n = 89)		DDWoR and MD (n = 9)		DDWoR and CH (n = 28)		MD and CH (n = 17)		DDWoR, MD and CH (n = 132)	
Code	Name	Code	Name	Code	Name	Code	Name	Code	Name	Code	Name	Code	Name
												TUBA1B	Tubulin Alpha 1b
												TUBA1C	Tubulin Alpha 1c
												TUBA3E	Tubulin Alpha 3e
												TUBA4A	Tubulin Alpha 4a
												TUBA8	Tubulin Alpha 8
												TUBB	Tubulin Beta Class I
												TUBB1	Tubulin Beta 1 Class VI
												TUBB2A	Tubulin Beta 2A Class IIa
												TUBB2B	Tubulin Beta 2B Class IIb
												TUBB3	Tubulin Beta 3 Class III
												TUBB4A	Tubulin Beta 4A Class IVa
												TUBB4B	Tubulin Beta 4B Class IVb
												TUBB6	Tubulin Beta 6 Class V
												TUBB8	Tubulin Beta 8 Class VIII
												TUBB8B	Tubulin Beta 8B

Table 4. Proteins expressed in both synovial fluid and TMJ disc samples of each group.

Protein Expressed in Each Group of TMJ Synovial Fluid and Disc Samples ($n = 11$)							
DDWoR ($n= 2$)	MD ($n = 3$)	CH ($n = 0$)	DDWoR and MD ($n = 0$)	DDWoR and CH ($n = 0$)	MD and CH ($n = 0$)	DDWoR, MD and CH ($n = 6$)
CHD8	FLNA					ENO1
MYL6B	PPFIA1					ENO2
	PPFIA2					ENO3
						MYH16
						RPL7L1
						SHLD3

Table 5. Gene code, protein name and function for each sample of TMJ synovial fluid.

Synovial Fluid Sample		
Code	Name	Function
DDWoR		
A2M	Alpha-2-Macroglobulin	Inhibits inflammatory cytokines.
APCS	Amyloid P Component, Serum	Binds to apoptotic cells at an early stage.
GPSM2	G Protein Signaling Modulator 2	Involved in the development of normal hearing.
KRT18	Keratin 18	Is involved in interleukin-6-mediated barrier protection.
MAP3K7	Mitogen-Activated Protein Kinase Kinase Kinase 7	Mediates signal transduction various cytokines including interleukin-1, transforming growth factor-beta, bone morphogenetic protein 2 and 4, Toll-like receptors, tumor necrosis factor receptor CD40 and B-cell receptor.
SERPINC1	Serpin Family C Member 1	This protein inhibits thrombin and it regulates the blood coagulation cascade.
MD		
ALDH1L1	Aldehyde Dehydrogenase 1 Family Member L1	Associated with decreased apoptosis, increased cell motility, and cancer progression.
C4A	Complement C4A (Rodgers Blood Group)	An antimicrobial peptide and a mediator of local inflammation.
HPX	Hemopexin	Acute phase protein that transports heme from the plasma to the liver and may be involved in protecting cells from oxidative stress.
IFT122	Intraflagellar Transport 122	Involved in cell cycle progression, signal transduction, apoptosis, and gene regulation.
MYO6	Myosin VI	This protein maintains the structural integrity of inner ear hair cells and mutations in this gene cause hearing loss.
PRDX1	Peroxiredoxin 1	Has an antioxidant protective role in cells and may contribute to the antiviral activity of CD8(+) T-cells.
SERPINH1	Serpin Family H Member 1	Plays a role in collagen biosynthesis as a collagen-specific molecular chaperone.
SMPD3	Sphingomyelin Phosphodiesterase 3	Mediates cellular functions, such as apoptosis and growth arrest.
CH		
ADH1	Alcohol Dehydrogenase Subunit Alpha	Catalyzes the oxidation of alcohols to aldehydes.
DDWoR and MD		
ANXA1	Annexin A1	Inhibits phospholipase A2 and has anti-inflammatory activity.

Table 5. Cont.

	Synovial Fluid Sample	
Code	Name	Function
	CH	
	DDWoR and MD	
ANXA2	Annexin A2	Functions as an autocrine factor which heightens osteoclast formation and bone resorption.
ASPN	Asporin	Regulate chondrogenesis by inhibiting transforming growth factor-beta 1-induced gene expression in cartilage. May induce collagen mineralization.
BGN	Biglycan	Plays a role in bone growth, muscle development and regeneration, and collagen fibril assembly in multiple tissues. This protein may also regulate inflammation and innate immunity.
CILP	Cartilage Intermediate Layer Protein	This protein is present in the cartilage intermediate layer protein (CILP), which increases in early osteoarthrosis cartilage.
CLU	Clusterin	Under stress conditions can be found in the cell cytosol. May be involved in cell death, tumor progression, and neurodegenerative disorders
COMP	Thrombospondin-5	Present in rheumatoid arthritis, is a noncollagenous extracellular matrix protein.
DCN	Decorin	Has a stimulatory effect on autophagy and inflammation and an inhibitory effect on angiogenesis and tumorigenesis.
FMOD	Fibromodulin	May also regulate TGF-beta activities by sequestering TGF-beta into the extracellular matrix.
FN1	Fibronectin 1	Fibronectin is involved in cell adhesion and migration processes including embryogenesis, wound healing, blood coagulation, host defense.
IGHG1	Immunoglobulin Heavy Constant Gamma 1 (G1m Marker)	Involved in pathways of Interleukin-4 and 13 signaling and IL4-mediated signaling events.
	DDWoR and CH	
x	x	x
	MD and CH	
x	x	x
	DDWoR, MD and CH	
ENO2	Enolase 2	Found in mature neurons and cells of neuronal origin.
ENO3	Enolase 3	May play a role in muscle development and regeneration.

Table 6. Gene code, protein name and function for each sample of TMJ discs.

	Disc Sample	
Code	Name	Function
	DDWoR	
AMBP	Alpha-1-Microglobulin/Bikunin Precursor	Regulation of the inflammatory process.
MMP10	Matrix Metallopeptidase 10	Breakdown of extracellular matrix.
MMP27	Matrix Metallopeptidase 27	Breakdown of extracellular matrix.
MMP3	Matrix Metallopeptidase 3	Breakdown of extracellular matrix.
PLA2G7	Phospholipase A2 Group VII	Inflammatory and oxidative stress response.

Table 6. Cont.

Code	Name	Function
	Disc Sample	
	DDWoR	
THADA	THADA Armadillo Repeat Containing	Apoptosis pathway.
THBS3	Thrombospondin 3	Matrix interactions.
	MD	
AKAP13	A-kinase anchor protein 13	Regulation of apoptotic process.
CCDC88A	Girdin	Vascular endothelial growth factor receptor 2 binding.
COL4A1	Collagen alpha-1(IV) chain	Extracellular matrix structural constituent.
ERAS	GTPase ERas	Tumor-like growth properties of embryonic stem cells.
ERBIN	Erbin	Inhibits NOD2-dependent NF-kappa-B signaling and proinflammatory cytokine secretion.
PARP10	Protein mono-ADP-ribosyltransferase PARP10	Negative regulation of fibroblast proliferation.
PPFIA1	Liprin-alpha-1	Cell–matrix adhesion.
PPFIA2	Liprin-alpha-2	Cell–matrix adhesion.
PTPN7	Tyrosine-protein phosphatase non-receptor type 7	Regulation of T and B-lymphocyte development and signal transduction.
UPK3A	Uroplakin-3a	Epithelial cell differentiation.
	CH	
ACTN4	Actinin Alpha 4	Transcriptional coactivator.
ADAM10	ADAM Metallopeptidase Domain 10	Responsible for the FasL ectodomain shedding.
COQ8B	Coenzyme Q8B	Biosynthesis of coenzyme Q.
HPX	Hemopexin	Protect cells from oxidative stress.
HSPA1A	Heat Shock Protein Family A (Hsp70) Member 1A	Protection of the proteome from stress.
NEK10	NIMA Related Kinase 10	Cellular response to UV irradiation.
PDLIM4	PDZ And LIM Domain 4	Involved in bone development.
SERPINH1	Serpin Family H Member 1	Chaperone in the biosynthetic pathway of collagen.
TTR	Transthyretin	Thyroid hormone-binding protein.
COL1A2	Collagen Type I Alpha 2 Chain	Fibril-forming collagen abundant in bone.
PRG4	Proteoglycan 4	This protein contains both chondroitin sulfate and keratan sulfate glycosaminoglycans.
PTPN13	Protein Tyrosine Phosphatase Non-Receptor Type 13	Regulates negatively FasL induced apoptosis.
	DDWoR and MD	
C4A	Complement C4A	Antimicrobial peptide and a mediator of local inflammation.
C4B	Complement C4B	Mediator of local inflammation.
C4B_2	Complement Component 4B	Mediator of local inflammatory process.
SEMA4F	Semaphorin 4F	Plays a role in neural development.
Code	Name	Function
	DDWoR and CH	
ACAN	Aggrecan	Part of the extracellular matrix that withstands compression in cartilage.
COL1A1	Collagen Type I Alpha 1 Chain	Collagen component.

Table 6. Cont.

Code	Name	Function
\multicolumn{3}{c}{Disc Sample}		
\multicolumn{3}{c}{DDWoR and CH}		
COL4A6	Collagen Type IV Alpha 6 Chain	Major structural component of basement membranes.
HSPA2	Heat Shock Protein Family A (Hsp70) Member 2	Protection of the proteome from stress.
POSTN	Periostin	Extracellular matrix protein that functions in tissue development and regeneration, including wound healing.
\multicolumn{3}{c}{MD and CH}		
KRT6A	Keratin 6A	Epidermis-specific type I keratin involved in wound healing.
\multicolumn{3}{c}{DDWoR, MD and CH}		
ANXA1	Annexin A1	Anti-inflammatory activity.
ANXA2	Annexin A2	Heightens osteoclast formation and bone resorption.
ANXA2P2	Annexin A2 Pseudogene 2	May be involved in heat-stress response.
APCS	Amyloid P Component	Is involved in dealing with apoptotic cells in vivo.
ASPN	Asporin	Regulates chondrogenesis by inhibiting transforming growth factor-beta 1-induced gene expression in cartilage
BGN	Biglycan	Plays a role in bone growth, and collagen fibril assembly in multiple tissues. This protein may also regulate inflammation and innate immunity.
C3	Complement C3	Modulates inflammation and possesses antimicrobial activity.
CILP	Cartilage Intermediate Layer Protein	Increases in early osteoarthrosis cartilage.
COL12A1	Collagen Type XII Alpha 1 Chain	Type XII collagen.
COL14A1	Collagen Type XIV Alpha 1 Chain	Type XIV collagen.
COL6A1	Collagen Type VI Alpha 1 Chain	Collagen VI.
COL6A2	Collagen Type VI Alpha 2 Chain	Type VI collagen.
COL6A3	Collagen Type VI Alpha 3 Chain	Ttype VI collagen.
COMP	Cartilage Oligomeric Matrix Protein	Degradation of the extracellular matrix.
ENO1	Enolase 1	Tumor suppressor.
ENO2	Enolase 2	Found in mature neurons and cells of neuronal origin.
ENO3	Enolase 3	Plays a role in muscle development and regeneration.
FN1	Fibronectin 1	Involved in wound healing, blood coagulation, host defense.
KRT7	Keratin 7	Co-expressed during differentiation of simple and stratified epithelial tissues.
LUM	Lumican	May regulate collagen fibril organization, epithelial cell migration and tissue repair.
MFAP4	Microfibril Associated Protein 4	Extracellular matrix protein which is involved in cell adhesion or intercellular interactions.
MFGE8	Milk Fat Globule EGF And Factor V/VIII Domain Containing	Promotes phagocytosis of apoptotic cells. This protein has also been implicated in wound healing, autoimmune disease, and cancer.
OGN	Osteoglycin	Induces ectopic bone formation in conjunction with transforming growth factor beta and may regulate osteoblast differentiation.

Table 6. *Cont.*

Code	Disc Sample	
	Name	Function
	MD and CH	
	DDWoR, MD and CH	
SOD3	Superoxide Dismutase 3	Antioxidant enzymes that protect tissues from oxidative stress.
TGFBI	Transforming Growth Factor Beta Induced	May be involved in endochondrial bone formation in cartilage.
TNC	Tenascin C	Modulation of inflammatory cytokine.
TNXB	Tenascin XB	Accelerates collagen fibril formation.
VCAN	Versican	A large chondroitin sulfate proteoglycan and is a major component of the extracellular matrix.
VIM	Vimentin	Involved in the stabilization of type I collagen mRNAs for CO1A1 and CO1A2.

The disc sample presented the following protein functions for each group (Table 6): the DDWoR group expressed proteins involved in inflammatory process, neurogenesis, cartilage formation, extracellular matrix degradation, oxidative stress and apoptosis. The MD group presented proteins related to apoptosis, vascular growth, inflammatory inhibitors, immunologic factors and epithelial growth, and the CH group showed protein expression implicated in apoptosis, apoptosis inhibition, oxidative stress, bone formation, chondroitin, bone and cartilage formation. The group with DDWoR and MD samples had proteins involved in inflammatory process; the group with DDWoR and CH samples showed proteins with collagen formation and wound healing functions; the group with MD and CH was involved in wound healing; and the group containing DDWoR, MD and CH samples was involved with inflammatory cascade modulation, osteoclastogenesis, chondrogenesis, apoptosis, bone formation, vascular and tissue repair, antioxidative activity.

There were proteins identified in both synovial fluid and TMJ disc samples, however, some of them in different pathology groups (Table 7).

Table 7. Name and function of expressed proteins in common between synovial fluid and TMJ disc sample, and the groups in each protein was expressed.

Name	Function	Disc	Synovial Fluid
Amyloid P Component, Serum	Is involved in dealing with apoptotic cells in vivo.	DDWoR, MD and CH	DDWoR
Annexin A1	Anti-inflammatory activity.	DDWoR, MD and CH	DDWoR and MD
Annexin A2	Heightens osteoclast formation and bone resorption.	DDWoR, MD and CH	DDWoR and MD
Asporin	Regulates chondrogenesis.	DDWoR, MD and CH	DDWoR and MD
Biglycan	Plays a role in bone growth, and collagen fibril assembly in multiple tissues.	DDWoR, MD and CH	DDWoR and MD
Cartilage Intermediate Layer Protein	Increases in early osteoarthrosis cartilage.	DDWoR, MD and CH	DDWoR and MD
Complement C4A	Antimicrobial peptide and a mediator of local inflammation.	DDWoR and MD	MD
Enolase 2	Found in mature neurons and cells of neuronal origin.	DDWoR, MD and CH	DDWoR, MD and CH

Table 7. Cont.

Name	Function	Disc	Synovial Fluid
Enolase 3	Play a role in muscle development and regeneration.	DDWoR, MD and CH	DDWoR, MD and CH
Fibronectin 1	Involved in wound healing, blood coagulation, host defense.	DDWoR, MD and CH	DDWoR and MD
Hemopexin	Protect cells from oxidative stress.	CH	MD
Lumican	May regulate collagen fibril organization, epithelial cell migration and tissue repair.	DDWoR, MD and CH	DDWoR and MD
Osteoglycin	Regulate osteoblast differentiation.	DDWoR, MD and CH	DDWoR and MD
Serpin Family H Member 1	Chaperones in the biosynthetic pathway of collagen.	CH	MD
Superoxide Dismutase 3	Antioxidant enzymes that protect tissues from oxidative stress.	DDWoR, MD and CH	DDWoR and MD
Tenascin XB	Modulation of inflammatory cytokine.	DDWoR, MD and CH	DDWoR and MD
Transforming Growth Factor Beta Induced	May be involved in endochondral bone formation in cartilage.	DDWoR, MD and CH	DDWoR and MD
Versican	A large chondroitin sulfate proteoglycan and is a major component of the extracellular matrix.	DDWoR, MD and CH	DDWoR and MD

Different types of collagen were identified in discs of the MD group, CH group, DDWoR and CH group, and in the group with all pathologies together (DDWoR, MD and CH). Besides the known collagen type I present in TMJ discs, collagen type IV, VI, XII and XIV were also identified (Table 8).

Table 8. Types of collagen identified in each TMJ disc group.

Type of Collagen Identified in Each Group										
DDWoR	MD		CH		DDWoR and MD	DDWoR and CH		MD and CH	DDWoR, MD and CH	
x	Code	Name	Code	Name	x	Code	Name	x	Code	Name
	COL4A1	Collagen Type IV Alpha 1 Chain	COL1A2	Collagen Type I Alpha 2 Chain		COL1A1	Collagen Type I Alpha 1 Chain		COL12A1	Collagen Type XII Alpha 1 Chain
						COL4A6	Collagen Type IV Alpha 6 Chain		COL14A1	Collagen Type XIV Alpha 1 Chain
									COL6A1	Collagen Type VI Alpha 1 Chain
									COL6A2	Collagen Type VI Alpha 2 Chain
									COL6A3	Collagen Type VI Alpha 3 Chain

All shared and group-specific proteins are indicated in a Venn diagram for the synovial fluid (Figure 1) and disc samples (Figure 2).

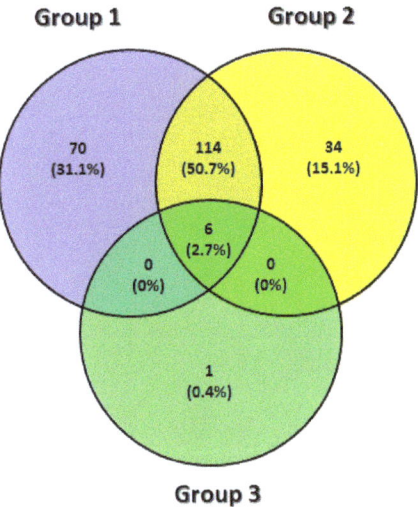

Figure 1. Venn diagram for synovial fluid: group 1—DDWoR, group 2—MD, group 3—CH.

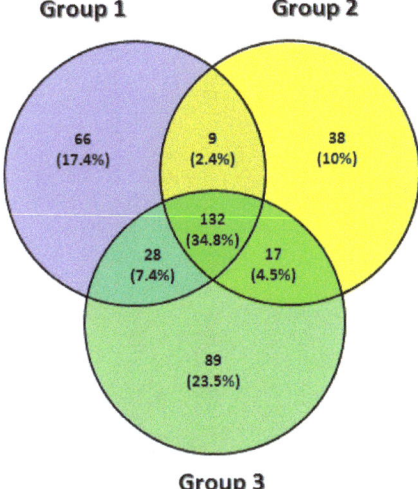

Figure 2. Venn diagram for the TMJ disc: group 1—DDWoR, group 2—MD, group 3—CH.

The interactions between the proteins were analyzed with Genemania (https://genemania.org—accessed on 5 September 2020), and its genetic network pointed out distinct protein cascades that might be modulating each pathology through the synovial fluid and disc samples. The physical and genetic interactions, co-expression and pathway of the proteins are shown in Figures 3 and 4.

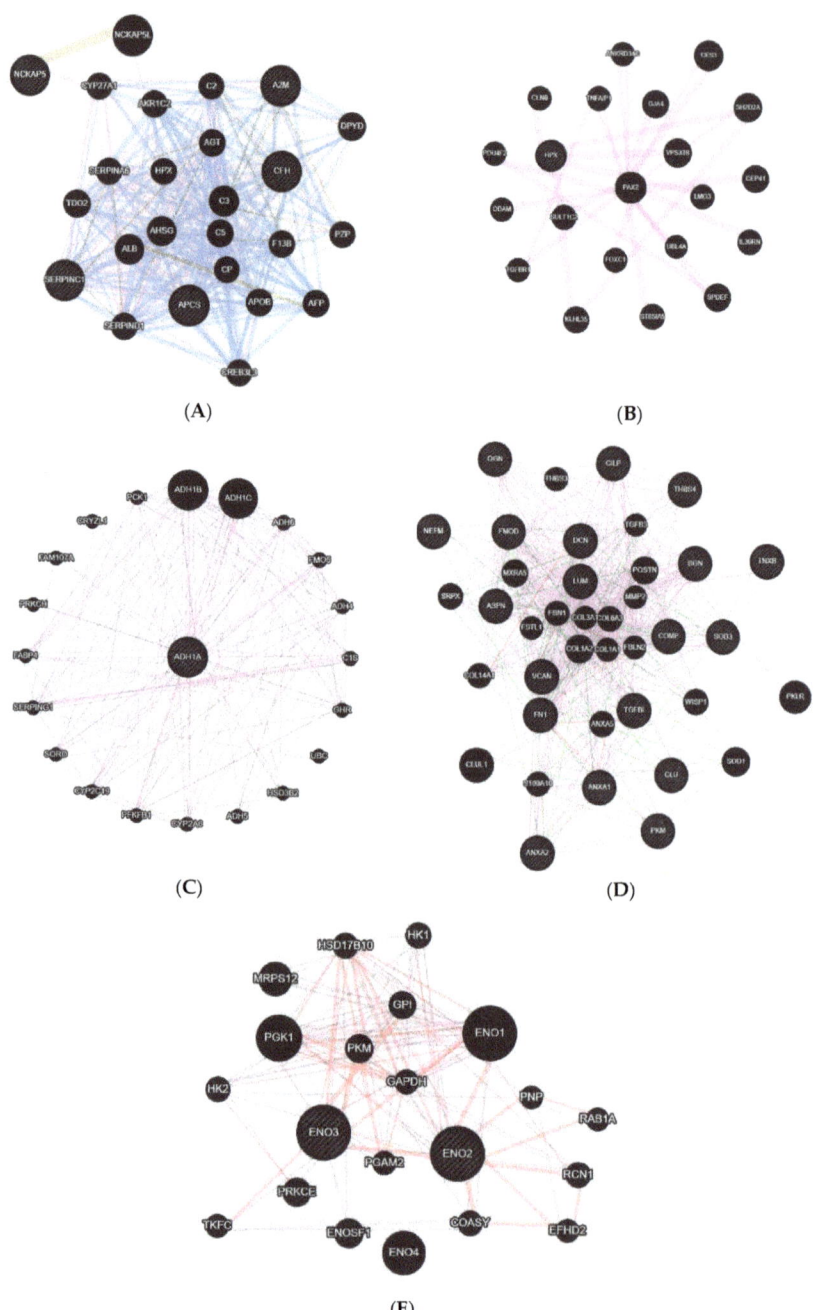

Figure 3. Gene interactions between the main functional proteins of synovial fluid. (**A**) showing the gene interactions of the DDWoR group. (**B**) showing the gene interactions of the MD group. (**C**) showing the gene interactions of the CH group. (**D**) showing the gene interactions of the DDWoR and MD group. (**E**) showing the gene interactions of the DDWoR, MD and CH group.

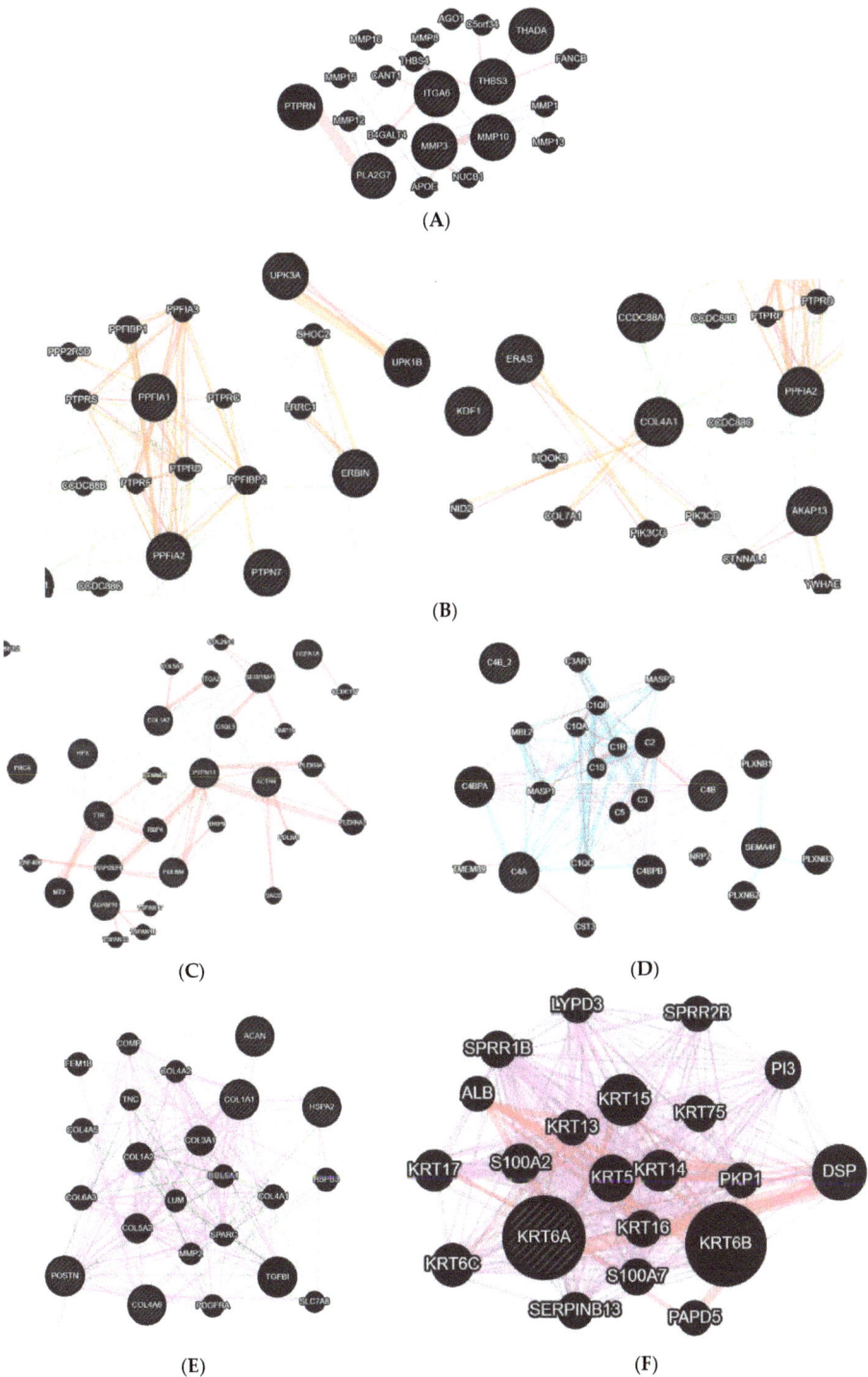

Figure 4. Cont.

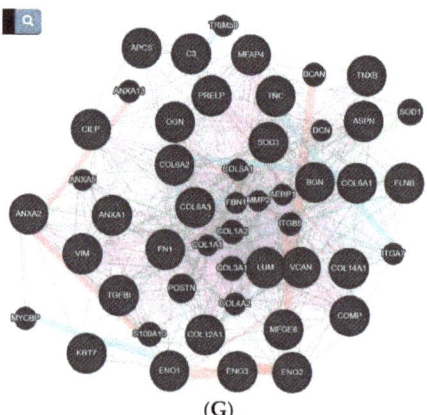

(G)

Figure 4. Gene interactions between the main functional proteins of the TMJ disc. (**A**) showing the gene interactions of the DDWoR group. (**B**) showing the gene interactions of the MD group. (**C**) showing the gene interactions of the CH group. (**D**) showing the gene interactions of the CH group. (**E**) showing the gene interactions of the DDWoR and CH group. (**F**) showing the gene interactions of the MD and CH group. (**G**) showing the gene interactions of the DDWoR, MD and CH group.

The main proteins with important functions and networks that were identified in the synovial fluid sample were analyzed for each group (Figure 3). A brief description of these findings are: in the DDWoR group (Figure 3A) alpha-2-macroglobulin (A2M) involved in inflammatory process, amyloid P component (APCS) involved with apoptosis and complement factor H (CFH) that modulates inflammatory cascade were highlighted in the Genemania interaction figure; in the MD group (Figure 3B), hemopexin (HPX) involved in protection against oxidative stress was present; in the CH group (Figure 3C), alcohol dehydrogenase subunit alpha (ADH1) that is responsible for alcohol degradation and interacts with growth hormone receptor (GHR) was present. In the group of DDWoR and MD (Figure 3D), annexin A1 (ANXA1), decorin (DCN), and immunoglobulin heavy constant gamma 1 (IGHG1) involved in inflammatory process, annexin A2 (ANXA2) involved with bone resorption, asporin (ASPN), biglycan (BGN), cartilage intermediate layer protein (CILP), osteoglycin (OGN), transforming growth factor beta induced (TGFBI) involved in bone and cartilage formation, fibronectin 1 (FN1), lumican (LUM) and tenascin XB (TNXB) involved in tissue repair, and neurofilament medium (NEFM) and thrombospondin 4 (THBS4) involved in neuropathic pain were included in the net. The DDWoR and CH group, and MD and CH group had no protein to be analyzed. The group with the three pathologies (DDWoR, MD and CH) showed an interaction of enolase 2 (ENO2) and 3 (ENO3), involved in muscle regeneration (Figure 3E).

The disc sample presented the following protein interactions in Genemania (Figure 4): group DDWoR (Figure 4A) presented mainly the matrix metalloproteinase protein (MMP) family (1,2,3,6,8,10,13,15,16), integrin subunit alpha 6 (ITGA6) and phospholipase A2 group VII (PLA2G7) that are involved in inflammatory cascade. Additionally, thrombospondin 3 (THBS3) and 4 (THBS4) involved in tissue remodeling, and THADA armadillo repeat containing (THADA) involved in apoptosis were present. In the MD group (Figure 4B), A-kinase anchor protein 13 (AKAP13), Erbin (ERBIN) and uroplakin-3a (UPK3A) involved in apoptosis, collagen alpha-1(IV) chain (COL4A1) and GTPase Eras (ERAS) involved in disc matrix constitution, and liprin-alpha-1 (PPFIA1) and (PPFIA2) 2 responsible for cell interactions were identified in the Genemania network. In the CH group (Figure 4C), the present proteins were ADAM metallopeptidase domain 10 (ADAM10), that regulates apoptosis, collagen type I alpha 2 chain (COL1A2) and serpin family H member 1 (SERPINH1) involved in collagen formation, actinin alpha 4 (ACTN4), PDZ Additionally, LIM domain 4 (PDLIM4), transthyretin (TTR) and protein tyrosine phosphatase non-receptor type 13

(PTPN13) involved in apoptosis, hormone modulation and bone formation. In the group of DDWoR and MD (Figure 4D), the complement C4A (C4A) and complement C4B (C4B) proteins that mediates the inflammatory process were identified. In the DDWoR and CH group (Figure 4E), mainly the proteins aggrecan (ACAN), collagen type I alpha 1 chain (COL1A1) and collagen type IV alpha 6 chain (COL4A6) that constitutes disc matrix, and periostin (POSTN) involved in wound healing were identified. In the MD and CH group (Figure 4F), keratin 6A (KRT6A) involved in wound healing was identified. Additionally, in the group with all three pathologies (DDWoR, MD and CH) the proteins that interacted were annexin A1 (ANXA1), complement C3 (C3) and tenascin C (TNC) involved in inflammatory cascade modulation, annexin A2 (ANXA2) and transforming growth factor beta induced (TGFBI) involved in osteoclastogenesis, asporin (ASPN), biglycan (BGN), collagen type VI alpha 1 chain (COL6A1), osteoglycin (OGN) and vimentin (VIM) involved in chondrogenesis and osteogenesis, amyloid P component (APCS) and complement C3 (C3) in apoptosis and lumican (LUM) involved in tissue repair (Figure 4G).

4. Discussion

The different types of TMD may jeopardize patients' quality of life, masticatory function and have a great impact on health expenses. The identification of its multifactorial etiological components will enhance the employment of specific treatments, diminishing the hazard it causes in the TMJ. Therefore, the identification of the proteins expressed on each pathology group of this study (DDWoR, MD, and CH) might elucidate the cascades involved in the progression and severity of each TMD, leading to an assertive handling of TMD.

A total of 225 proteins were identified in the synovial fluid sample, and 379 in the TMJ disc sample (Table 2). It is important to highlight that the synovial fluid sample is very complex to obtain, therefore some proteins might not have been identified due to the technique that advocates the dilution of the synovial fluid. Nevertheless, the sample was collected according to worldwide employed standard methods previously described by other research groups [21,25]. Additionally, even though few proteins' expression might not have been observed, the expression of new proteins were identified for each pathology group, which enriches the global analysis of this study.

In our analysis, we found that all proteins expressed in the DDWoR group (synovial fluid and disc sample) (Tables 2 and 3) presented many proteins related to inflammatory process (MMP-3, -10, -27 in the disc sample) and apoptosis (mitogen-activated protein kinase 7—MAP3K7) and THADA in synovial fluid). Only the MMP-3 protein was previously associated with TMD [26,27]. These are proteins that highly impact the degeneration process in the TMJ of patients with DDWoR [26,28]. In the MD group, ERBIN protein was found in the disc sample, and it modulates TGFB, which was previously associated with TMJ degeneration [29]. Additionally, unprecedented proteins were seen in the synovial fluid associated with apoptosis (aldehyde dehydrogenase 1 family member L—ALDH1L1) and protection against oxidative stress (HPX), which probably helps diminish the mechanical overload consequences of the dislocation in the TMJ. Regarding CH proteins in the synovial fluid sample, ADH1 catalyzes the oxidation of alcohols to aldehydes, but as seen in Genemania (Figure 3C), it interacts with GHR, which might be involved with the condylar overgrowth. In a previous study, GHR has been injected in rabbits' TMJ to increase cartilage thickness [30], but it has not been studied as a possible etiology of condylar overgrowth yet.

Additionally, we also found a set of proteins to be common in both synovial fluid and disc samples (Table 4) in the groups DDWoR (chromodomain-helicase-DNA-binding protein 8 and myosin light chain 6B), MD (filamin A and liprin-alpha-1), and in the three groups (enolase 1, 2, 3, myosin heavy chain 16, ribosomal protein L7 like 1 and component of the shield in complex). These proteins were involved in cell matrix adhesion, cellular motor protein, reorganization of cytoskeleton, muscle development and regeneration. Additionally, another group of proteins were identified in both synovial fluid and disc samples (Table 7), being prevalent in all groups of disc samples. In the DDWoR and MD groups of synovial fluid samples, proteins implicated in apoptosis, inflammatory process, bone formation and resorption, chondrogenesis, wound healing, tissue repair and protection against oxidative stress were found. CH disc samples and MD synovial fluid samples presented, as common proteins, HPX (protection against oxidative stress) and SERPINC1 (biosynthetic pathway of collagen).

LUM is associated with the regulation of collagen fibers and with cell migration. In this study, LUM was present in all disc samples, and it has been pointed out to be elevated when the disc is under stress, as it enhances tissue repair [31]. Ulmner [32] reported that higher levels of LUM in synovial tissue might diminish TMD surgical success. On the other hand, TNC was present in all disc samples and in DDWoR and MD synovial fluid sample, being an important protein in wound healing [33].

Temporomandibular joint discs are fibrocartilaginous discs composed mainly by collagen, glycosaminoglycan and proteoglycans [34]. Studies in human adults and fetuses showed the expression of mainly collagen type I and III in TMJ discs, with type I collagen observed in the posterior band of the articular disc and collagen type III on the inferior surface of the articular disc [35,36]. Moreover, collagen type II synthesis was expressed on the external layer of the TMJ disc [37]. In this study, collagen type IV was identified in MD and CH samples (Table 8), and a previous study observed the presence of collagen type IV in the middle part of fetuses' TMJ disc, indicating the development of blood vessels [38]. The TMJ disc is an avascular tissue, although under stress it may undergo metaplasia, forming a vascularized fibrous tissue. Collagen type VII was present in all samples, and along with collagen type IV, it has chondroprotective effects against inflammation [39]. Collagen type XII and XIV were present in the disc samples of this study, which have never been identified in this region before in humans. A study identified collagen type XII only in bovine disc samples, which helps maintain collagen type I integrity [40]. Nevertheless, collagen type XIV was also observed in all TMJ disc samples, and it plays an essential structural role in the integrity of collagen type I, mechanical properties, organization, and shape of articular cartilage, which has never been described in the TMJ disc before [41]. This is important information to understand the composition's strength and weakness of the TMJ disc.

5. Conclusions

In conclusion, many proteins were identified for the first time in the TMJ disc and synovial fluid of the groups DDWoR, MD and CH, leading to the enlightenment of each pathology's etiology, modulation and progression. Further studies with a greater sample are necessary to evaluate other proteins that might be present in these pathologies as well.

Author Contributions: Conceptualization: A.D.D., P.C.T., R.H.H.; methodology: A.D.D., P.C.T., R.H.H., M.A.R.B.; software: A.D.D., R.H.H., M.A.R.B.; validation: A.D.D., P.C.T., R.H.H., M.A.R.B.; formal Analysis: A.D.D., P.C.T., R.H.H., M.A.R.B.; investigation: A.D.D., P.C.T., R.H.H., M.A.R.B.; resources: A.D.D., P.C.T., R.H.H.; data curation: A.D.D., P.C.T., R.H.H., M.A.R.B.; writing—original draft preparation A.D.D., R.H.H.; writing—review and editing: A.D.D., P.C.T., R.H.H., M.A.R.B.; supervision: P.C.T., R.H.H., M.A.R.B.; project administration: A.D.D.; funding acquisition: A.D.D., P.C.T., R.H.H. All authors have read and agreed to the published version of the manuscript.

Funding: P.C.T. is supported by the National Council for Scientific and Technological Development, Chamada MCTIC/CNPq N° 28/2018—Universal, Process: 426505/2018-2 for this research. R.H.H. is supported by Fundação Araucária (grant FA#09/2016).

Institutional Review Board Statement: The study was conducted according to the guidelines of the Declaration of Helsinki, and approved by the Ethics Committee of Pontifical Catholic University of Paraná, Brazil, according to Resolution 196/96 of the National Health Council and approved under registration number 1.863.521, on the 20 May 2016.

Informed Consent Statement: Written informed consent was obtained from all subjects involved in the study.

Data Availability Statement: Data is contained within the article.

Acknowledgments: We thank all individuals that were volunteers for agreeing to participate in this study. A.D.D. was supported by Fundação Araucária scholarship. P.C.T. is supported by the National Council for Scientific and Technological Development, Chamada MCTIC/CNPq N° 28/2018—Universal, Process: 426505/2018-2 for this research. R.H.H. is supported by Fundação Araucária (grant FA#09/2016). We thank Alexandra Senegaglia and Paulo R. S. Brofman for the laboratory support at Pontifícia Universidade Católica do Paraná, Brazil.

Conflicts of Interest: The authors declare no conflict of interest.

References

1. Slade, G.D.; Ohrbach, R.; Greenspan, J.D.; Fillingim, R.B.; Bair, E.; Sanders, A.E.; Dubner, R.; Diatchenko, L.; Meloto, C.B.; Smith, S.; et al. Painful Temporomandibular Disorder: Decade of Discovery from OPPERA Studies. *J. Dent. Res.* **2016**, *95*, 1084–1092. [CrossRef]
2. National Institute of Health. Available online: https://www.nidcr.nih.gov/health-info/tmj (accessed on 3 October 2019).
3. Ohrbach, R.; Dworkin, S.F. The Evolution of TMD Diagnosis: Past, Present, Future. *J. Dent. Res.* **2016**, *95*, 1093–1101. [CrossRef]
4. Minervini, G.; Lucchese, A.; Perillo, L.; Serpico, R.; Minervini, G. Unilateral superior condylar neck fracture with disloca-tion in a child treated with an acrylic splint in the upper arch for functional repositioning of the mandible. *Case Rep. Cranio* **2017**, *35*, 337–341.
5. Eberhard, D.; Bantleon, H.; Steger, W. The efficacy of anterior repositioning splint therapy studied by magnetic resonance imaging. *Eur. J. Orthod.* **2002**, *24*, 343–352. [CrossRef]
6. Supplement, D.; Minervini, G.; Nucci, L.; Lanza, A.; Femiano, F.; Contaldo, M.; Grassia, V. Temporomandibular disc displacement with reduction treated with anterior repositioning splint: A 2-year clinical and magnetic resonance imaging (MRI) follow-up. *Case Rep. J. Biol. Regul. Homeost. Agents* **2020**, *34*, 151–160.
7. Talaat, W.M.; Adel, O.I.; Al Bayatti, S. Prevalence of temporomandibular disorders discovered incidentally during routine dental examination using the Research Diagnostic Criteria for Temporomandibular Disorders. *Oral Surg. Oral Med. Oral Pathol. Oral Radiol.* **2018**, *125*, 250–259. [CrossRef] [PubMed]
8. Cakarer, S.; Isler, S.; Yalcin, B.; Şitilci, T. Management of the bilateral chronic temporomandibular joint dislocation. *Ann. Maxillofac. Surg.* **2018**, *8*, 154. [CrossRef] [PubMed]
9. Poluha, R.L.; Canales, G.D.L.T.; Costa, Y.M.; Grossmann, E.; Bonjardim, L.R.; Conti, P.C.R. Temporomandibular joint disc displacement with reduction: A review of mechanisms and clinical presentation. *J. Appl. Oral Sci.* **2019**, *27*, e20180433. [CrossRef]
10. Fayed, M.M.S.; El-Mangoury, N.H.; El-Bokle, D.N.; Belal, I.A. Occlusal splint therapy and magnetic resonance imaging. *World J. Orthod.* **2004**, *5*, 133–140.
11. Prechel, U.; Ottl, P.; Ahlers, O.M.; Neff, A. The Treatment of Temporomandibular Joint Dislocation: A Systematic Review. *Dtsch. Arztebl. Int.* **2018**, *115*, 59–64.
12. Nitzan, D.W.; Katsnelson, A.; Bermanis, I.; Brin, I.; Casap, N. The clinical characteristics of condylar hyperplasia: Expe-rience with 61 patients. *J. Oral Maxillofac. Surg.* **2008**, *66*, 312–318. [CrossRef] [PubMed]
13. Raijmakers, P.G.; Karssemakers, L.H.; Tuinzing, D.B. Female Predominance and Effect of Gender on Unilateral Condylar Hyperplasia: A Review and Meta-Analysis. *J. Oral Maxillofac. Surg.* **2012**, *70*, 72–76. [CrossRef]
14. Mahajan, M. Unilateral condylar hyperplasia—A genetic link? Case reports. *Nat. J. Maxillofacial Surg.* **2017**, *8*, 58–63. [CrossRef]
15. Herr, M.M.; Fries, K.M.; Upton, L.G.; Edsberg, L.E. Potential Biomarkers of Temporomandibular Joint Disorders. *J. Oral Maxillofac. Surg.* **2011**, *69*, 41–47. [CrossRef]
16. Demerjian, G.G.; Sims, A.B.; Stack, B.C. Proteomic signature of Temporomandibular Joint Disorders (TMD): Toward di-agnostically predictive biomarkers. *Bioinformation* **2011**, *6*, 282–284. [CrossRef] [PubMed]
17. DuPree, E.J.; Jayathirtha, M.; Yorkey, H.; Mihasan, M.; Petre, B.A.; Darie, C.C. A Critical Review of Bottom-Up Proteomics: The Good, the Bad, and the Future of this Field. *Proteomes* **2020**, *8*, 14. [CrossRef] [PubMed]
18. Murphy, M.K.; MacBarb, R.F.; Wong, M.E.; Athanasiou, K.A. Temporomandibular Joint Disorders: A Review of Etiology, Clinical Management, and Tissue Engineering Strategies. *Int. J. Oral Maxillofac. Implant.* **2013**, *28*, 393–414. [CrossRef] [PubMed]
19. Olate, S.; Netto, H.D.; Rodriguez-Chessa, J.; Alister, J.P.; Albergaria-Barbosa, J.P.; de Moraes, J. Mandible condylar hy-perplasia: A review of diagnosis and treatment protocol. *Int J. Clin. Exp. Med.* **2013**, *6*, 727–737. [PubMed]
20. Mehra, P.; Wolford, L.M. Serum nutrient deficiencies in the patient with complex temporomandibular joint problems. *Bayl. Univ. Med. Cent. Proc.* **2008**, *21*, 243–247. [CrossRef]
21. Alstergren, P.; Benavente, C.; Kopp, S. Interleukin-1beta, interleukin-1 receptor antagonist, and interleukin-1 soluble receptor II in temporomandibular joint synovial fluid from patients with chronic polyarthritides. *J. Oral Maxillofac. Surg.* **2003**, *61*, 1171–1178. [CrossRef]
22. Cassiano, L.P.; Ventura, T.M.; Silva, C.M.; Leite, A.L.; Magalhães, A.C.; Pessan, J.P.; Buzalaf, M.A.R. Protein Profile of the Acquired Enamel Pellicle after Rinsing with Whole Milk, Fat-Free Milk, and Water: An in vivo Study. *Caries Res.* **2018**, *52*, 288–296. [CrossRef]
23. Universal Protein Resource. Available online: http://www.uniprot.org (accessed on 5 September 2020).

24. Warde-Farley, D.; Donaldson, S.L.; Comes, O.; Zuberi, K.; Badrawi, R.; Chao, P.; Franz, M.; Grouios, C.; Kazi, F.; Lopes, C.T.; et al. The GeneMANIA prediction server: Biological network integration for gene prioritization and predicting gene function. *Nucleic Acids Res.* **2010**, *38*, 214–220. [CrossRef]
25. Fredriksson, L.; Alstergren, P.; Kopp, S. Tumor Necrosis Factor-α in Temporomandibular Joint Synovial Fluid Predicts Treatment Effects on Pain by Intra-Articular Glucocorticoid Treatment. *Mediat. Inflamm.* **2006**, *2006*, 59425. [CrossRef]
26. Fujita, H.; Morisugi, T.; Tanaka, Y.; Kawakami, T.; Kirita, T.; Yoshimura, Y. MMP-3 activation is a hallmark indicating an early change in TMJ disorders, and is related to nitration. *Int. J. Oral Maxillofac. Surg.* **2009**, *38*, 70–78. [CrossRef]
27. Tiilikainen, P.; Pirttiniemi, P.; Kainulainen, T.; Pernu, H.; Raustia, A. MMP-3 and -8 expression is found in the condylar surface of temporomandibular joints with internal derangement. *J. Oral Pathol. Med.* **2005**, *34*, 39–45. [CrossRef] [PubMed]
28. Loreto, C.; Filetti, V.; Almeida, L.E.; Rosa, G.R.; Leonardi, R.; Grippaudo, C.; Giudice, A. MMP-7 and MMP-9 are over-expressed in the synovial tissue from severe temporomandibular joint dysfunction. *Eur. J. Histochem.* **2020**, *64*, 3113. [CrossRef]
29. Da Costa, G.F.A.; Souza, R.D.C.; de Araújo, G.M.; Gurgel, B.C.V.; Barbosa, G.A.S.; Calderon, P.D.S. Does TGF-beta play a role in degenerative temporomandibular joint diseases? A systematic review. *Cranio* **2017**, *35*, 228–232. [CrossRef] [PubMed]
30. Ulmner, M.; Sugars, R.; Naimi-Akbar, A.; Tudzarovski, N.; Kruger-Weiner, C.; Lund, B. Synovial Tissue Proteins and Patient-Specific Variables as Predictive Factors for Temporomandibular Joint Surgery. *Diagnostics* **2020**, *11*, 46. [CrossRef] [PubMed]
31. Feizbakhsh, M.; Razavi, M.; Minaian, M.; Teimoori, F.; Dadgar, S.; Maghsoodi, S. The effect of local injection of the human growth hormone on the mandibular condyle growth in rabbit. *Dent. Res. J.* **2014**, *11*, 436–441.
32. Koyama, E.; Saunders, C.; Salhab, I.; Decker, R.; Chen, I.; Um, H.; Pacifici, M.; Nah, H. Lubricin is Required for the Structural Integrity and Post-natal Maintenance of TMJ. *J. Dent. Res.* **2014**, *93*, 663–670. [CrossRef] [PubMed]
33. Stocum, D.L.; Roberts, W.E. Part I: Development and Physiology of the Temporomandibular Joint. *Curr. Osteoporos. Rep.* **2018**, *16*, 360–368. [CrossRef]
34. Berkovitz, B.K.B.; Holland, G.R.; Moxham, B.J. *Oral Anatomy, Histology and Embryology*, 4th ed.; Mosby: St. Louis, MD, USA, 2009.
35. Gage, J.; Virdi, A.; Triffitt, J.; Howlett, C.; Francis, M. Presence of type III collagen in disc attachments of human temporomandibular joints. *Arch. Oral Biol.* **1990**, *35*, 283–288. [CrossRef]
36. De Moraes, L.O.; Lodi, F.R.; Gomes, T.S.; Marques, S.R.; Oshima, C.T.; Lancellotti, C.L.; Rodríguez-Vázquez, J.F.; Mé-rida-Velasco, J.R.; Alonso, L.G. Immunohistochemical expression of types I and III collagen antibodies in the tem-poromandibular joint disc of human foetuses. *Eur. J. Histochem.* **2011**, *55*, 24. [CrossRef]
37. Kondoh, T.; Hamada, Y.; Iino, M.; Takahashi, T.; Kikuchi, T.; Fujikawa, K.; Seto, K. Regional differences of type II collagen synthesis in the human temporomandibular joint disc: Immunolocalization study of carboxy-terminal type II procollagen peptide (chondrocalcin). *Arch. Oral Biol.* **2003**, *48*, 621–625. [CrossRef]
38. De Moraes, L.O.; Lodi, F.R.; Gomes, T.S.; Marques, S.R.; Fernandes Junior, J.A.; Oshima, C.T.; Alonso, L.G. Immuno-histochemical expression of collagen type IV antibody in the articular disc of the temporomandibular joint of human fe-tuses. *Ital. J. Anat. Embryol.* **2008**, *113*, 91–95. [PubMed]
39. Chu, W.C.; Zhang, S.; Sng, T.J.; Ong, Y.J.; Tan, W.-L.; Ang, V.Y.; Foldager, C.B.; Toh, W.S. Distribution of pericellular matrix molecules in the temporomandibular joint and their chondroprotective effects against inflammation. *Int. J. Oral Sci.* **2017**, *9*, 43–52. [CrossRef] [PubMed]
40. Deng, M.H.; Xu, J.; Cai, H.X.; Fang, W.; Long, X. Effect of temporomandibular joint disc perforation on expression of type ? collagen in temporomandibular joint disc cells. *Chin. J. Stomatol.* **2017**, *52*, 274–277.
41. Ciavarella, D.; Mastrovincenzo, M.; Sabatucci, A.; Campisi, G.; Di Cosola, M.; Suriano, M.; Muzio, L.L. Primary and secondary prevention procedures of temporo-mandibular joint disease in the evolutive age. *Minerva Pediatr.* **2009**, *61*, 93–97.

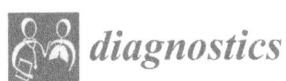

Review

Is There an Association between Temporomandibular Disorders and Articular Eminence Inclination? A Systematic Review

Xiao-Chuan Fan [1], Diwakar Singh [2], Lin-Sha Ma [1], Eva Piehslinger [3], Xiao-Feng Huang [1,*] and Xiaohui Rausch-Fan [2,*]

1 Department of Stomatology, Beijing Friendship Hospital, Capital Medical University, Beijing 100050, China; foxtail_09@hotmail.com (X.-C.F.); malinthe@yeah.net (L.-S.M.)
2 Division of Conservative Dentistry and Periodontology, School of Dentistry, Medical University of Vienna, Vienna 1090, Austria; dentistdiwakarsingh@gmail.com
3 Division of Prosthodontics, School of Dentistry, Medical University of Vienna, Vienna 1090, Austria; eva.piehslinger@meduniwien.ac.at
* Correspondence: huangxf1998@163.com (X.-F.H.); xiaohui.rausch-fan@meduniwien.ac.at (X.R.-F.)

Abstract: (1) Background: In order to determine the correlation between the inclination of articular eminence (AEI) and the development of temporomandibular disorders (TMDs), a systematic review was performed. (2) Methods: A systematic literature research was conducted between 1946 and January 2020, based on the following electronic databases: PubMed, Cochrane Library, Embase, Medline, Scope, SciELO, and Lilacs. Observational studies, analytical case-control studies, and cohort studies written in English were identified. The articles were selected and analyzed by two authors independently. The PICO format was used to analyze the studies and the Newcastle-Ottawa Scale (NOS) was used to verify the quality of the evidence. (3) Results: Sixteen articles were included in this review, ten case-control studies and six cohort studies. Eight articles (50%) established a positive relation between AEI and TMDs and eight (50%) did not. The scientific quality was medium-low, mainly influenced by the exposure to the risk of bias and the lack of clinical methods with adequate consistency and sensitivity on the diagnosis of TMDs. (4) Conclusions: It is controversial to establish a causal relationship between the TMDs and the AEI in the field of stomatology, due to limited and inconclusive evidence. However, it is suggested that the AEI defined by some specific methods may be associated with some special pathological stages of TMDs. High-quality prospective studies are required to draw any definitive conclusions.

Keywords: temporomandibular disorders; inclination of articular eminence; temporomandibular joint; glenoid fossa

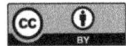

1. Introduction

The temporomandibular joint (TMJ) is one of the most complex articular systems in human beings, which is formed by the glenoid fossa of the temporal bone (the superior component of the joint), and the mandibular condyle (the inferior component of the joint) and the two are separated by the articular disk [1,2]. The anatomy of the TMJ can provide capacity in both hinging movement and gliding movements of the mandible within the three planes of space. The TMJ is critical to the craniomandibular system because it can achieve the mandibular functions with a dynamic balance mechanism [3]. Over the years, numerous studies have focused on the relation of the change of anatomical and physiological characteristics to stomatognathic dysfunctions [4], especially in cases of joint disorders [5].

Temporomandibular disorders (TMDs) are one of the most prevalent pathologies, which are defined as a comprehensive term of disorders affecting the TMJ, the muscles involved in mastication and/or the related structures [6]. Epidemiological studies of non-patient adult populations have shown that about 40–75% of patients have at least one sign of joint dysfunction, such as joint clicking, abnormal movement, and 33% of them have joint or facial pain [6]. Although the prevalence of TMDs in the population has attracted more attention from clinicians and researchers over the years, the etiology of TMDs is still poorly understood and remains to be elucidated [7,8].

Numerous factors that contribute to the development of TMDs have been proposed, such as traumatic injuries, occlusal disharmony, psychological factors, luxation of the joints, loss of posterior teeth, spine and postural alterations, and muscle hyperactivity [9–12]. Beside these factors, the features of the anatomic structure of the TMJ are also considered to be a local factor involved in the development of TMDs. During functional movements of the mandibular, the condylar process slides along the posterior slope of the articular eminence. A change of inclination of articular eminence might result in biomechanical variations of the TMJ because its characteristics determine the trajectory of functional movement [13]. Therefore, we speculate that articular eminence steepness and mandibular fossa morphology may have some connections with certain diseases that induce TMJ.

The relationship between the TMDs with the articular eminence inclination (AEI) has been investigated by previous studies. However, the associations between these two indicators have been found to be inconsistent and definitive conclusions cannot be drawn [14–20]. On the basis of these premises, a well-designed systematic review is needed to clarify this opening question. This study attempts to systematically review the literature to find out the correlation between the inclination of articular eminence and the development of TMDs, analyzing the quality of the methodological soundness of previous studies.

2. Materials and Methods

In order to answer the research question about the relationship between the AEI and TMDs, a systematic search of the medical literature was performed on 17 June 2019 and updated on 27 January 2020. Databases used were as follows: PubMed, Cochrane Library, Embase, Medline, Scope, SciELO, and Lilacs.

2.1. Protocol

This systematic review was reported following the guidelines of the Preferred Reporting Items for Systematic Reviews and Meta-Analysis (PRISMA) checklist [21].

2.2. Types of Studies

Observational studies, analytical case-control studies, or cohort studies aimed to determine the relationship of the inclination of articular eminence to the occurrence of TMDs.

2.3. Language Studies

The search was limited to articles in peer-reviewed journals and written in the English language.

2.4. Types of Participants

The studies selected for this review included subjects of both genders without the limitation of age.

2.5. Intervention Type

Studies without intervention in order to correlate AEI and TMDs.

2.6. Type of Results

The primary outcome was to determine the relationship between AEI and TMDs.

The secondary outcome was to determine AEI and the morphology of glenoid fossa related to the different pathological stages of TMDs.

2.7. Data Collection

For TMDs, the data were collected from studies that showed the diagnosis of TMDs with a clear reference to the concept and diagnosis of temporomandibular pathology in any method without limitation. Diagnostic criteria for TMD was based on research diagnostic criteria for temporomandibular disorders (RDC/TMD), diagnostic criteria for temporomandibular disorders (DC/TMD) [22,23], evaluation according to the American Academy of Orofacial Pain (AAOP) guide [6], radiology studies (including magnetic resonance imaging (MRI), computed tomography (CT), cone-beam computed tomography (CBCT), sagittal corrected tomography, arthrography, and other methods), Helkimo index, surveys' studies, and/or clinical examination based on signs and symptoms with reference to TMD and others.

For AEI, the data were collected from studies that showed a clear method for measuring the AEI in degrees. The AEI is defined as the angle between the articular eminence and the Frankfort horizontal (FH) plane or any other horizontal reference plane, such as the palatal plane, the occlusion plane, the anterior nasal spine to the posterior nasal plane (ANS-PNS), and other defined reference planes. Data were collected based on MRI, CT, CBCT, tomography, dry skulls, autopsy, and other methods.

2.8. Databases Used

1. PubMed database (article types, clinical trials, randomized controlled trials, controlled clinical trials; language, English; publication dates, 1 January 1966 to 27 January 2020);
2. Cochrane Library (database, Trials; publication dates, 1966 to 2020);
3. Embase (publication dates, 1974 to 2020)
4. Medline (publication dates, 1946 to 2020)
5. Scope (document type, article; language, English; publication dates, 1970 to 2020)
6. SciELO (publication dates, to 2020)
7. Lilacs (publication dates, to 2020).

2.9. Search Strategy

A systematic search of the computerized database was performed to identify and select the potentially eligible literature that examined the association between AEI and TMDs for this systematic review. The semantic field related to the term "TMDs" (temporomandibular disorders, TMJ dysfunction, disk displacement, muscular pain, clicking) was crossed search with the semantic field related to the term "AEI" (glenoid fossa, posterior slope, articular eminence). For details regarding the specific search terms and combinations, see Table 1.

2.10. Study Selection

For article selection or first approach, all potentially eligible articles were listed by title and abstract and evaluated by two researchers independently (X-C.F. and D.S.). Then, the full text of articles, which may meet the inclusion criteria based on the first stage of selection, was assessed independently by the same two researchers (X-C.F. and D.S.). When no agreement was found during the first and second stage of selection, the data was discussed with a third researcher (X.R.F.), to reach final decision for including it or not. When the full-text version of the study was not directly available, the paper was requested from the corresponding author by email. Articles that met all inclusion and exclusion criteria were selected in the review for the final analysis. The reasons for the exclusion of the articles were recorded in an adjacent column and presented in the results (Table 2).

Table 1. Search strategy and terms used for the search.

Database and Limits	Search Strategy and Terms		
	Semantic Fields: Temporomandibular Disorders		Semantic Fields: Articular Eminence Inclination
PubMed (n = 574) Article types, clinical trials, randomized controlled trials, controlled clinical trials Language, English Publication dates, 01 January 1966 to 27 January 2020	Temporomandibular disorder [tiab] OR TMJ Dysfunction [tiab] OR disk displacement [tiab] OR Muscular pain [tiab] OR clicking [tiab]	AND	glenoid fossa [tiab] OR posterior slope [tiab] OR articular eminence [tiab]
Cochrane Library (n = 26) Database, trials Publication dates, 1966 to 2020	Temporomandibular disorder OR TMJ Dysfunction OR disk displacement OR Muscular pain OR clicking	AND	glenoid fossa OR posterior slope OR articular eminence
Embase and Medline (n = 274) Publication dates, Embase 1974 to 2020 and Medline 1946 to 2020	Temporomandibular disorder OR TMJ Dysfunction OR disk displacement OR Muscular pain OR clicking	AND	glenoid fossa OR posterior slope OR articular eminence
Scope (n = 330) Document type, article Language, English Publication dates, 1970 to 2020.	(TITLE-ABS-KEY (temporomandibular AND disorders) OR TITLE-ABS-KEY (tmj AND dysfunction) OR TITLE-ABS-KEY (disk AND displacement) OR TITLE-ABS-KEY (clicking) OR TITLE-ABS-KEY (muscular AND pain) AND TITLE-ABS-KEY (articular AND eminence) OR TITLE-ABS-KEY (glenoid AND fossa)) AND (LIMIT-TO (DOCTYPE, "ar")) AND (LIMIT-TO (LANGUAGE, "English"))		
SciELO (n = 10) Publication dates, to 2020	(Temporomandibular disorder OR TMJ Dysfunction OR disk displacement OR Muscular pain OR clicking)	AND	(glenoid fossa OR articular eminence)
Lilacs (n = 21) Publication dates, to 2020	(Temporomandibular disorder OR TMJ Dysfunction OR disk displacement OR Muscular pain OR clicking)	AND	(glenoid fossa OR articular eminence)

Table 2. Studies retrieved in full text and excluded from the review.

First Author and Year	Reason for Exclusion
de Pontes, 2019 [24]	Morphological research
Shokri, 2019 [25]	Quantitative data of AEI is not shown
Piancino, 2020 [16]	Concerning on TMDs patients with or without condylar asymmetry
Sa, 2017 [26]	Patients with degenerative bone diseases
Rabelo, 2017 [27]	No direct relationship between fossa shape and TMDs
Türp, 2016 [28]	No direct relationship between AEI and TMDs
Su, 2014 [29]	Grouping of the glenoid fossa is not clear
İlgüy, 2014 [30]	The diagnosis of participates is not clear
Çağlayan, 2014 [31]	Same data as Sümbüllü, 2012 [3]
Learreta, 2013 [32]	Group divided based on alterations in the condylar axis
Robinson de Senna, 2009 [33]	No description of the morphology of the fossa
Hirata, 2007 [34]	Sample size is too small
Kurita, 2006 [35]	Morphological research
Tanaka, 2004 [8]	Dry skull study, no TMDs diagnosis
Pullinger, 2001 [36]	Same data as Pullinger, 2002 [19]
Kurita, 2000 [37]	Grouping is not clear
Toyama, 1999 [38]	Only the relationship between disk and fossa

2.11. Extracting Data from the Studies

The methodological features of the selected articles were assessed according to a format, the PICO criteria, which enabled a structured summary of the analyzed articles in relation to four main issues, namely, population, intervention, comparison, and outcome. For each article, we defined the following analysis variables in detail: population (sample size, distribution by gender, mean age, and age range); intervention (type of method used for the diagnosis of TMDs, main variables to compare, statistical analysis); comparison (assessed the presence of any comparison groups); outcomes (the answer to the hypothesis, the presence of causal relationship between AEI and TMD). Some studies investigating more items were reported in two or more groups of correlation.

2.12. Quality Assessment

Critical appraisal of studies included in the review was determined by the Newcastle-Ottawa Scale (NOS), which was used to assess the quality of case-control and cohort studies [39]. To determine the quality of case-control studies, there were three categories with a level of evidence score ranging from 0 to 9 points as follows: (1) selection (four points), (2) comparability (two points), and (3) exposure (three points). For cohort studies, there were also three categories assigning a score ranging from 0 to 9 points as follows: (1) selection (four points), (2) comparability (two points), and (3) outcome (three points).

The quality was determined by the same two researchers (X-C.F. and D.S.) in charge of the search, where the highest quality achieved was obtained by those items that were assigned a maximum score of 9.

3. Results

In total, 1235 potentially eligible articles were examined in the first approach in the seven databases used (Table 1). However, 299 of these articles were excluded due to duplication. On the basis of the title and abstract of the remaining 936 studies, 904 of them were eliminated due to their lack of relevance. Of the 32 articles left, after reading the full text, a consensus decision was to eliminate 17 articles that did not fulfill the inclusion criteria for this systematic review. Table 2 reveals the list of excluded studies including the reason for exclusion. Search expansion strategies allowed including one additional paper, thus, accounting for a total of 16 studies that were analyzed in the review and prepared according to the PICO criteria (Tables 3–5). Figure 1 summarizes the search strategy and results described.

Table 3. Summary of findings from studies of TMDs and AEI with MRI.

First Author & Year	Type of Study	Population	Intervention	Comparison (Control Group)	Outcome	Conclusions
Poluha, 2020 [40]	Case-control study	36 individuals: 12 DDWR and arthralgia (12F, m.a.: 33.58 ± 9.75), DDWR and no arthralgia (4M, 8F, m.a.: 32.58 ± 10.9), asymptomatic individuals (3M, 9F, m.a.: 29 ± 6.86)	TMDs: symptoms & signs, RDC/TMD AEI: best-fit line 1-way ANOVA, Logistic regression analysis, $p < 0.05$	Case: Unilateral DDWR and arthralgia (n = 12) Bilateral DDWR and no arthralgia (n = 12) Control: asymptomatic individuals (n = 12)	No significant differences ($p > 0.05$) between groups for AEI	No factors associated with the concomitant presence of arthralgia in patients with DDWR
Rabelo, 2017 [17]	Cohort study	199 joints of 104 patients (86F, 18M) m.a.:40.92 a.r.:18-88	TMDs: with TMD symptom AEI: top-roof line 1-way ANOVA, Mann-Whitney rank-sum test, Tukey post hoc test, $p < 0.05$	Classified by shape of fossa (Flattened n = 45; Sigmoid n = 78; Box n = 57; Deformed n = 19) Classified by position of disc (Normal n = 86, Displaced n = 113) Classified into 8 groups based on types of DD Displaced group (n = 113) divided into 2 subgroups (DDWR n = 85, DDWOR n = 28)	AEI was higher in box shaped group AEI were not related to the presence or absence of DD AEI were not related to the type of DD and AEI AEI was higher for DDWR group	Disc position is not influenced by articular eminence morphology AEI has an influence on disk reduction
Aydin, 2012 [41]	Cohort study	70 joints of 35 selected patients (17F, 18M)	TMDs: signs and symptoms AEI: best-fit line Mann–Whitney U- test	DDWR (n = 51) DDWOR (n = 19) Two groups then subdivided by distributions of AEI (shallow (15°–30°), moderate (30°–60°), steep (60°–90°))	No correlation between the 2 groups and AEI ($p > 0.05$) For the distributions of AEI in both groups, moderate was the most frequent, followed by shallow and steep	The AEI may not have a predisposing effect on development of DD

Table 3. *Cont.*

First Author & Year	Type of Study	Population	Intervention	Comparison (Control Group)	Outcome	Conclusions
Sülün, 2001 [42]	Case-control study	112 joints of 56 symptomatic patients (44F, 12M, m.a.: 33.35) 50 joints of 25 symptom-free volunteers (14F, 11M, m.a.: 23.87)	TMDs: symptoms, confirmed disk malpositions by MRI AEI: best-fit line Mann-Whitney U test, Wilcoxon matched pairs test, $p < 0.05$	Case: DDWR: n = 61, DDWOR: n = 28, Asymptomatic side of the patients: n = 23 Control: AV: n = 50	The AEI on the central and the medial slices in the DDWR group were steeper than those in the AV joints and in DDWOR joints The AEI of the medial slice was larger than the central and lateral slices in DDWR group	A steeper slope is a factor of DD. The flattening observed in the bone surface during the DDWOR stage

M: male; F: female; a.r.: age range; m.a.: mean age; ANOVA: analysis of variance; DD: disk displacement; DDWR: disk displacement with reduction; DDWOR: disk displacement without reduction; AV: asymptomatic volunteer; RDC/TMD: research diagnostic criteria for temporomandibular disorders; AEI: articular eminence inclination.

Table 4. Summary of findings from studies of TMDs and AEI with CBCT or Helical CT.

First Author & Year	Type of Study	Population	Intervention	Comparison (Control Group)	Outcome	Conclusions
Al-Rawi, 2017 [43]	Case-control study	70 participants (a.r.: 16–44): 35 TMD patients (19M, 16F, m.a.: 27.9), 35 patients without TMD history (19M, 16F, m.a.: 24.7)	TMDs: RDC/TMD; AEI: top-roof line; Paired sample t-test, independent sample t-test, $p < 0.05$	Case: TMD patients (n = 35); Control: patients without TMD history (n = 35)	AEI was significantly greater in the affected joints in male group, but no difference between affected and normal joints in female group	The condyles of the affected joints may rotate inward
Paknahad, 2016 [14]	Case-control study	40 patients (28F, 12M) with TMD, a.r: 21–57; 23 participants (18F, 5M) without TMD, a.r.: 25–50	TMDs: according to the Helkimo index; AEI: top-roof line; Paired t-test, Student's t-test, $p \leq 0.05$	Case: patients with signs and symptoms of TMDs; Control: participants without signs and symptoms of TMDs	AEI was higher in patient group than in control group ($p = 0.001$) No significant difference between the two genders in control group and patient group ($p > 0.05$)	AEI was steeper in patients with TMD
Imanimoghaddam, 2016 [44]	Case-control study	50 patients: 25 TMD patients (5M, 20F, m.a.: 28.84 ± 9.84), 25 normal patients (8M, 17F, m.a.: 28.43 ± 3.24)	TMDs: symptoms & signs, RDC/TMD; AEI: tangent line from the uppermost point of the glenoid fossa; independent t-test, $p < 0.05$	Case: patients suffering from TMD (n = 25); Control: patients with normal TMJs and Class I occlusion (n = 25)	AEI did not differ between the normal and TMD patients	CBCT could be considered a useful diagnostic imaging modality for TMD patients
Shahidi, 2013 [18]	Cohort study	60 joints of 30 patients (21 F, 9M), m.a.: 31.89, a.r: 18–52	TMDs: according to the Helkimo index; AEI: top-roof line; Spearman's correlation test, paired t test, $p < 0.05$	Classified into 3 groups regarding the clinical Di of the Helkimo index (Di I (n = 5), Di II (n = 18), Di III (n = 7)	No correlation between the 3 groups (Di I, II, and III) and AEI in either joint ($p > 0.05$)	No apparent relationship between the AEI and the clinical Di in patients with TMD

Table 4. *Cont.*

First Author & Year	Type of Study	Population	Intervention	Comparison (Control Group)	Outcome	Conclusions
Sümbüllü, 2012 [3]	Case-control study	104 joints of 52 patients (41F, 11M) with TMDs and 82 joints of 41 patients (24F, 17M) without TMDs	TMDs: clinical signs and symptoms; AEI: top-roof line, best-fit line; One-way ANOVA, student's t-test, $p < 0.05$	Case: patients with TMJ dysfunction; Control: patients without TMJ dysfunction	There was a difference in AEI between the patient and control groups ($p < 0.05$) No differences in AEI according to gender and age in TMD group ($p > 0.05$)	AEI was steeper in healthy control group than in TMDs group
Estomaguio, 2005 [45]	Cohort study	39 female orthodontic patients with TMDs	TMDs: signs and symptoms; AEI: best-fit line; Unpaired t-test, $p < 0.05$	NBC: n = 18, m.a.: 19.1 ± 4.7, a.r.: 15-23; BCBC: n = 21, m.a.: 22.7 ± 7.5, a.r.: 14-30	Lateral and central sections of AEI was steeper in NBC than in BCBC	Flattening of the eminence accompany condylar change
Yamada, 2004 [46]	Cohort study	42 joints of 21 female TMD patients scheduled for orthognathic surgery	TMDs: signs and symptoms; AEI: best-fit line; Mann–Whitney U-test, one-factor ANOVA, $p < 0.05$	Classified by bone change (NBC: n = 20, m.a.: 21.44, a.r.: 17.9-24.6; BCBC: n = 22, m.a.: 22.8, a.r.: 17.5-24.3) BCBC subdivided by types of bone change (erosion: n = 10; osteophyte: n = 12), NBC: n = 20 Classified by DD (normal: n = 15; displacement: n = 27) Displacement group then subdivided into 2 groups (DDWR: n = 7; DDWOR: n = 20)	AEI in the lateral and central sections were steeper in NBC group than BCBC group AEI in all three sections of the osteophyte group were less than in the NBC group No significant differences between the normal group and displacement group AEI of central and lateral sections in DDWR were steeper than DDWOR	Flattening of the eminence seems to occur during changes from erosion to osteophyte, and from DDWR to DDWOR.

M: male; F: female; a.r.: age range; m.a.: mean age; ANOVA: analysis of variance; DD: disk displacement; DDWR: disk displacement with reduction; DDWOR: disk displacement without reduction; NBC: no bone change; BCBC: bilateral condylar bone change; AEI: articular eminence inclination.

Table 5. Summary of findings from studies of TMDs and AEI with two-dimensional radiographs.

First Author & Year	Type of Study	Population	Intervention	Comparison (Control group)	Outcome	Conclusions
Pullinger, 2002 [19]	Case-control study	162 female patients with unilateral disk disorders (m.a.: 33.68 ± 13.89); 21 asymptomatic female subjects (m.a.: 24.2 ± 2.9)	TMDs: RDC/TMD; AEI: best-fit line; Classification tree analysis, independent samples t test, $p < 0.05$	Case: patients with unilateral disk disorders (DDWR: n = 84; DDWOR: n = 78;) Control: asymptomatic female subjects (n = 21)	No difference in eminence slope angle between 2 groups	
Sato, 1996 [47]	Case-control study	91 joints of 79 females with ADD (m.a.: 24.5 ± 4.90); 48 joints of 24 females without TMDs (m.a.: 21.5 ± 2.45)	TMDs: clinical sign, confirmed with arthrography; AEI: top-roof line, best-fit line; Student's t-test, $p < 0.05$	Case: joints with ADD (n = 91), then subdivided into DDWR (n = 46) and DDWOR (n = 45); Control: joints without TMJ dysfunction (n = 48)	AEI (best-fit line) of joints with ADD was significantly larger than control joints ($p < 0.01$); No difference of AEI (top-roof line) between the joints with ADD and the control joints; No difference in any variable studied (best-fit line and top-roof line) between DDWR and DDWOR	A steep AEI appears to be partly responsible for the genesis of ADD
Ren, 1995 [20]	Case-control study	34 joints of 34 asymptomatic volunteers (18F, 16M, m.a.: 28, a.r: 18–44); 85 joints of 71 patients (50F, 21M, m.a.: 38, a.r: 21–70)	TMDs: pain in TMJ area, confirmed with arthrography; AEI: best-fit line; ANOVA, paired t-test, $p < 0.05$	Case: ADD joints (n = 85) divided into DDWR (n = 37) and DDWOR (n = 48). Then subdivided by OC: with OC (DDWR = 7, DDWOR = 27), without OC (ADR = 30, ADNR = 21); Control: asymptomatic joints (n = 34)	No difference in the AEI between normal joints and joints with DD in the central and medial sections. ($p > 0.05$). A tendency of a flat eminence in the joints with DDWOR; Normal joints steeper than OC joints in lateral ($p < 0.01$) and medial ($p < 0.05$) section. Joints without OC steeper than Joints with OC ($p < 0.05$)	A steep eminence could not be verified as a predisposing factor for DD; Flattening of the eminence was not related to the DD but OC

Table 5. *Cont.*

First Author & Year	Type of Study	Population	Intervention	Comparison (Control group)	Outcome	Conclusions
Galante, 1995 [48]	Case-control study	74 patients (62F, 12M); 35 asymptomatic volunteers (15F, 14M)	TMDs: with TMD symptom AEI: best-fit line; Chi-square tests, Student-Newman-Keuls tests, $p < 0.05$	Case: patients are classified by MRI into 4 groups (SN, DDWR, DDWOR, DDN/DJD, the simple size of different groups was not mentioned); Control: volunteers are classified by MRI into 2 groups (AV: n = 29, ABN: n = 6)	No difference among the six diagnostic groups.	AEI may not represent a predisposing factor for the development of internal derangement of the TMJ
Panmekiate, 1991 [49]	Cohort study	60 joint of 54 patients	TMDs: Disk position classified by arthrography; AEI: top-roof line; Two-tailed t test, $p < 0.05$.	Superior disc position (20 joints from 17 patients, m.a.: 38); DDWR (20 joints from 19 patients, m.a.: 32); DDWOR (20 joints from 18 patients, m.a.: 33)	No differences in angulation among 3 section in each 3 group	No correlation between a steep articular eminence and ADD.

M: male; F: female; a.r.: age range; m.a.: mean age; ANOVA: analysis of variance; RDC/TMD: research diagnostic criteria for temporomandibular disorders; DDWR: disk displacement with reduction; DDWOR: disk displacement without reduction; ADD: anterior disk displacement; AEI: articular eminence inclination; DD: disk displacement; DDN/DJD: disk displacement without reduction with degenerative joint disease; TMJ: temporomandibular joint.

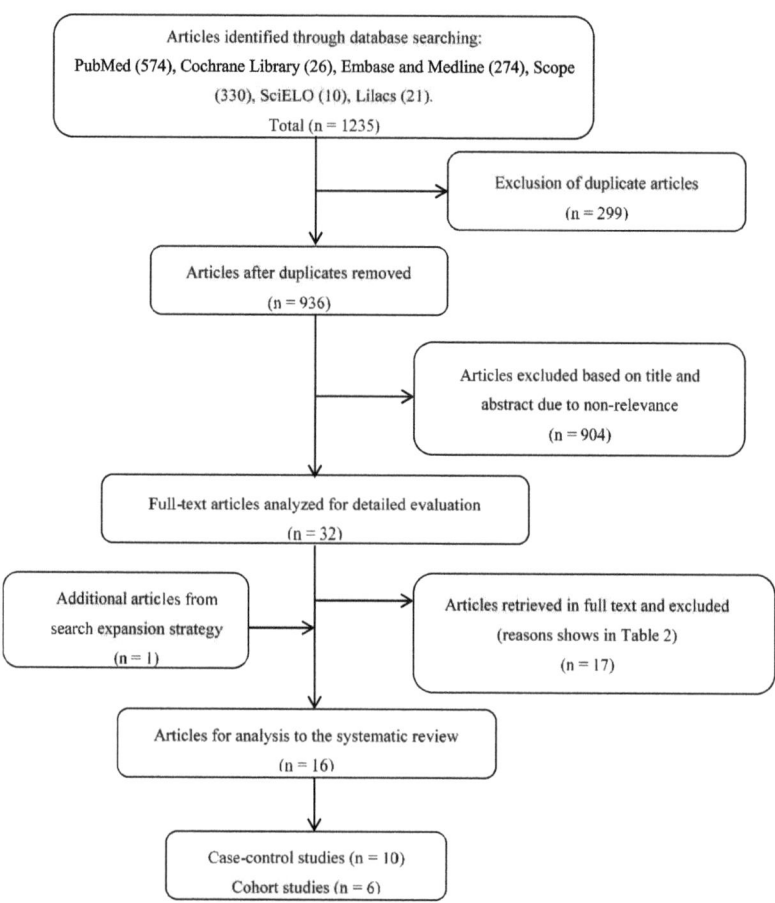

Figure 1. Search method, identification, selection, and inclusion of articles.

3.1. Characteristics of Studies

In all, 16 articles were included in this systematic review. ten case-control studies and six cohort studies were identified. According to the radiological methods, four are MRI studies, seven are CT or CBCT studies, and the other five articles used two-dimensional (2D) radiographs (sagittal corrected tomography or lateral oblique transcranial radiographs). Among these articles, two of them used both three-dimensional (3D) (CT or MRI) and two-dimensional (2D) radiographs (lateral cephalogram or laminography) [45,48] (Tables 3–5). We selected these two articles for a single group, because the other radiological methods were not used to evaluate the AEI after reading of the full text.

3.2. Characteristics of Participants

The age range of patients was between 14 and 88 years; the average age was from 19.1 ± 4.7 to 40.92 years. Three studies did not specify the age of the participants clearly [3,41,48]. In relation to gender, four studies included only females in their sample [19,45–47].

3.3. Quality Assessment

Among the total 16 articles selected in this review, eight studies presented correlations between TMDs and the AEI, however, the other eight studies did not find any correlations between the TMDs and the AEI. None of the included studies obtained the highest score based on NOS. The range of scores was between two and six (Table 6).

Table 6. Studies retrieved in full text and excluded from the review.

Positive			Negative		
First Author & Year	Radiological Method	NOS Score	First Author & Year	Radiological Method	NOS Score
Rabelo, 2017 [17]	MRI	4	Poluha, 2020 [40]	MRI	6
Al-Rawi, 2017 [43]	CBCT	4	Imanimoghaddam M, 2016 [42]	CBCT	5
Paknahad, 2016 [14]	CBCT	5	Shahidi, 2013 [18]	CBCT	5
Sümbüllü, 2012 [3]	CBCT	5	Aydin, 2012 [41]	MRI	4
Estomaguio, 2005 [44]	Helical CT	4	Pullinger, 2002 [19]	2D (tomograms)	5
Yamada, 2004 [45]	Helical CT	3	Ren, 1995 [20]	2D (tomograms)	4
Sülün, 2001 [46]	MRI	4	Galante, 1995 [48]	2D (laminagraph)	2
Sato, 1996 [47]	2D (transcranial radiographs)	3	Panmekiate, 1991 [49]	2D (tomograms)	3

NOS score, Newcastle-Ottawa Scale, three categories with a score of level of evidence ranging from 0 to 9 points to determine the quality of case-control and cohort studies.

4. Discussion

A review of literature can help us gain knowledge more effectively, however, it is necessary to carefully analyze the quality, to avoid erroneous conclusions from their results. The objective of this systematic review was to select and analyze the studies that verify the correlation between the inclination of articular eminence and specific TMD signs and symptoms, presenting real applicability to clinical practice.

According to the inclusion and exclusion criteria of this review, the search was conducted with the limitation of peer-reviewed English language papers, although this strategy may lead to the possibility that some publications in other languages and/or publications included in databases were unjustly excluded. However, it is a way to improve the methodological rigor and the conclusion drawn to a certain extent. Case reports and reviews are also excluded, as they do not have uniform standards that could increase the risk of bias.

From a methodological point of view, all the articles selected in this systematic review were retrospective observational studies with or without control groups verifying the correlation between AEI and TMDs. The scientific quality of evidence of the analyzed studies included in the present review was medium-low, mainly influenced by the exposure to the risk of bias and the lack of clinical methods with adequate consistency and sensitivity used for the diagnosis of TMDs. One of the methods created with the purpose of clinical and epidemiological research used for the diagnosis of evidence-based TMDs is the RDC/TMD, and the other method is the DC/TMD, which results in an evidence-based system with greater validity for clinical use [23]. The RDC/TMD criteria and the DC/TMD criteria are emphasized as the international standard for examination of patients, which have existed since 1992 or 2014. Therefore, the qualities of all studies before that time are evaluated as weak. All of the selected articles in this systematic review, except for one (Panmekiate, 1991 [49]), were published after 1992. The types of method used for the diagnosis of TMDs of the selected articles were shown in the "intervention" part of Table 3. However, only four studies, included in the review, diagnosed TMDs and classified samples according to RDC/TMD criteria [19,40,43,44], two studies diagnosed TMDs based on Helkimo index [14,18], and others diagnosed TMDs only by clinical sign and symptoms or then further confirmed by MRI or arthrography. That means the inclusion criteria of the papers are not consistent. The lack of introduction of uniform diagnostic criteria, such as RDC/TMD or DC/TMD defining the different categories of TMDs, decreases the level of consistency, resulting in a low quality of studies, and therefore comparisons between different studies could not be established. Without consistency, may imply that the observed correlations between two variables appeared because of chance or error [50]. Furthermore, TMDs are considered to be a heterogeneous group of different diseases involving the craniomandibular system, other than a single pathology [51]. It is difficult to control for all of the other variables when evaluating the relative importance of single risk factors for disorders with a multifactorial etiology [52,53]. Some studies that still seem to continue to use "TMDs" as a collective term of all TMD signs and symptoms during the clinical examinations, pooled them in a unique dependent variable in the statistical analysis and the results [3,43,44]. Nevertheless, the evaluation of the multifactorial complex pathologies, such as TMDs, should use multivariate statistical analyses, as univariate models may overestimate some resulting associations and possibly produce misleading conclusions [54,55]. This could be shown from the study of Rabelo KA et al. [17], who found an important correlation among the type of disk displacement of the AEI ($p < 0.001$), but there was no statistical correlation between the presence and absence of disk displacement of AEI measurements ($p > 0.05$). Similarly, the AEI was steeper in the no condyle bone change group than in those of the bilateral condylar bone change (centre section $p < 0.05$, lateral section $p < 0.01$). However, these differences were only seen in the joints with osteophyte (all three sections $p < 0.05$) but not with erosion (all three sections $p > 0.05$), based on the study of Yamada K et al. [46].

Many radiographic methods have been selected to measure the AEI in previous studies. In the early days, conventional radiographs, such as tomography or arthrography, were used for diagnosing the morphology of TMJ, but these modalities proved to have certain limitations [1] and were replaced by helical CT, which evaluates osseous components in 3D without superimposition or distortion. The CBCT, which has high dimensional accuracy in measuring maxillofacial structures including TMJ, is considered to be one of the preferred ways to evaluate bone structure in the stomatological area [3,14,18]. Nowadays, CBCT was selected rather than helical CT because of lower radiation dose, better spatial resolution, shorter scanning time, and more cost effective [56]. The MRI also allows a tridimensional analysis of the TMJ, and this technology can provide hard tissue and also soft tissue imaging, such as articular disk, related muscles, and ligaments. It has already been considered to be the gold standard imaging method for the diagnosis of internal derangement and the disk displacements with or without reduction. The radiographic methods are very important factors for angular and linear measurements as it influences the results. The articles included in this systematic review involve five imaging methods, from two-dimensional methods to three-dimensional methods. Using 3D imaging, the steepness of the eminence may be influenced by the location of the image (more laterally, centrally, more medially), whereas the 2D images show a summarization of the whole articular eminence as a three-dimensional structure. It is hard for us to establish comparisons of the values of AEI between different studies with different imaging methods because the consistencies of them still need more studies to support.

The AEI is defined as the angle formed by one of the lines that passes through the articular eminence and the horizontal reference plane [57]. In previous articles, two main methods have been described for evaluating the AEI, i.e., the "top-roof line" method and the "best-fit line" method, which are reliable and have already been used in studies. The "top-roof line" is obtained by connecting the crest point of the articular eminence and the roof of the mandibular fossa (Figure 2). The angle between the "top-roof line" and the horizontal reference plane is related to the height of articular eminence, which focuses on the localization of the tubercle in relation to the mandibular fossa and depicts the morphology of articular eminence better. The "best-fit line" method was defined as the angle between the tangent line drawn to the posterior slope of the articular eminence and the horizontal reference plane, which is directly related to the movement direction of the condyle-disk complex and reflects the actual condylar path (Figure 3) [26,30,31,41,57,58]. Five of 16 articles selected in this systematic review used the "top-roof line" method [14,17,18,43,49]; eight articles used the "best-fit line" method [19,20,40–42,45,46,48]; two articles used both the "top-roof line" method and the "top-roof line" method to evaluate the AEI [3,47], and the other article used the angle between tangent line from the uppermost point of the glenoid fossa and the true horizontal line as AEI [44]. Although the three mentioned methods all represent the inclination of the articulator eminence, the features they focus on are different. Therefore, they should be considered separately.

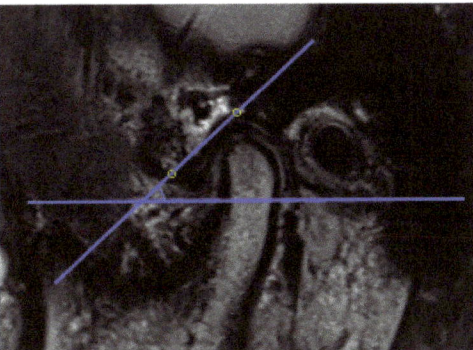

Figure 2. Representative images of "top-roof line" method, the articular eminence inclination (AEI) defined as the angle between the line connecting the crest point of the articular eminence and the roof of the mandibular fossa and the horizontal reference plane.

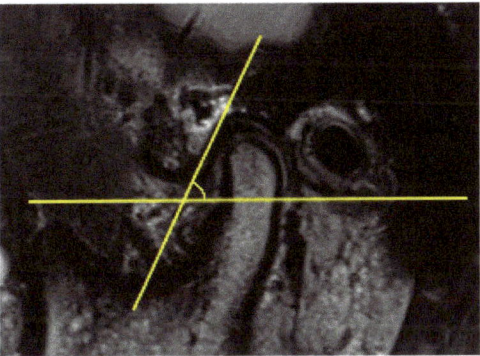

Figure 3. Representative images of the "best-fit line" method, the articular eminence inclination (AEI) defined as the angle between the tangent line drawn to the posterior slope of the articular eminence and the horizontal reference plane.

The horizontal reference plane is the other important factor affecting the AEI, which determines the degree of the angle directly. At the stage of the literature selection, the reference planes used were not limited, which can be FH plane, palatal plane, occlusion plane, and other defined reference planes. Except for three studies (one study used the true horizontal line [44], one study used the line tangent to the anterior and posterior articular eminences [19], one study used the line tangent to the curve of articular eminence and the point of squamotympanic fissure [47]), and the remaining 13 studies included in this review all used the FH plane as horizontal reference planes. It has been generally recognized as an important reference plane and has proved to be of great value in cephalometric analysis and the three dimensions measurement since the Frankfurt agreement concluded in Germany in 1884, which is defined by a line drawn from the lowest point on the inferior orbital margin (Or) to the most superior point of the outline of the external auditory meatus (Po) [59,60]. A stable and comparable horizontal reference plane is very essential, and the FH plane seems to be a relatively ideal reference plane for evaluating AEI because the landmarks of the FH plane are independent of TMJ structure, which are not affected by the changes of mandibular fossa and articular eminence. However, although FH is well defined, the external auditory meatus changes its shape looking on a more lateral, central, or medial slice of MRI, CT, or CBCT, which may also influence the steepness of the articular eminence.

Another important confounding factor in the analysis of the correlation between TMDs and AEI may be represented by the selection of the samples. Some of the studies were based on orthodontic patients [45,46], who may be alerted to the potential role of malocclusion as a risk factor of TMD. The control group or the asymptomatic volunteers of some studies was selected from the dental students [42], who can be aware of the risk factors of the TMDs and avoid them. In such cases, the samples selected may hardly represent the general population. The genders of the samples included also have such a problem. The groups of symptomatic patients in most studies included in this systematic review contain more female than male, which has a significant difference in gender distribution from the general population [3,14,17,18,20,42,45,48,49]. However, TMDs affect approximately 40% to 75% of the general adult population, 80% of which seeking for TMD are females. Milano et al. reported that disk displacements of TMJ appeared considerably more often in females than in males because of altered collagen metabolism associated with joint laxity of genetic origin [61]. Peroz et al. also found that females present a greater correlation with disk displacements than males [62]. According to Warren and Fried, estrogen may influence the development and metabolism of the TMJ and associated structures (include bone, cartilage, and articular disk), and it may also influence the pain regulation mechanism [63]. The evidence in the previous articles suggested that the pathogenesis of TMDs may have a possible link with estrogen and that TMDs is more prevalent in the female. Therefore, we also included four articles containing only female subjects [19,45–47].

The development stage of the articulation may also influence the AEI. According to the previous studies [64,65], from newborn to infancy, the articular surface was largely flat and the articular eminence was poorly developed. From the stage of the end of the primary dentition to mixed dentition, the fossa and the articular eminence had clearly developed and completed approximately 45% of its development, but the articular eminence was still fairly flat. Around the age of 10 years old, articular eminence completed approximately 70–72% of its development. The fully developed time of the articular eminence is still controversial. From the study by Katsavrias and Dibbets [65], articular eminence was 90–94% complete by the age of 20 years. However, based on the autopsy study published in 1971 [64], tubercle and the fossa were well developed at the age of 14–15 years. This review presents a high variability in the age range of 14–88 years. A poorly developed fossa may show a flatter tendency, which may possibly produce misleading conclusions.

This systematic review retrieves and analyzes the medical literature about the relationships between the TMDs and the AEI published in seven databases over the past 74 years, 50% of the studies showed a positive correlation between the TMDs and AEI, but the evidence is not in high quality. In relation to the findings in this review, the following suggestions can be drawn:

1. The correlation between TMDs and AEI is still an unsolved issue. Definitive conclusions cannot be drawn based on the present studies.
2. Evidence-based diagnosis with TMDs was not uniform. It is suggested to use multivariate statistical analyses for the evaluation of multifactorial complex pathologies such as TMDs.
3. The insufficient number of articles considered of high methodological quality is a factor that hinders the acceptance or denial of this correlation.

4. More quality and carefully designed prospective studies are required by future researchers to determine the causal relationship between TMDs and AEI.

5. Conclusions

Definitive conclusions cannot be drawn based on the quality of evidence available, since the definition and clinical methods were very heterogeneous and presented a high risk of bias. The insufficient number of articles considered of high methodological quality is another factor that hinders the acceptance or denial of this correlation. However, it is suggested that the AEI defined by some specific methods may be related to some special pathological stages of TMDs to a certain extent. Well-designed prospective studies are required to draw any further definitive conclusions.

Author Contributions: Literature search, X.-C.F., D.S. and X.R.-F.; conceptualization, X.-C.F. and L.-S.M.; methodology, X.-C.F., D.S. and E.P.; formal analysis, X.-C.F., X.-F.H. and X.R.-F.; data curation, E.P. and L.-S.M.; writing—original draft preparation, X.-C.F. and L.-S.M.; writing—review and editing, X.-F.H. and X.R.-F.; supervision, X.-F.H. and X.R.-F. All authors have read and agreed to the published version of the manuscript.

Funding: This study was supported by the Natural Science Foundation of Beijing Municipality (grant No. 7202036) and the Capital Health Research and Development of Special Funding (grant No. 2018-2-1102).

Institutional Review Board Statement: Not applicable.

Informed Consent Statement: Not applicable.

Data Availability Statement: No new data were created or analyzed in this study. Data sharing is not applicable to this article.

Conflicts of Interest: The authors declare no conflict of interest.

References

1. Wu, C.-K.; Hsu, J.-T.; Shen, Y.-W.; Chen, J.-H.; Shen, W.-C.; Fuh, L.-J. Assessments of inclinations of the mandibular fossa by computed tomography in an Asian population. *Clin. Oral Investig.* **2012**, *16*, 443–450. [CrossRef] [PubMed]
2. Som, P.M.; Curtin, H.D. *Head and Neck Imaging*, 5th ed.; Mosby, Inc.: St. Louis, MI, USA, 2011; p. 1547.
3. Sümbüllü, M.A.; Çağlayan, F.; Akgül, H.M.; Yilmaz, A.B. Radiological examination of the articular eminence morphology using cone beam CT. *Dentomaxillofac. Radiol.* **2012**, *41*, 234–240. [CrossRef] [PubMed]
4. Granados, J.I. The influence of the loss of teeth and attrition on the articular eminence. *J. Prosthet. Dent.* **1979**, *42*, 78–85. [CrossRef]
5. Gedrange, T.; Gredes, T.; Hietschold, V.; Kunert-Keil, C.; Dominiak, M.; Gerber, H.; Spassov, A.; Laniado, M. Comparison of reference points in different methods of temporomandibular joint imaging. *Adv. Med. Sci.* **2012**, *57*, 157–162. [CrossRef] [PubMed]
6. De Leeuw, R.; Klasser, G.D. The American Academy of Orofacial Pain. In *Orofacial Pain: Guidelines for Assessment, Diagnosis, and Management*; Quintessence Publishing: Chicago, IL, USA, 2013.
7. Manfredini, D.; Guarda-Nardini, L.; Winocur, E.; Piccotti, F.; Ahlberg, J.; Lobbezoo, F. Research diagnostic criteria for temporomandibular disorders: A systematic review of axis I epidemiologic findings. *Oral Surg. Oral Med. Oral Pathol. Oral Radiol. Endodontology* **2011**, *112*, 453–462. [CrossRef] [PubMed]
8. Tanaka, T.; Morimoto, Y.; Tanaka, Y.; Kobayashi, S.; Okumura, Y.; Kito, S.; Okabe, S.; Ohba, T. Radiographic examination of the mandibular (glenoid) fossa in ancient and modern man. *Oral Dis.* **2004**, *10*, 369–377. [CrossRef] [PubMed]
9. Pullinger, A.; Seligman, D. Trauma history in diagnostic groups of temporomandibular disorders. *Oral Surg. Oral Med. Oral Pathol.* **1991**, *71*, 529–534. [CrossRef]
10. Pullinger, A.; Seligman, D. Overbite and overjet characteristics of refined diagnostic groups of temporomandibular disorder patients. *Am. J. Orthod. Dentofac. Orthop.* **1991**, *100*, 401–415. [CrossRef]
11. Melis, M.; Di Giosia, M. The role of genetic factors in the etiology of temporomandibular disorders: A review. *Cranio®* **2016**, *34*, 43–51. [CrossRef]
12. Juniper, R.P. Temporomandibular joint dysfunction: A theory based upon electromyographic studies of the lateral pterygoid muscle. *Br. J. Oral Maxillofac. Surg.* **1984**, *22*, 1–8. [CrossRef]
13. Isberg, A.; Westesson, P.-L. Steepness of articular eminence and movement of the condyle and disk in asymptomatic temporomandibular joints. *Oral Surg. Oral Med. Oral Pathol. Oral Radiol. Endodontol.* **1998**, *86*, 152–157. [CrossRef]
14. Paknahad, M.; Shahidi, S.; Akhlaghian, M.; Abolvardi, M. Is Mandibular Fossa Morphology and Articular Eminence Inclination Associated with Temporomandibular Dysfunction? *J. Dent. (Shiraz Iran)* **2016**, *17*, 134–141.
15. Atkinson, W.B.; Bates, R.E. The effects of the angle of the articular eminence on anterior disk displacement. *J. Prosthet. Dent.* **1983**, *49*, 554–555. [CrossRef]

16. Piancino, M.G.; Tepedino, M.; Cavarra, F.; Bramanti, E.; Laganà, G.; Chimenti, C.; Cirillo, S. Condylar long axis and articular eminence in MRI in patients with temporomandibular disorders. *Cranio®* **2018**, *38*, 1–9. [CrossRef] [PubMed]
17. Rabelo, K.A.; Melo, S.L.S.; Torres, M.G.G.; Campos, P.S.F.; Bentoe, P.M.; de Melo, D.P. Condyle Excursion Angle, Articular Eminence Inclination, and Temporomandibular Joint Morphologic Relations with Disc Displacement. *J. Oral Maxillofac. Surg.* **2017**, *75*, 938.e1–938.e10. [CrossRef] [PubMed]
18. Shahidi, S.; Vojdani, M.; Paknahad, M. Correlation between articular eminence steepness measured with cone-beam computed tomography and clinical dysfunction index in patients with temporomandibular joint dysfunction. *Oral Surg. Oral Med. Oral Pathol. Oral Radiol.* **2013**, *116*, 91–97. [CrossRef] [PubMed]
19. Pullinger, A.G.; Seligman, D.A.; John, M.T.; Harkins, S. Multifactorial modeling of temporomandibular anatomic and orthopedic relationships in normal versus undifferentiated disk displacement joints. *J. Prosthet. Dent.* **2002**, *87*, 289–297. [CrossRef]
20. Ren, Y.F.; Isberg, A.; Westesson, P.L. Steepness of the articular eminence in the temporomandibular joint: Tomographic comparison between asymptomatic volunteers with normal disk position and patients with disk displacement. *Oral Surg. Oral Med. Oral Pathol. Oral Radiol. Endodontol.* **1995**, *80*, 258–266. [CrossRef]
21. Moher, D.; Liberati, A.; Tetzlaff, J.; Altman, D.G. Preferred reporting items for systematic reviews and meta-analyses: The PRISMA statement. *BMJ* **2009**, *339*, b2535. [CrossRef]
22. Dworkin, S.F.; LeResche, L. Research diagnostic criteria for temporomandibular disorders: Review, criteria, examinations and specifications, critique. *J. Craniomandib. Disord.* **1992**, *6*, 301–355.
23. Ohrbach, R.; Dworkin, S.F. The Evolution of TMD Diagnosis: Past, Present, Future. *J. Dent. Res.* **2016**, *95*, 1093–1101. [CrossRef] [PubMed]
24. Pontes, M.L.C.; Melo, S.L.S.; Bento, P.M.; Campos, P.S.F.; de Melo, D.P. Correlation between temporomandibular joint morphometric measurements and gender, disk position, and condylar position. *Oral Surg. Oral Med. Oral Pathol. Oral Radiol.* **2019**, *128*, 538–542. [CrossRef] [PubMed]
25. Shokri, A.; Zarch, H.H.; Hafezmaleki, F.; Khamechi, R.; Amini, P.; Ramezani, L. Comparative assessment of condylar position in patients with temporomandibular disorder (TMD) and asymptomatic patients using cone-beam computed tomography. *Dent. Med Probl.* **2019**, *56*, 81–87. [CrossRef] [PubMed]
26. Sa, S.C.; Melo, S.L.S.; de Melo, D.P.; Freitas, D.Q.; Campos, P.S.F. Relationship between articular eminence inclination and alterations of the mandibular condyle: A CBCT study. *Braz. Oral Res.* **2017**, *31*, 25. [CrossRef] [PubMed]
27. Rabelo, K.A.; Melo, S.L.S.; Torres, M.G.G.; Peixoto, L.R.; Campos, P.S.F.; Rebello, I.M.C.R.; de Melo, D.P. Assessment of condyle position, fossa morphology, and disk displacement in symptomatic patients. *Oral Surg. Oral Med. Oral Pathol. Oral Radiol.* **2017**, *124*, 199–207. [CrossRef]
28. Türp, J.C.; Schlenker, A.; Schröder, J.; Essig, M.; Schmitter, M. Disk displacement, eccentric condylar position, osteoarthrosis—Misnomers for variations of normality? Results and interpretations from an MRI study in two age cohorts. *Bmc Oral Health* **2016**, *16*, 1–10. [CrossRef] [PubMed]
29. Su, N.; Liu, Y.; Yang, X.; Luo, Z.; Shi, Z. Correlation between bony changes measured with cone beam computed tomography and clinical dysfunction index in patients with temporomandibular joint osteoarthritis. *J. Cranio Maxillofac. Surg.* **2014**, *42*, 1402–1407. [CrossRef]
30. İlgüy, D.; İlgüy, M.; Fişekçioğlu, E.; Dölekoğlu, S.; Ersan, N. Articular eminence inclination, height, and condyle morphology on cone beam computed tomography. *Sci. World J.* **2014**, *2014*, 761714. [CrossRef]
31. Çağlayan, F.; Sümbüllü, M.A.; Akgül, H.M. Associations between the articular eminence inclination and condylar bone changes, condylar movements, and condyle and fossa shapes. *Oral Radiol.* **2013**, *30*, 84–91. [CrossRef]
32. Learreta, J.A.; Barrientos, E.E. Application of a Cephalometric Method to the Temporomandibular Joint in Patients with or without Alteration in the Orientation of the Mandibular Condyle Axis. *Cranio®* **2013**, *31*, 46–55. [CrossRef]
33. De Senna, B.R.; Marques, L.S.; França, J.P.; Ramos-Jorge, M.L.; Pereira, L.J. Condyle-disk-fossa position and relationship to clinical signs and symptoms of temporomandibular disorders in women. *Oral Surg. Oral Med. Oral Pathol. Oral Radiol. Endodontol.* **2009**, *108*, e117–e124. [CrossRef] [PubMed]
34. Hirata, F.H.; Guimarães, A.S.; de Oliveira, J.X.; Moreira, C.R.; Ferreira, E.T.T.; Cavalcanti, M.G.P. Evaluation of TMJ articular eminence morphology and disc patterns in patients with disc displacement in MRI. *Braz. Oral Res.* **2007**, *21*, 265–271. [CrossRef] [PubMed]
35. Kurita, H.; Uehara, S.; Yokochi, M.; Nakatsuka, A.; Kobayashi, H.; Kurashina, K. A long-term follow-up study of radiographically evident degenerative changes in the temporomandibular joint with different conditions of disk displacement. *Int. J. Oral Maxillofac. Surg.* **2006**, *35*, 49–54. [CrossRef] [PubMed]
36. Pullinger, A.G.; Seligman, D.A. Multifactorial analysis of differences in temporomandibular joint hard tissue anatomic relationships between disk displacement with and without reduction in women. *J. Prosthet. Dent.* **2001**, *86*, 407–419. [CrossRef]
37. Kurita, H.; Ohtsuka, A.; Kobayashi, H.; Kurashina, K. Flattening of the articular eminence correlates with progressive internal derangement of the temporomandibular joint. *Dentomaxillofac. Radiol.* **2000**, *29*, 277–279. [CrossRef]
38. Toyama, M.; Kurita, K.; Westesson, P.-L.; Sakuma, S.; Ariji, E.; Rivera, R. Decreased disk-eminence ratio is associated with advanced stages of temporomandibular joint internal derangement. *Dentomaxillofac. Radiol.* **1999**, *28*, 301–304. [CrossRef]
39. Newcastle Ottawa Scale. Available online: http://www.ohri.ca/programs/clinical_epidemiology/oxford.asp (accessed on 12 October 2005).

40. Poluha, R.L.; Cunha, C.O.; Bonjardim, L.R.; Conti, P.C.R. Temporomandibular joint morphology does not influence the presence of arthralgia in patients with disk displacement with reduction: A magnetic resonance imaging–based study. *Oral Surg. Oral Med. Oral Pathol. Oral Radiol.* **2020**, *129*, 149–157. [CrossRef]
41. Aydin, O.; Ayberk, A.H.; Metin, S.; Bugra, S. Evaluation of articular eminence morphology and inclination in tmj internal derangement patients with MRI. *Int. J. Morphol.* **2012**, *30*, 740–744.
42. Sulun, T.; Cemgil, A.T.; Duc, J.-M.P.; Rammelsberg, P.; Jäger, L.; Gernet, W. Morphology of the mandibular fossa and inclination of the articular eminence in patients with internal derangement and in symptom-free volunteers. *Oral Surg. Oral Med. Oral Pathol. Oral Radiol. Endodontol.* **2001**, *92*, 98–107. [CrossRef]
43. Al-Rawi, N.H.; Uthman, A.T.; Sodeify, S.M. Spatial analysis of mandibular condyles in patients with temporomandibular disorders and normal controls using cone beam computed tomography. *Eur. J. Dent.* **2017**, *11*, 099–105. [CrossRef]
44. Imanimoghaddam, M.; Madani, A.S.; Mahdavi, P.; Bagherpour, A.; Darijani, M.; Ebrahimnejad, H. Evaluation of condylar positions in patients with temporomandibular disorders: A cone-beam computed tomographic study. *Imaging Sci. Dent.* **2016**, *46*, 127–131. [CrossRef] [PubMed]
45. Estomaguio, G.A.; Yamada, K.; Ochi, K.; Hayashi, T.; Hanada, K. Craniofacial Morphology and Inclination of the Posterior Slope of the Articular Eminence in Female Patients With and Without Condylar Bone Change. *Cranio®* **2005**, *23*, 257–263. [CrossRef] [PubMed]
46. Yamada, K.; Tsuruta, A.; Hanada, K.; Hayashi, T. Morphology of the articular eminence in temporomandibular joints and condylar bone change. *J. Oral Rehabil.* **2004**, *31*, 438–444. [CrossRef] [PubMed]
47. Sato, S.; Kawamura, H.; Motegi, K.; Takahashi, K. Morphology of the mandibular fossa and the articular eminence in temporomandibular joints with anterior disk displacement. *Int. J. Oral Maxillofac. Surg.* **1996**, *25*, 236–238. [CrossRef]
48. Galante, G.; Paesani, D.; Tallents, R.; Hatala, M.; Katzberg, R.; Murphy, W. Angle of the articular eminence in patients with temporomandibular joint dysfunction and asymptomatic volunteers. *Oral Surg. Oral Med. Oral Pathol. Oral Radiol. Endodontol.* **1995**, *80*, 242–249. [CrossRef]
49. Panmekiate, S.; Petersson, A.; Åkerman, S. Angulation and prominence of the posterior slope of the eminence of the temporomandibular joint in relation to disc position. *Dentomaxillofac. Radiol.* **1991**, *20*, 205–208. [CrossRef]
50. Türp, J.C.; Schindler, H. The dental occlusion as a suspected cause for TMDs: Epidemiological and etiological considerations. *J. Oral Rehabil.* **2012**, *39*, 502–512. [CrossRef]
51. De Boever, J.A.; Carlsson, G.E.; Klineberg, I.J. Need for occlusal therapy and prosthodontic treatment in the management of temporomandibular disorders. Part I. Occlusal interferences and occlusal adjustment. *J. Oral Rehabil.* **2000**, *27*, 367–379. [CrossRef]
52. Greene, C.S. Relationship between occlusion and temporomandibular disorders: Implications for the orthodontist. *Am. J. Orthod. Dentofac. Orthop.* **2011**, *139*, 11–15. [CrossRef]
53. Slade, G.D.; Diatchenko, L.; Ohrbach, R.; Maixner, W. Orthodontic Treatment, Genetic Factors, and Risk of Temporomandibular Disorder. *Semin. Orthod.* **2008**, *14*, 146–156. [CrossRef]
54. Landi, N.; Manfredini, D.; Tognini, F.; Romagnoli, M.; Bosco, M. Quantification of the relative risk of multiple occlusal variables for muscle disorders of the stomatognathic system. *J. Prosthet. Dent.* **2004**, *92*, 190–195. [CrossRef] [PubMed]
55. Pullinger, A.; Seligman, D.; Gornbein, J. A Multiple Logistic Regression Analysis of the Risk and Relative Odds of Temporomandibular Disorders as a Function of Common Occlusal Features. *J. Dent. Res.* **1993**, *72*, 968–979. [CrossRef] [PubMed]
56. Honey, O.B.; Scarfe, W.C.; Hilgers, M.J.; Klueber, K.; Silveira, A.M.; Haskell, B.S.; Farman, A.G. Accuracy of cone-beam computed tomography imaging of the temporomandibular joint: Comparisons with panoramic radiology and linear tomography. *Am. J. Orthod. Dentofac. Orthop.* **2007**, *132*, 429–438. [CrossRef] [PubMed]
57. Katsavrias, E.G. Changes in articular eminence inclination during the craniofacial growth period. *Angle Orthod.* **2002**, *72*, 258–264. [PubMed]
58. Kikuchi, K.; Takeuchi, S.; Tanaka, E.; Shibaguchi, T.; Tanne, K. Association between condylar position, joint morphology and craniofacial morphology in orthodontic patients without temporomandibular joint disorders. *J. Oral Rehabil.* **2003**, *30*, 1070–1075. [CrossRef] [PubMed]
59. Kollmann, J.; Ranke, J.; Virchow, R. Verständigung über ein gemeinsames craniometrisches Verfahren: Frankfurter Verständigung. *Arch. Anthr.* **1883**, *15*, 1–8.
60. Schmidt, E. Die horizontalebene des menschlichen schädels. *Arch. Anthr.* **1876**, *25*, 9–60.
61. Milano, V.; Desiate, A.; Bellino, R.; Garofalo, T. Magnetic resonance imaging of temporomandibular disorders: Classification, prevalence and interpretation of disc displacement and deformation. *Dentomaxillofac. Radiol.* **2000**, *29*, 352–361. [CrossRef]
62. Peroz, I.; Seidel, A.; Griethe, M.; Lemke, A.-J. MRI of the TMJ: Morphometric comparison of asymptomatic volunteers and symptomatic patients. *Quintessence Int.* **2011**, *42*, 659–667.
63. Warren, M.P.; Fried, J.L. Temporomandibular Disorders and Hormones in Women. *Cells Tissues Organs* **2001**, *169*, 187–192. [CrossRef]

64. Öberg, T.; Carlsson, G.E.; Fajers, C.-M. The Temporomandibular Joint: A Morphologic Study on a Human Autopsy Material. *Acta Odontol. Scand.* **1971**, *29*, 349–384. [CrossRef] [PubMed]
65. Katsavrias, E.G.; Dibbets, J. The growth of articular eminence height during craniofacial growth period. *Cranio®* **2001**, *19*, 13–20. [CrossRef] [PubMed]

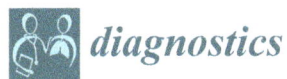

Review

Temporomandibular Disorders: Current Concepts and Controversies in Diagnosis and Management

Dion Tik Shun Li and Yiu Yan Leung *

Department of Oral and Maxillofacial Surgery, Faculty of Dentistry, The University of Hong Kong, Hong Kong, China; diontsli@hku.hk
* Correspondence: mikeyyleung@hku.hk; Tel.: +852-28890511

Abstract: Temporomandibular disorders (TMD) are a group of orofacial pain conditions which are the most common non-dental pain complaint in the maxillofacial region. Due to the complexity of the etiology, the diagnosis and management of TMD remain a challenge where consensus is still lacking in many aspects. While clinical examination is considered the most important process in the diagnosis of TMD, imaging may serve as a valuable adjunct in selected cases. Depending on the type of TMD, many treatment modalities have been proposed, ranging from conservative options to open surgical procedures. In this review, the authors discuss the present thinking in the etiology and classification of TMD, followed by the diagnostic approach and the current trend and controversies in management.

Keywords: temporomandibular disorders; temporomandibular joint; TMD; facial pain; craniomandibular disorders

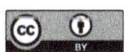

1. Introduction

The diagnosis and management of the most common cause of non-dental pain in the maxillofacial region, namely temporomandibular disorders (TMD), remains a challenge for clinicians to this day, despite extensive clinical research into the topic. This is because TMD is a broad term comprising of different conditions with complex etiologies, with symptoms that vary in intensity. Intriguingly, some signs and symptoms resolve spontaneously even without treatment, whereas others persist for years despite all treatment options having been exhausted. More perplexing is that while some may have a recognizable physical basis, many cases of TMD also involve a significant biopsychosocial component [1–3] with various associated psychological symptoms, such as depression and anxiety [4–6]. Numerous treatment modalities have been proposed over the years, with some becoming obsolete while others are gaining in popularity. Nevertheless, it seems that there is no single solution for every case as many different symptoms are included in TMD. Controversies exist in the literature regarding the diagnosis and the management protocol for TMD, hence the selection of treatment modality may often be largely influenced by the expertise of the treating healthcare provider.

In general, TMD is believed to affect anywhere between 5 and 15% of adults in the population [7–10], yet TMD related symptoms have been reported to be present in up to 50% of adults [11]. Interestingly, there is evidence that the prevalence of TMD appears to be on the rise in recent years [12–16]. A recent systematic review and meta-analysis in 2021 concluded that the prevalence of TMD was 31% for adults and 11% for children and adolescence [17]. The fact that TMD encompasses a broad assortment of clinical diseases is partially responsible for the wide range of prevalence rate estimates among studies, as the classification of different types of TMD, the distinction between disease and non-disease, as well as whether to include those with inactive disease as having TMD, may all be subject to the partialities of the assessing clinical researchers. In addition, studies that are questionnaire-based might over-estimate the prevalence of TMD, as the symptoms of many other conditions, such as headache not caused by TMD, dental pain, neuropathic conditions, and otological diseases, can mimic the presentation of TMD.

TMD represents a significant and complex health problem, with opinions regarding the appropriate course of management often equivocal. In this review, we discuss the current concepts in the etiology and diagnosis of TMD, followed by an up-to-date management approach from a surgeons' perspective.

2. Etiologies and Classifications

As an umbrella term for pain and dysfunction of the temporomandibular regions, TMD encompasses a wide variety of clinical conditions. The etiologies of TMD are multifactorial and can be attributed to both physical and psychosocial factors [18–20]. The physical causes can broadly be divided into arthrogenous, and the more common myogenous origins. Many believe that TMD symptoms of arthrogenous origin may be related to internal derangement of the TMJ, which can be defined as a disruption of the internal aspect of the joint, and usually pertains to an articular disc that has been displaced. Although internal derangement does not necessarily lead to pain, it is generally believed that internal derangement precedes degenerative joint diseases, namely osteoarthritis [21]. Osteoarthritis is associated with pain and functional impairment of the TMJ, and is characterized by subchondral bony changes such as cortical erosion and marginal lipping, secondary to pathological changes of the cartilaginous articular disc [22]. Note that the term "osteoarthrosis" has been used as a synonym of osteoarthritis, but also has been used to describe degenerative joint changes of non-inflammatory cause [22]. The severity of internal derangement has been classified by Wilkes into five stages with relations to pain, mouth opening, disc location and anatomy [21]. The classification ranges from painless clicking of the joint (Stage I) to severe pain of the joint with severe degenerative bony changes (Stage V), which has served as an aid to guide treatment options in the management of arthrogenous TMD.

While structural anomalies of the TMJ may predispose the patients to symptoms of TMD [23], it should be noted that not all those with structural abnormalities suffer from the same level of clinical symptoms. Apart from physical causes, the association between biopsychosocial factors and TMD has been described by many [1–4,19,24]. Similar to other chronic pain conditions, such as back pain and headache, it appears that there are those in the population who are at risk for developing symptomatic TMD, who also share a certain psychological profile and dysfunction [25,26]. Higher levels of depression and somatization are associated with TMD of arthrogenous and myogenous origins [27]. Moreover, in those with pre-existing TMD, symptoms may be exacerbated during times of stressful events. For example, recent studies have suggested that the during periods of lockdown and social isolation due to the ongoing COVID-19 pandemic, an impact was found on the prevalence of depressive symptoms, stress, as well as pain related to TMD [28,29]. The finding that psychological variables are closely tied to the development of TMD has been confirmed by the Orofacial Pain: Prospective Evaluation and Risk Assessment (OPPERA) study, which found that TMD onset was strongly associated with somatic symptoms, while previous life events, perceived stress and negative affect were also associated with the incidence of TMD [30].

What makes the diagnosis and classification of TMD complicated at times is that many patients present with multiple diagnoses of TMD simultaneously, and it is impossible to isolate the condition to a single particular cause. When discussing about TMD, most clinical researchers refer to those pain conditions that are most commonly seen. However, one must not forget that disorders related to the TMJ include those that are less routinely encountered. Importantly, the presentation of these uncommon conditions of the TMJ may initially mimic those of the more common TMD, yet the management approach may be completely different. For example, a patient who presents with ankylosis of the TMJ may initially present with signs and symptoms similar to closed-lock due to disc displacement, but the standard treatment for ankylosis is surgical release of ankylosis, while conservative or minimally invasive options, such as arthrocentesis, are usually indicated for closed-lock of the TMJ due to disc displacement.

The crude classification of the most common diagnoses of TMD into arthrogenous, myogenous, or of mixed origin is helpful in steering the clinician into the appropriate path in the initial phases of management. However, more specific diagnoses are usually required, especially if the management progresses beyond conservative options. In the past, classification was often confusing, with many different terminologies referring to similar entities. Today, the Diagnostic Criteria for Temporomandibular Disorders (DC/TMD) is the most widely accepted and standardized tool for assessment and classification of TMD, with sensitivity and specificity established for the most common diagnoses of TMD [31]. Recognizing that TMD contains a structural as well as a biopsychosocial component, the DC/TMD consists of two Axes in its assessment. Axis-I contains a protocol for a prescribed physical examination to arrive at specific physical diagnoses of TMD with regard to the joint and musculature, while Axis-II contains several instruments to assess the psychological state of the patient.

There are 12 most common diagnoses of TMD described in Axis-I of the DC/TMD, which are divided into painful conditions (myalgia, local myalgia, myofascial pain, myofascial pain with referral, arthralgia, headache attributed to TMD) and non-painful conditions (disc displacement with reduction, disc displacement with reduction with intermittent locking, disc displacement without reduction with limited opening, disc displacement without reduction without limited opening, degenerative joint disease, subluxation) [31] (Table 1). Note that in many cases, multiple diagnoses are present at any timepoint in a single patient, and that diagnoses may change as the disease progresses or resolves. For example, a patient with complaints of joint clicking with pain in the TMJ and masseter muscle, and headache during mouth opening may be diagnosed with having local myalgia, arthralgia, disc displacement with reduction, and headache attributed to TMD. The classification of TMD also includes those that are less common, but clinically important diseases [32]. Some of these less common diagnoses include fractures of the TMJ, manifestations of systemic diseases, as well as rare conditions such as neoplasms and developmental disorders (Table 2) [32]. However, when these diagnoses do not fit the clinical symptoms, other conditions should also be considered.

Table 1. Common diagnoses of temporomandibular disorders (TMD) and their clinical findings.

Painful Conditions	Clinical Findings
Myalgia	Familiar pain in the masseter or temporalis upon palpation or mouth opening
Local Myalgia	Familiar pain in the masseter or temporalis localized to the site of palpation
Myofascial pain	Pain in the masseter or temporalis spreading beyond the site of palpation but within the confines of the muscle
Myofascial pain with referral	Pain in the masseter or temporalis beyond the confines of the muscle being palpated
Arthralgia	Familiar pain in the TMJ upon palpation or during function
Headache attributed to TMD	Headache in the temple upon palpation of the temporalis muscle or during function

Table 1. *Cont.*

Non-Painful Conditions	Clinical Findings
Disc displacement with reduction	Clicking in the TMJ upon function
Disc displacement with reduction with intermittent locking	Clicking in the TMJ with reported episodes of limited mouth opening
Disc displacement without reduction with limited opening	Limited mouth opening affecting function, with maximum assisted opening < 40mm
Disc displacement without reduction without limited opening	Limited mouth opening affecting function, with maximum assisted opening of $\geq$ 40mm
Degenerative joint disease	Crepitus of the TMJ upon function
Subluxation	History of jaw locking in an open mouth position, cannot close without a self-maneuver

Modified from Schiffman et al., 2014 [31].

Table 2. Some less common diagnoses of temporomandibular disorders (TMD).

I. TMJ
A. Joint pain
1. Arthritis
B. Joint disorders
1. Hypomobility disorders other than disc disorders
a. Adhesions/Adherence
b. Ankylosis (Fibrous or Osseous)
2. TMJ dislocations
C. Joint diseases
1. Systemic arthritides
2. Condylysis/Idiopathic condylar resorption
3. Osteochondritis dissecans
4. Osteonecrosis
5. Neoplasm
6. Synovial Chondromatosis
D. Fractures
E. Congenital/Developmental disorders
1. Aplasia
2. Hypoplasia
3. Hyperplasia
II. Masticatory Muscles
A. Muscle pain
1. Tendonitis
2. Myositis
3. Spasm
B. Contracture
C. Hypertrophy
D. Neoplasm
E. Movement Disorders
1. Orofacial dyskinesia
2. Oromandibular dystonia
F. Masticatory muscle pain related to central/systemic pain disorder
1. Fibromyalgia/widespread pain
III. Associated Structures
A. Coronoid hyperplasia

Modified from Peck et al., 2014 [32].

3. Diagnostic Approach

The signs and symptoms of TMD may mimic other orofacial pain conditions. Although precise physical diagnosis into the type of TMD is helpful in developing an appropriate treatment plan, it might not be straight forward in every case. Taking a patients' history is an important part of diagnosing the TMJ condition. The acquisition of history follows the usual format. Apart from the chief complaint, inquiries should be made regarding any history of trauma or previous episodes, aggravating factors, such as eating, talking, yawning or spontaneous background pain, and any previous investigations or treatment. The severity of pain should also be graded using a visual analogue scale (VAS), so treatment progress can be quantitatively monitored. A past and current medical history, including a full medications list, may reveal any comorbidities that may be related to TMD. The clinician should note any habits such as smoking, drinking and recreational drug use, and any history of clenching or bruxism as complained by the patients' bed partner. Additionally, the clinician should ask questions regarding stress and level of life satisfaction, and whether there are any recent life events, such as change of job or loss of a loved one. Although most clinicians treating TMD may be experienced with acquiring a clinical history, some may not be comfortable with taking a psychological history. If desired, the clinician may employ the numerous psychosocial instruments available to aid in their diagnosis, such as those in Axis-II of DC/TMD [31]. When necessary, the patient may be referred for a psychological assessment.

Most clinicians who treat orofacial pain believe clinical examination is the most crucial process of diagnosing TMD. The location of pain, and whether the pain is localized, remains within or spreads beyond the confines of the muscle, should be confirmed with palpation, which is done at rest and during mandibular function. Clicking or crepitus upon mandibular function might be quite obvious in some cases, and the detection might be aided by the use of a stethoscope. Intriguingly, the presence or location of clicking detected by the clinician might be different from that reported by the patient, and this should be documented. The range of mouth opening measured should include pain-free maximum mouth opening, maximum unassisted mouth opening, and maximum assisted mouth opening. Any deviation of the mandible may indicate differential obstruction of the movement of the mandibular condyle in rotation and/or translation. An intra-oral examination is performed to rule out any mucosal pathologies of the oral cavity and oropharyngeal region, as well as to assess the state of the dentition.

3.1. Imaging and Other Investigations

Imaging is considered to be a useful adjunct in the diagnosis of TMD. Although the diagnostic information provided by plain radiographs like orthopantomogram is limited, they are convenient, simple and serve to rule out some of the differential diagnoses of the bony TMJ, such as fractures, ankylosis, growth disturbances, as well as neoplasms. For the most common types of TMD which clinical presentation is typical, many units might not routinely employ additional imaging. This is due to availability and cost, and that additional imaging might not alter the initial management plan. However, when further information is desired, magnetic resonance imaging (MRI) is the gold standard for TMJ imaging, and is useful in assessing the status of the osseous, as well as the non-osseous structures of the TMJ, such as the masticatory muscles, ligaments and the cartilaginous disc [33] (Figure 1). Classification systems, such as Wilkes [21], combine clinical and MRI findings to stage the extent of internal derangement in order to guide treatment protocol. MRI is therefore considered mandatory prior to any surgical intervention.

While MRI is the most commonly used diagnostic imaging for the common diagnoses of TMD, other imaging modalities are also employed for specific indications. Cone-beam computed tomography (CBCT) has been used to further assess the osseous structure of the TMJ [34–36]. This may be desirable in cases of TMJ ankylosis, benign bony neoplasms or overgrowth, or for the planning of osseous surgery, such as for eminectomy for recurrence TMJ dislocation. However, for most other diagnoses of TMJ, the value of CBCT is not well-established since the information provided in terms of soft tissues is limited [36]. Moreover, the use of ultrasound as a diagnostic tool for TMD has been suggested [15,37,38]. Ultrasound has the advantages of being non-invasive, cheap, and widely available in many health institutions, yet the effectiveness as a diagnostic method remains to be confirmed [15]. For some inflammatory conditions of the TMJ, such as osteoarthritis and joint inflammation, bone scintigraphy may be of value as a diagnostic tool [39–43]. Moreover, bone scintigraphy has been proposed as a method for the evaluation of active TMJ condylar growth, but it has been shown that both the sensitivity and specificity are low for this indication [44].

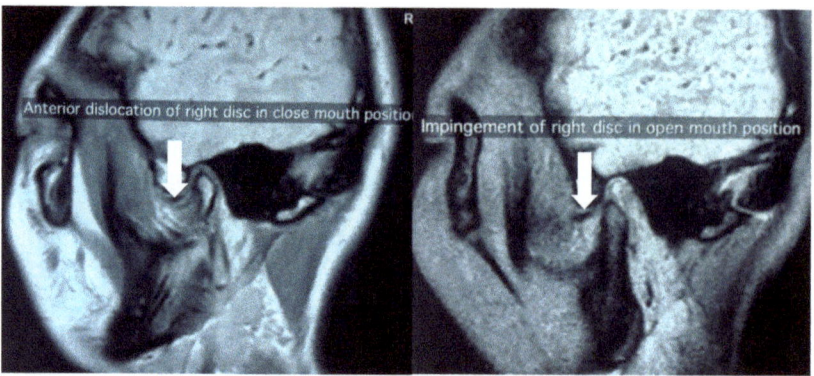

Figure 1. Magnetic resonance imaging (MRI) showing anteriorly displaced disc in both the close and open mouth position in a patient presented with lock jaw.

Apart from the different imaging modalities available, other investigations are not commonly done for most diagnoses of TMD, except in specific indications. For example, blood investigations may be done for TMD related to systemic conditions, such as rheumatoid arthritis or gout. In the case of uncertain diagnoses of rare diseases or neoplasms, tissue biopsies might be taken, which may be done by fine-needle aspiration, arthroscopic or open joint approach.

3.2. Diagnosis of TMD

Recognizing the causes of pain and dysfunction related to TMD is important in order to guide treatment decisions. For instance, different treatment options are often employed for the treatment of myogenous versus arthrogenous TMD. Moreover, in those patients who present with TMD symptoms without an obvious physical cause, who also suffer from psychological comorbidities, may be best treated by counselling and psychological intervention.

The most important part of the diagnosis of TMD is to differentiate the common diseases from those clinically significant, but unusual conditions, as well as conditions that are more serious which urgent attention is needed. For example, some neoplasms, such as chondrosarcoma of the TMJ may initially share signs and symptoms as some of the common diagnoses of TMD, such as pain at the preauricular region and limited opening. Another example that requires urgent attention is temporal arteritis, which is an inflammatory condition of the temporal vessels with some TMD-like symptoms, such as headache, pain in the temporal region, and limited mouth opening. However, temporal arteritis is a medical emergency which may cause permanent blindness if not treated promptly. Some of the differential diagnoses of orofacial pain that may mimic TMD are listed in Table 3 [45].

Table 3. Differential diagnosis of temporomandibular disorders (TMD).

Neuropathic Pain
Trigeminal neuralgia
Glossopharyngeal neuralgia
Postherpetic neuralgia
Traumatic neuralgia
Burning mouth syndrome
Atypical odontalgia
Atypical facial pain
Odontogenic Pain
Dental caries
Periodontal disease
Dental abscess
Dental sensitivity
Cracked tooth syndrome
Pericoronitis
Intracranial Pain
Tumours
Aneurysms
Bleeding
Infection
Pain from Other Adjacent Structures
Ear
Nose
Throat
Eyes
Sinus
Salivary glands
Lymph nodes
Vasculature
Cervical region
Headaches not Attributed to TMD
Migraine
Cluster headache
Tension-type headache
Temporal arteritis
Referred Pain
Psychogenic Pain

Modified from Kumar et al. (2013) [45].

4. Treatment Modalities—A Change in Paradigm?

The goals of treatment for TMD include reduction of pain and improvement of jaw function. Additionally, treatment with the goal of behavioural change may be important in the reduction of tension and parafunction. Currently, physically restoring the disc position in the case of internal derangement is not the primary treatment objective as it may not be relevant to clinical improvement [46,47], unless of course if there is inflammation related to disc displacement then it should be addressed. Symptoms of TMD should be addressed promptly, as chronic pain becomes more difficult to manage due to psychological deterioration and somatization [2,19]. Since conservative options are less likely to cause any harm, they are usually indicated in the early stages of treatment. This is especially true when definitive diagnosis is difficult to ascertain and treatment is performed empirically. However, there is no agreement on how long conservative treatment should be attempted before progressing to other options when clear benefits are not observed. Although the treatment of TMD has shifted away from open procedures which were once popular, the demonstrated success of minimally invasive options may indicate that they may be considered as an early option for those cases refractory to conservatory approaches.

4.1. Conservative Options

The initial management of TMD may include various medications, such as analgesics, non-steroidal anti-inflammatory drugs (NSAIDs), anxiolytics, and anti-depressants. Occlusal appliances of various designs are routinely prescribed, which represent a non-invasive option with minimal risks (Figure 2). The use of occlusal splint therapy has been shown to reduce pain intensity and increase maximal mouth opening [48]. However, whether the effect of an occlusal splint is due to the placebo effect has been questioned, and that the evidence of its efficacy remains to be low [49,50]. A systematic review in 2018 by Alkhutari et al. has suggested that the use of occlusal splint may improve patient-centred treatment outcomes, which may be more than merely a placebo effect [51]. Multiple designs are available, such as hard, soft, and anterior repositioning splint. At present, there is no consensus on which design is superior, as results from different studies are equivocal in terms of the efficacy of different designs of occlusal splints [50,52].

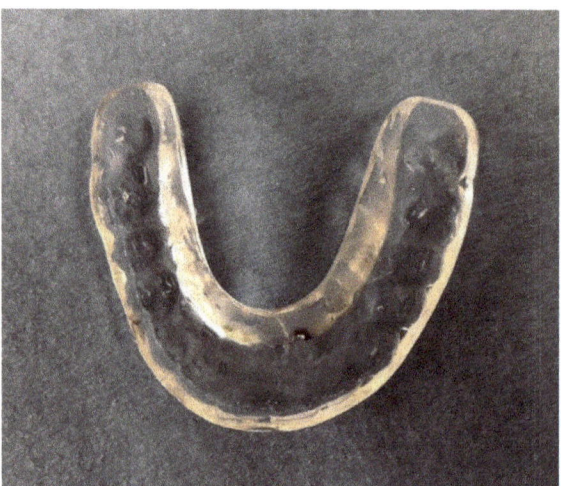

Figure 2. Occlusal splint for the management of temporomandibular disorders (TMD) and bruxism.

Physiotherapy has been suggested to be an important part in the management of TMD [53,54], which may be particularly useful for myalgia or myofascial pain. Understanding the loading of the stomatognathic system, and the existence of any tension and parafunctions, is important in delivering physiotherapy such as muscle training and changing of behaviour. Evidence shows that physiotherapy is effective in treatment of TMD, in particular the headache symptoms associated with the condition; future research into this area will further ascertain these findings [54]. For myogenous TMD, Botox injection and dry-needling techniques have been suggested [55,56]. Note that Botox is not considered a standard treatment option for TMD, while dry-needling, or acupuncture, may be an effective method to reduce tension in some patients. Additionally, initial results regarding extracorporeal shock wave therapy for myogenous TMD appear to show positive results [57,58].

There has been increasing evidence demonstrating that psychosocial assessment serves as a powerful tool in terms of predicting treatment outcome [59,60]. For those patients with a significant psychosocial component, counselling seems to be a promising treatment adjunct [50,61–63], which might be most beneficial when included in a multimodal approach [50]. Other conservative treatment options for TMD include stress reduction techniques and diet modification. In the past, a causative relationship between occlusion and TMD had been suggested, but it is now considered an outdated theory not supported by robust evidence, and occlusal adjustment is an irreversible treatment which is no longer supported by the recent literature [64–67].

4.2. Minimally Invasive Options—Arthroscopy, Arthrocentesis and Intra-Articular Injections

In the 1980s, the availability of MRI has led clinicians to acknowledge the structural anomalies related to TMD. This has resulted in a boom of open joint surgeries, which were unfortunately ineffective in the most part. For those cases of TMD that are arthrogenous and not responsive to conservative treatment, more focus has since been shifted to minimally invasive procedures which have shown promising clinical results.

Arthroscopy of the TMJ was initially pioneered by the Japanese in the 1970s [68,69], and later popularized by the Americans [70–72]. TMJ arthroscopy may involve lysis and lavage of the superior joint space, as well as operative procedures, such as repositioning of a displaced disc, arthroplasty, and removal of inflamed tissues and adhesions. The efficacy of arthroscopy has since been well-recognized [73–79], and has been found that the therapeutic effect was mainly due to lysis and lavage but not disc position [80]. It was due to this finding that a modification was made, where lysis and lavage was performed without arthroscopic view. This was termed arthrocentesis which was first described by Nitzan et al., in 1991 [81], with efficacy that has since been well-documented [46,82–94] (Figure 3).

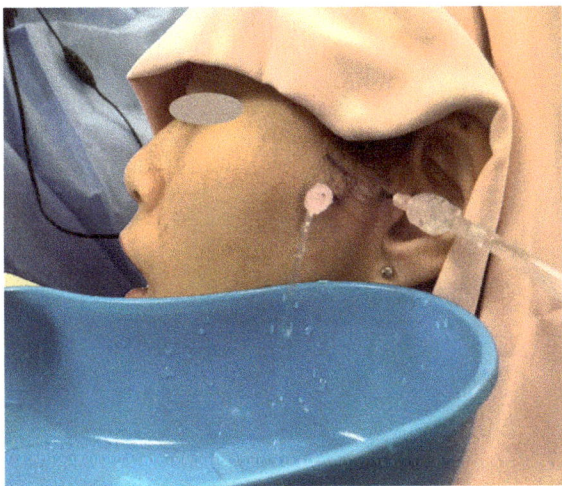

Figure 3. Arthrocentesis performed under local anaesthesia.

In addition to the shift from open joint surgery to minimally invasive treatment for those cases not responsive to conservative treatment, recent literature seems to support that minimally invasive options may be attempted early for arthrogenous TMD [95,96], and this may represent a paradigm shift in the management protocol. A recent integrated review and meta-analysis performed by the authors of this article showed that arthrocentesis was beneficial, whether it was performed as an initial treatment, as an early or late treatment with regard to conservative treatment [97]. However, the best timing to perform arthrocentesis is still unclear due to the paucity of research on the topic, which warrants more future well-designed clinical trials [97].

Although both arthroscopy and arthrocentesis have been shown to be beneficial in the treatment of TMD, it is unclear which method produces better clinical results. In a systematic review and meta-analysis by Al-Moraissi, it was revealed that arthroscopy was superior to arthrocentesis in pain reduction and jaw function improvement, with similar complication rates for both methods [78]. However, other studies have shown comparable results with the two procedures [98,99]. Nevertheless, arthrocentesis has been suggested to be attempted first due to simplicity and cost-effectiveness, with a similar or potentially lower complication rate [99].

Several modifications have been suggested for the conventional arthrocentesis, which involves two puncture needles into the superior joint space guided by landmarks in relations to adjacent structures, followed by lavage with an irrigation solution. For example, single-puncture techniques employ specially designed devices, and may have both the inflow and outflow fluid going through a single cannula but with different ports. Although single-puncture techniques may appear more simple than double-puncture arthrocentesis, most studies to date have shown a similar clinical outcome between the two techniques [83,100–102]. In addition, ultrasound-guided arthrocentesis has been proposed to increase the accuracy of puncture into the superior joint space [103–106]. However, a recent systematic review by Leung et al. has shown that no additional benefit is seen with ultrasound-guided arthrocentesis compared to conventional arthrocentesis [107]. Furthermore, different pharmacological agents for intra-articular injection have been proposed, with the common ones including hyaluronic acid, corticosteroid, analgesics, and platelet-rich plasma [93,96,108,109]. Although promising results are seen in some studies, there is currently no consensus regarding which intra-articular injection agent is superior over the others.

Despite the reported efficacy, arthroscopy is seldom required in TMD patients, even in cases of true arthrogenous disorders. Additionally, arthrocentesis is still considered to be a controversial procedure [87], despite the documented efficacy and low complication rates. The reasons for this controversy are as follows. Firstly, some cases of TMD improve with mere conservative options, or even without treatment. Additionally, many cases of TMD are due to multiple etiologies, which may require a multimodal approach before any clear clinical improvement can be appreciated. In addition, intra-articular injection of corticosteroids is a simple and very effective treatment, which may be attempted prior to arthrocentesis. In short, minimally invasive procedures may be the answer in those patients with true arthrogenous TMD not responsive to conservative treatment options, whose condition also lack a significant biopsychosocial component.

4.3. Open Joint Surgery

Open surgical treatment for TMD is now uncommon, and is reserved for specific indications as well as end-stage diseases. Though, surgery may be the only viable option in some conditions, such as ankylosis and neoplasms, which require release of ankylosis and removal of tumour, respectively. Pending on the availability of equipment and skills, there is now an option of arthroscopic surgery for procedures that were only performed with an open-joint approach in the past. These procedures include disc repositioning procedures, removal of osteophyte, removal of pathologic tissue, and biopsy of the TMJ. In recent years, much work has been done regarding replacement of the TMJ with alloplastic prosthesis [110–116] with an observed improvement in prognosis and longevity. Due to this success, it is likely that we will see a continuous increase in popularity of alloplastic replacement of the TMJ for conditions such as end stage arthritic conditions, ankylosis, post-tumour resection, and developmental anomalies of the TMJ.

5. Conclusions

TMD represents a divergent group of orofacial pain symptoms which shares similarities with other chronic pain conditions. The etiology of TMD is often multi-factorial, and precise causes for the symptoms may be difficult to pinpoint. In the past, focus has been placed on the physical origins of TMD, but an at least equally significant psychosocial factor is now well-recognized. Consequently, a multimodal approach, which might include counselling and psychological therapy, is being increasingly advocated. Most instances of

TMD are managed conservatively and empirically during the early phases of treatment, yet lingering in the conservative phase for an extended period when clinical improvement is unclear is not recommended. Though open joint surgery is rare nowadays and is reserved for specific situations, we may be in the midst of a changing paradigm which favours early minimally invasive procedures.

Author Contributions: Both authors are responsible for all parts of the work. All authors have read and agreed to the published version of the manuscript.

Funding: This research received no external funding.

Conflicts of Interest: The authors declare no conflict of interest.

References

1. Von Korff, M.; Ormel, J.; Keefe, F.J.; Dworkin, S.F. Grading the severity of chronic pain. *Pain* **1992**, *50*, 133–149. [CrossRef]
2. Ismail, F.; Eisenburger, M.; Lange, K.; Schneller, T.; Schwabe, L.; Strempel, J.; Stiesch, M. Identification of psychological comorbidity in TMD-patients. *Cranio* **2016**, *34*, 182–187. [CrossRef] [PubMed]
3. List, T.; Jensen, R.H. Temporomandibular disorders: Old ideas and new concepts. *Cephalalgia* **2017**, *37*, 692–704. [CrossRef] [PubMed]
4. Bitiniene, D.; Zamaliauskiene, R.; Kubilius, R.; Leketas, M.; Gailius, T.; Smirnovaite, K. Quality of life in patients with temporomandibular disorders. A systematic review. *Stomatologija* **2018**, *20*, 3–9. [PubMed]
5. Resende, C.; Rocha, L.; Paiva, R.P.; Cavalcanti, C.D.S.; Almeida, E.O.; Roncalli, A.G.; Barbosa, G.A.S. Relationship between anxiety, quality of life, and sociodemographic characteristics and temporomandibular disorder. *Oral Surg. Oral Med. Oral Pathol. Oral Radiol.* **2020**, *129*, 125–132. [CrossRef] [PubMed]
6. Dahlstrom, L.; Carlsson, G.E. Temporomandibular disorders and oral health-related quality of life. A systematic review. *Acta Odontol. Scand.* **2010**, *68*, 80–85. [CrossRef]
7. Goncalves, D.A.; Camparis, C.M.; Speciali, J.G.; Franco, A.L.; Castanharo, S.M.; Bigal, M.E. Temporomandibular disorders are differentially associated with headache diagnoses: A controlled study. *Clin. J. Pain* **2011**, *27*, 611–615. [CrossRef]
8. Lim, P.F.; Smith, S.; Bhalang, K.; Slade, G.D.; Maixner, W. Development of temporomandibular disorders is associated with greater bodily pain experience. *Clin. J. Pain* **2010**, *26*, 116–120. [CrossRef] [PubMed]
9. Facial Pain. Available online: http://www.nidcr.nih.gov/DataStatistics/FindDataByTopic/FacialPain/ (accessed on 9 June 2019).
10. Lipton, J.A.; Ship, J.A.; Larach-Robinson, D. Estimated prevalence and distribution of reported orofacial pain in the United States. *J. Am. Dental Assoc.* **1993**, *124*, 115–121. [CrossRef] [PubMed]
11. Locker, D.; Slade, G. Prevalence of symptoms associated with temporomandibular disorders in a Canadian population. *Community Dent. Oral Epidemiol.* **1988**, *16*, 310–313. [CrossRef]
12. Magnusson, T.; Egermark, I.; Carlsson, G.E. A longitudinal epidemiologic study of signs and symptoms of temporomandibular disorders from 15 to 35 years of age. *J. Orofac. Pain* **2000**, *14*, 310–319.
13. Ebrahimi, M.; Dashti, H.; Mehrabkhani, M.; Arghavani, M.; Daneshvar-Mozafari, A. Temporomandibular Disorders and Related Factors in a Group of Iranian Adolescents: A Cross-sectional Survey. *J. Dent. Res. Dent. Clin. Dent. Prospect.* **2011**, *5*, 123–127. [CrossRef]
14. Manfredini, D.; Piccotti, F.; Ferronato, G.; Guarda-Nardini, L. Age peaks of different RDC/TMD diagnoses in a patient population. *J. Dent.* **2010**, *38*, 392–399. [CrossRef] [PubMed]
15. Klatkiewicz, T.; Gawriolek, K.; Pobudek Radzikowska, M.; Czajka-Jakubowska, A. Ultrasonography in the Diagnosis of Temporomandibular Disorders: A Meta-Analysis. *Med. Sci. Monit.* **2018**, *24*, 812–817. [CrossRef] [PubMed]
16. Sena, M.F.; Mesquita, K.S.; Santos, F.R.; Silva, F.W.; Serrano, K.V. Prevalence of temporomandibular dysfunction in children and adolescents. *Rev. Paul. Pediatr.* **2013**, *31*, 538–545. [CrossRef] [PubMed]
17. Valesan, L.F.; Da-Cas, C.D.; Reus, J.C.; Denardin, A.C.S.; Garanhani, R.R.; Bonotto, D.; Januzzi, E.; de Souza, B.D.M. Prevalence of temporomandibular joint disorders: A systematic review and meta-analysis. *Clin. Oral Investig.* **2021**. [CrossRef] [PubMed]
18. Rollman, G.B.; Gillespie, J.M. The role of psychosocial factors in temporomandibular disorders. *Curr. Rev. Pain* **2000**, *4*, 71–81. [CrossRef] [PubMed]
19. Auerbach, S.M.; Laskin, D.M.; Frantsve, L.M.; Orr, T. Depression, pain, exposure to stressful life events, and long-term outcomes in temporomandibular disorder patients. *J. Oral Maxillofac. Surg.* **2001**, *59*, 628–633. [CrossRef]
20. Toh, A.Q.J.; Chan, J.L.H.; Leung, Y.Y. Mandibular asymmetry as a possible etiopathologic factor in temporomandibular disorder: A prospective cohort study of 134 patients. *Clin. Oral Investig.* **2021**. [CrossRef] [PubMed]
21. Wilkes, C.H. Internal Derangements of the Temporomandibular Joint: Pathological Variations. *Arch. Otolaryngol. Head Neck Surg.* **1989**, *115*, 469–477. [CrossRef]
22. Mercuri, L.G. Osteoarthritis, osteoarthrosis, and idiopathic condylar resorption. *Oral Maxillofac. Surg. Clin. N. Am.* **2008**, *20*, 169–183. [CrossRef]
23. Bertram, S.; Rudisch, A.; Innerhofer, K.; Pümpel, E.; Grubwieser, G.; Emshoff, R. Diagnosing TMJ internal derangement and osteoarthritis with magnetic resonance imaging. *J. Am. Dent. Assoc.* **2001**, *132*, 753–761. [CrossRef]

24. Turk, D.C.; Gatchel, R.J. *Psychological Approaches to Pain Management: A Practitioner's Hand Book*; The Gilford Press: New York, NY, USA, 2002.
25. Dworkin, S.F.; Massoth, D.L. Temporomandibular disorders and chronic pain: Disease or illness? *J. Prosthet. Dent.* **1994**, *72*, 29–38. [CrossRef]
26. Suvinen, T.I.; Reade, P.C. Temporomandibular disorders: A critical review of the nature of pain and its assessment. *J. Orofac. Pain* **1995**, *9*, 317–339. [PubMed]
27. Yap, A.U.; Tan, K.B.; Chua, E.K.; Tan, H.H. Depression and somatization in patients with temporomandibular disorders. *J. Prosthet. Dent.* **2002**, *88*, 479–484. [CrossRef] [PubMed]
28. Saccomanno, S.; Bernabei, M.; Scoppa, F.; Pirino, A.; Mastrapasqua, R.; Visco, M.A. Coronavirus Lockdown as a Major Life Stressor: Does It Affect TMD Symptoms? *Int. J. Environ. Res. Public Health* **2020**, *17*, 8907. [CrossRef]
29. Medeiros, R.A.; Vieira, D.L.; Silva, E.; Rezende, L.; Santos, R.W.D.; Tabata, L.F. Prevalence of symptoms of temporomandibular disorders, oral behaviors, anxiety, and depression in Dentistry students during the period of social isolation due to COVID-19. *J. Appl. Oral Sci.* **2020**, *28*, e20200445. [CrossRef]
30. Fillingim, R.B.; Ohrbach, R.; Greenspan, J.D.; Knott, C.; Diatchenko, L.; Dubner, R.; Bair, E.; Baraian, C.; Mack, N.; Slade, G.D.; et al. Psychological factors associated with development of TMD: The OPPERA prospective cohort study. *J. Pain Off. J. Am. Pain Soc.* **2013**, *14*, T75–T90. [CrossRef] [PubMed]
31. Schiffman, E.; Ohrbach, R.; Truelove, E.; Look, J.; Anderson, G.; Goulet, J.P.; List, T.; Svensson, P.; Gonzalez, Y.; Lobbezoo, F.; et al. Diagnostic Criteria for Temporomandibular Disorders (DC/TMD) for Clinical and Research Applications: Recommendations of the International RDC/TMD Consortium Network* and Orofacial Pain Special Interest Groupdagger. *J. Oral Facial Pain Headache* **2014**, *28*, 6–27. [CrossRef] [PubMed]
32. Peck, C.C.; Goulet, J.P.; Lobbezoo, F.; Schiffman, E.L.; Alstergren, P.; Anderson, G.C.; de Leeuw, R.; Jensen, R.; Michelotti, A.; Ohrbach, R.; et al. Expanding the taxonomy of the diagnostic criteria for temporomandibular disorders. *J. Oral Rehabil.* **2014**, *41*, 2–23. [CrossRef] [PubMed]
33. Al-Saleh, M.A.; Alsufyani, N.A.; Saltaji, H.; Jaremko, J.L.; Major, P.W. MRI and CBCT image registration of temporomandibular joint: A systematic review. *J. Otolaryngol. Head Neck Surg.* **2016**, *45*, 30. [CrossRef]
34. Al-Saleh, M.A.; Jaremko, J.L.; Alsufyani, N.; Jibri, Z.; Lai, H.; Major, P.W. Assessing the reliability of MRI-CBCT image registration to visualize temporomandibular joints. *Dentomaxillofac. Radiol.* **2015**, *44*, 20140244. [CrossRef] [PubMed]
35. Ladeira, D.B.; da Cruz, A.D.; de Almeida, S.M. Digital panoramic radiography for diagnosis of the temporomandibular joint: CBCT as the gold standard. *Braz. Oral Res.* **2015**, *29*, S1806-83242015000100303. [CrossRef]
36. Larheim, T.A.; Abrahamsson, A.K.; Kristensen, M.; Arvidsson, L.Z. Temporomandibular joint diagnostics using CBCT. *Dentomaxillofac. Radiol.* **2015**, *44*, 20140235. [CrossRef]
37. Su, N.; van Wijk, A.J.; Visscher, C.M.; Lobbezoo, F.; van der Heijden, G. Diagnostic value of ultrasonography for the detection of disc displacements in the temporomandibular joint: A systematic review and meta-analysis. *Clin. Oral Investig.* **2018**, *22*, 2599–2614. [CrossRef]
38. Talmaceanu, D.; Lenghel, L.M.; Bolog, N.; Popa Stanila, R.; Buduru, S.; Leucuta, D.C.; Rotar, H.; Baciut, M.; Baciut, G. High-resolution ultrasonography in assessing temporomandibular joint disc position. *Med. Ultrason.* **2018**, *1*, 64–70. [CrossRef]
39. Choi, B.H.; Yoon, S.H.; Song, S.I.; Yoon, J.K.; Lee, S.J.; An, Y.S. Comparison of Diagnostic Performance Between Visual and Quantitative Assessment of Bone Scintigraphy Results in Patients With Painful Temporomandibular Disorder. *Medicine* **2016**, *95*, e2485. [CrossRef]
40. Epstein, J.B.; Rea, A.; Chahal, O. The use of bone scintigraphy in temporomandibular joint disorders. *Oral Dis.* **2002**, *8*, 47–53. [CrossRef] [PubMed]
41. Kang, J.H.; An, Y.S.; Park, S.H.; Song, S.I. Influences of age and sex on the validity of bone scintigraphy for the diagnosis of temporomandibular joint osteoarthritis. *Int. J. Oral Maxillofac. Surg.* **2018**, *47*, 1445–1452. [CrossRef] [PubMed]
42. Lee, Y.H.; Hong, I.K.; Chun, Y.H. Prediction of painful temporomandibular joint osteoarthritis in juvenile patients using bone scintigraphy. *Clin. Exp. Dent. Res.* **2019**, *5*, 225–235. [CrossRef] [PubMed]
43. Park, K.S.; Song, H.C.; Cho, S.G.; Kang, S.R.; Kim, J.; Jun, H.M.; Song, M.; Jeong, G.C.; Park, H.J.; Kwon, S.Y.; et al. Open-Mouth Bone Scintigraphy Is Better than Closed-Mouth Bone Scintigraphy in the Diagnosis of Temporomandibular Osteoarthritis. *Nucl. Med. Mol. Imaging* **2016**, *50*, 213–218. [CrossRef]
44. Chan, B.H.; Leung, Y.Y. SPECT bone scintigraphy for the assessment of condylar growth activity in mandibular asymmetry: Is it accurate? *Int. J. Oral Maxillofac. Surg.* **2018**, *47*, 470–479. [CrossRef] [PubMed]
45. Kumar, A.; Brennan, M.T. Differential diagnosis of orofacial pain and temporomandibular disorder. *Dent. Clin. N. Am.* **2013**, *57*, 419–428. [CrossRef]
46. Alpaslan, G.H.; Alpaslan, C. Efficacy of temporomandibular joint arthrocentesis with and without injection of sodium hyaluronate in treatment of internal derangements. *J. Oral Maxillofac. Surg.* **2001**, *59*, 613–618. [CrossRef]
47. Nitzan, D.W.; Dolwick, M.F.; Heft, M.W. Arthroscopic lavage and lysis of the temporomandibular joint: A change in perspective. *J. Oral Maxillofac. Surg.* **1990**, *48*, 798–801. [CrossRef]
48. Zhang, C.; Wu, J.Y.; Deng, D.L.; He, B.Y.; Tao, Y.; Niu, Y.M.; Deng, M.H. Efficacy of splint therapy for the management of temporomandibular disorders: A meta-analysis. *Oncotarget* **2016**, *7*, 84043–84053. [CrossRef] [PubMed]

49. Riley, P.; Glenny, A.M.; Worthington, H.V.; Jacobsen, E.; Robertson, C.; Durham, J.; Davies, S.; Petersen, H.; Boyers, D. Oral splints for temporomandibular disorder or bruxism: A systematic review. *Br. Dent. J.* **2020**, *228*, 191–197. [CrossRef]
50. Al-Moraissi, E.A.; Farea, R.; Qasem, K.A.; Al-Wadeai, M.S.; Al-Sabahi, M.E.; Al-Iryani, G.M. Effectiveness of occlusal splint therapy in the management of temporomandibular disorders: Network meta-analysis of randomized controlled trials. *Int. J. Oral Maxillofac. Surg.* **2020**, *49*, 1042–1056. [CrossRef]
51. Alkhutari, A.S.; Alyahya, A.; Rodrigues Conti, P.C.; Christidis, N.; Al-Moraissi, E.A. Is the therapeutic effect of occlusal stabilization appliances more than just placebo effect in the management of painful temporomandibular disorders? A network meta-analysis of randomized clinical trials. *J. Prosthet. Dent.* **2020**. [CrossRef] [PubMed]
52. Seifeldin, S.A.; Elhayes, K.A. Soft versus hard occlusal splint therapy in the management of temporomandibular disorders (TMDs). *Saudi Dent. J.* **2015**, *27*, 208–214. [CrossRef]
53. Incorvati, C.; Romeo, A.; Fabrizi, A.; Defila, L.; Vanti, C.; Gatto, M.R.A.; Marchetti, C.; Pillastrini, P. Effectiveness of physical therapy in addition to occlusal splint in myogenic temporomandibular disorders: Protocol of a randomised controlled trial. *BMJ Open* **2020**, *10*, e038438. [CrossRef]
54. van der Meer, H.A.; Calixtre, L.B.; Engelbert, R.H.H.; Visscher, C.M.; Nijhuis-van der Sanden, M.W.; Speksnijder, C.M. Effects of physical therapy for temporomandibular disorders on headache pain intensity: A systematic review. *Musculoskelet. Sci. Pract.* **2020**, *50*, 102277. [CrossRef] [PubMed]
55. Kutuk, S.G.; Ozkan, Y.; Kutuk, M.; Ozdas, T. Comparison of the Efficacies of Dry Needling and Botox Methods in the Treatment of Myofascial Pain Syndrome Affecting the Temporomandibular Joint. *J. Craniofacial Surg.* **2019**, *30*, 1556–1559. [CrossRef]
56. Connelly, S.T.; Myung, J.; Gupta, R.; Tartaglia, G.M.; Gizdulich, A.; Yang, J.; Silva, R. Clinical outcomes of Botox injections for chronic temporomandibular disorders: Do we understand how Botox works on muscle, pain, and the brain? *Int. J. Oral Maxillofac. Surg.* **2017**, *46*, 322–327. [CrossRef]
57. Kim, Y.H.; Bang, J.I.; Son, H.J.; Kim, Y.; Kim, J.H.; Bae, H.; Han, S.J.; Yoon, H.J.; Kim, B.S. Protective effects of extracorporeal shockwave on rat chondrocytes and temporomandibular joint osteoarthritis; preclinical evaluation with in vivo(99m)Tc-HDP SPECT and ex vivo micro-CT. *Osteoarthr. Cartil.* **2019**, *27*, 1692–1701. [CrossRef]
58. Schenk, I.; Vesper, M.; Nam, V.C. Initial results using extracorporeal low energy shockwave therapy ESWT in muscle reflex-induced lock jaw. *Mund Kiefer Gesichtschir.* **2002**, *6*, 351–355. [CrossRef] [PubMed]
59. Dworkin, S.F.; Turner, J.A.; Mancl, L.; Wilson, L.; Massoth, D.; Huggins, K.H.; LeResche, L.; Truelove, E. A randomized clinical trial of a tailored comprehensive care treatment program for temporomandibular disorders. *J. Orofac. Pain* **2002**, *16*, 259–276.
60. Türp, J.C.; Jokstad, A.; Motschall, E.; Schindler, H.J.; Windecker-Gétaz, I.; Ettlin, D.A. Is there a superiority of multimodal as opposed to simple therapy in patients with temporomandibular disorders? A qualitative systematic review of the literature. *Clin. Oral Implant. Res.* **2007**, *18* (Suppl. 3), 138–150. [CrossRef]
61. Conti, P.C.; Correa, A.S.; Lauris, J.R.; Stuginski-Barbosa, J. Management of painful temporomandibular joint clicking with different intraoral devices and counseling: A controlled study. *J. Appl. Oral Sci.* **2015**, *23*, 529–535. [CrossRef]
62. de Resende, C.; de Oliveira Medeiros, F.G.L.; de Figueiredo Rego, C.R.; Bispo, A.S.L.; Barbosa, G.A.S.; de Almeida, E.O. Short-term effectiveness of conservative therapies in pain, quality of life, and sleep in patients with temporomandibular disorders: A randomized clinical trial. *Cranio* **2019**, 1–9. [CrossRef]
63. de Barros Pascoal, A.L.; de Freitas, R.; da Silva, L.F.G.; Oliveira, A.; Dos Santos Calderon, P. Effectiveness of Counseling on Chronic Pain Management in Patients with Temporomandibular Disorders. *J. Oral Facial Pain Headache* **2020**, *34*, 77–82. [CrossRef]
64. Delgado-Delgado, R.; Iriarte-Álvarez, N.; Valera-Calero, J.A.; Centenera-Centenera, M.B.; Garnacho-Garnacho, V.E.; Gallego-Sendarrubias, G.M. Association between temporomandibular disorders with clinical and sociodemographic features: An observational study. *Int. J. Clin. Pract* **2021**, e13961. [CrossRef]
65. Al-Ani, Z. Occlusion and Temporomandibular Disorders: A Long-Standing Controversy in Dentistry. *Prim. Dent. J.* **2020**, *9*, 43–48. [CrossRef]
66. Manfredini, D.; Lombardo, L.; Siciliani, G. Temporomandibular disorders and dental occlusion. A systematic review of association studies: End of an era? *J. Oral Rehabil.* **2017**, *44*, 908–923. [CrossRef]
67. Kakudate, N.; Yokoyama, Y.; Sumida, F.; Matsumoto, Y.; Gordan, V.V.; Gilbert, G.H.; Velly, A.M.; Schiffman, E.L. Dentist Practice Patterns and Therapeutic Confidence in the Treatment of Pain Related to Temporomandibular Disorders in a Dental Practice-Based Research Network. *J. Oral Facial Pain Headache* **2017**, *31*, 152–158. [CrossRef] [PubMed]
68. Onishi, M. Arthroscopy of the temporomandibular joint (author's transl). *Kokubyo Gakkai Zasshi* **1975**, *42*, 207–213. [CrossRef] [PubMed]
69. Murakami, K.; Ono, T. Temporomandibular joint arthroscopy by inferolateral approach. *Int. J. Oral Maxillofac. Surg.* **1986**, *15*, 410–417. [CrossRef]
70. Sanders, B. Arthroscopic surgery of the temporomandibular joint: Treatment of internal derangement with persistent closed lock. *Oral Surg. Oral Med. Oral Pathol.* **1986**, *62*, 361–372. [CrossRef]
71. Sanders, B.; Buoncristiani, R. Diagnostic and surgical arthroscopy of the temporomandibular joint: Clinical experience with 137 procedures over a 2-year period. *J. Craniomandib. Disord.: Facial Oral Pain* **1987**, *1*, 202–213.
72. McCain, J.P. Arthroscopy of the human temporomandibular joint. *J. Oral Maxillofac. Surg.* **1988**, *46*, 648–655. [CrossRef]
73. McCain, J.P.; Sanders, B.; Koslin, M.G.; Quinn, J.H.; Peters, P.B.; Indresano, A.T. Temporomandibular joint arthroscopy: A 6-year multicenter retrospective study of 4,831 joints. *J. Oral Maxillofac. Surg.* **1992**, *50*, 926–930. [CrossRef]

74. Reston, J.T.; Turkelson, C.M. Meta-analysis of surgical treatments for temporomandibular articular disorders. *J. Oral Maxillofac. Surg.* **2003**, *61*, 3–10. [CrossRef]
75. Schiffman, E.L.; Velly, A.M.; Look, J.O.; Hodges, J.S.; Swift, J.Q.; Decker, K.L.; Anderson, Q.N.; Templeton, R.B.; Lenton, P.A.; Kang, W.; et al. Effects of four treatment strategies for temporomandibular joint closed lock. *Int. J. Oral Maxillofac. Surg.* **2014**, *43*, 217–226. [CrossRef]
76. Dimitroulis, G. Outcomes of temporomandibular joint arthroscopy in patients with painful but otherwise normal joints. *J. Craniomaxillofac. Surg.* **2015**, *43*, 940–943. [CrossRef]
77. McCain, J.P.; Hossameldin, R.H.; Srouji, S.; Maher, A. Arthroscopic discopexy is effective in managing temporomandibular joint internal derangement in patients with Wilkes stage II and III. *J. Oral Maxillofac. Surg.* **2015**, *73*, 391–401. [CrossRef]
78. Al-Moraissi, E.A. Arthroscopy versus arthrocentesis in the management of internal derangement of the temporomandibular joint: A systematic review and meta-analysis. *Int. J. Oral Maxillofac. Surg.* **2015**, *44*, 104–112. [CrossRef]
79. Liu, X.; Zheng, J.; Cai, X.; Abdelrehem, A.; Yang, C. Techniques of Yang's arthroscopic discopexy for temporomandibular joint rotational anterior disc displacement. *Int. J. Oral Maxillofac. Surg.* **2019**, *48*, 769–778. [CrossRef]
80. Machoň, V.; Levorová, J.; Hirjak, D.; Beňo, M.; Drahoš, M.; Foltán, R. Does arthroscopic lysis and lavage in subjects with Wilkes III internal derangement reduce pain? *Oral Maxillofac. Surg.* **2021**. [CrossRef] [PubMed]
81. Nitzan, D.W.; Dolwick, M.F.; Martinez, G.A. Temporomandibular joint arthrocentesis: A simplified treatment for severe, limited mouth opening. *J. Oral Maxillofac. Surg.* **1991**, *49*, 1163–1167. [CrossRef]
82. Alpaslan, C.; Kahraman, S.; Guner, B.; Cula, S. Does the use of soft or hard splints affect the short-term outcome of temporomandibular joint arthrocentesis? *Int J. Oral Maxillofac. Surg.* **2008**, *37*, 424–427. [CrossRef] [PubMed]
83. Bayramoglu, Z.; Tozoglu, S. Comparison of single- and double-puncture arthrocentesis for the treatment of temporomandibular joint disorders: A six-month, prospective study. *Cranio* **2019**, 1–6. [CrossRef]
84. Carvajal, W.A.; Laskin, D.M. Long-term evaluation of arthrocentesis for the treatment of internal derangements of the temporomandibular joint. *J. Oral Maxillofac. Surg.* **2000**, *58*, 852–855. [CrossRef]
85. Diracoglu, D.; Saral, I.B.; Keklik, B.; Kurt, H.; Emekli, U.; Ozcakar, L.; Karan, A.; Aksoy, C. Arthrocentesis versus nonsurgical methods in the treatment of temporomandibular disc displacement without reduction. *Oral Surg. Oral Med. Oral Pathol. Oral Radiol. Endod.* **2009**, *108*, 3–8. [CrossRef] [PubMed]
86. Emshoff, R.; Rudisch, A. Determining predictor variables for treatment outcomes of arthrocentesis and hydraulic distention of the temporomandibular joint. *J. Oral Maxillofac. Surg.* **2004**, *62*, 816–823. [CrossRef]
87. Monje-Gil, F.; Nitzan, D.; Gonzalez-Garcia, R. Temporomandibular joint arthrocentesis. Review of the literature. *Med. Oral Patol Oral Cir. Bucal* **2012**, *17*, e575–e581. [CrossRef] [PubMed]
88. Neeli, A.S.; Umarani, M.; Kotrashetti, S.M.; Baliga, S. Arthrocentesis for the treatment of internal derangement of the temporomandibular joint. *J. Maxillofac. Oral Surg.* **2010**, *9*, 350–354. [CrossRef] [PubMed]
89. Nitzan, D.W.; Price, A. The use of arthrocentesis for the treatment of osteoarthritic temporomandibular joints. *J. Oral Maxillofac. Surg.* **2001**, *59*, 1154–1159. [CrossRef]
90. Nitzan, D.W.; Samson, B.; Better, H. Long-term outcome of arthrocentesis for sudden-onset, persistent, severe closed lock of the temporomandibular joint. *J. Oral Maxillofac. Surg.* **1997**, *55*, 151–157. [CrossRef]
91. Nitzan, D.W.; Svidovsky, J.; Zini, A.; Zadik, Y. Effect of Arthrocentesis on Symptomatic Osteoarthritis of the Temporomandibular Joint and Analysis of the Effect of Preoperative Clinical and Radiologic Features. *J. Oral Maxillofac. Surg.* **2017**, *75*, 260–267. [CrossRef]
92. Polat, M.E.; Yanik, S. Efficiency of arthrocentesis treatment for different temporomandibular joint disorders. *Int. J. Oral Maxillofac. Surg.* **2020**, *49*, 621–627. [CrossRef]
93. Toameh, M.H.; Alkhouri, I.; Karman, M.A. Management of patients with disk displacement without reduction of the temporomandibular joint by arthrocentesis alone, plus hyaluronic acid or plus platelet-rich plasma. *Dent. Med. Probl.* **2019**, *56*, 265–272. [CrossRef]
94. Yilmaz, O.; Korkmaz, Y.T.; Tuzuner, T. Comparison of treatment efficacy between hyaluronic acid and arthrocentesis plus hyaluronic acid in internal derangements of temporomandibular joint. *J. Craniomaxillofac. Surg.* **2019**, *47*, 1720–1727. [CrossRef]
95. Vos, L.M.; Huddleston Slater, J.J.; Stegenga, B. Arthrocentesis as initial treatment for temporomandibular joint arthropathy: A randomized controlled trial. *J. Craniomaxillofac. Surg.* **2014**, *42*, e134–e139. [CrossRef] [PubMed]
96. Al-Moraissi, E.A.; Wolford, L.M.; Ellis, E., 3rd; Neff, A. The hierarchy of different treatments for arthrogenous temporomandibular disorders: A network meta-analysis of randomized clinical trials. *J. Craniomaxillofac. Surg.* **2020**, *48*, 9–23. [CrossRef] [PubMed]
97. Li, D.T.S.; Wong, N.S.M.; Li, S.K.Y.; McGrath, C.P.; Leung, Y.Y. Timing of Arthrocentesis in the Management of Temporomandibular Disorders: An Integrative Review and Meta-analysis. *Int. J. Oral Maxillofac. Surg.* **2021**. [CrossRef]
98. Hobeich, J.B.; Salameh, Z.A.; Ismail, E.; Sadig, W.M.; Hokayem, N.E.; Almas, K. Arthroscopy versus arthrocentesis. A retrospective study of disc displacement management without reduction. *Saudi Med. J.* **2007**, *28*, 1541–1544. [PubMed]
99. Laskin, D.M. Arthroscopy Versus Arthrocentesis for Treating Internal Derangements of the Temporomandibular Joint. *Oral Maxillofac. Surg. Clin. N. Am.* **2018**, *30*, 325–328. [CrossRef]
100. Monteiro, J.; de Arruda, J.A.A.; Silva, E.; Vasconcelos, B. Is Single-Puncture TMJ Arthrocentesis Superior to the Double-Puncture Technique for the Improvement of Outcomes in Patients With TMDs? *J. Oral Maxillofac. Surg.* **2020**, *78*, 1319.e1311–1319.e1315. [CrossRef] [PubMed]

101. Nagori, S.A.; Roy Chowdhury, S.K.; Thukral, H.; Jose, A.; Roychoudhury, A. Single puncture versus standard double needle arthrocentesis for the management of temporomandibular joint disorders: A systematic review. *J. Oral Rehabil.* **2018**, *45*, 810–818. [CrossRef]
102. Folle, F.S.; Poluha, R.L.; Setogutti, E.T.; Grossmann, E. Double puncture versus single puncture arthrocentesis for the management of unilateral temporomandibular joint disc displacement without reduction: A randomized controlled trial. *J. Craniomaxillofac. Surg.* **2018**, *46*, 2003–2007. [CrossRef] [PubMed]
103. Bhargava, D.; Thomas, S.; Pawar, P.; Jain, M.; Pathak, P. Ultrasound-guided arthrocentesis using single-puncture, double-lumen, single-barrel needle for patients with temporomandibular joint acute closed lock internal derangement. *Oral Maxillofac. Surg.* **2019**, *23*, 159–165. [CrossRef]
104. Antony, P.G.; Sebastian, A.; Annapoorani, D.; Varghese, K.G.; Mohan, S.; Jayakumar, N.; Dominic, S.; John, B. Comparison of clinical outcomes of treatment of dysfunction of the temporomandibular joint between conventional and ultrasound-guided arthrocentesis. *Br. J. Oral Maxillofac. Surg.* **2019**, *57*, 62–66. [CrossRef]
105. Bilgir, E.; Yildirim, D.; Senturk, M.F.; Orhan, H. Clinical and ultrasonographic evaluation of ultrasound-guided single puncture temporomandibular joint arthrocentesis. *Cranio* **2020**, 1–10. [CrossRef]
106. Hu, Y.; Zhang, X.; Liu, S.; Xu, F. Ultrasound-guided vs conventional arthrocentesis for management of temporomandibular joint disorders: A systematic review and meta-analysis. *Cranio* **2020**. [CrossRef]
107. Leung, Y.Y.; Wu, F.H.W.; Chan, H.H. Ultrasonography-guided arthrocentesis versus conventional arthrocentesis in treating internal derangement of temporomandibular joint: A systematic review. *Clin. Oral Investig.* **2020**, *24*, 3771–3780. [CrossRef]
108. Haigler, M.C.; Abdulrehman, E.; Siddappa, S.; Kishore, R.; Padilla, M.; Enciso, R. Use of platelet-rich plasma, platelet-rich growth factor with arthrocentesis or arthroscopy to treat temporomandibular joint osteoarthritis: Systematic review with meta-analyses. *J. Am. Dent. Assoc.* **2018**, *149*, 940–952.e942. [CrossRef]
109. Liu, Y.; Wu, J.S.; Tang, Y.L.; Tang, Y.J.; Fei, W.; Liang, X.H. Multiple Treatment Meta-Analysis of Intra-Articular Injection for Temporomandibular Osteoarthritis. *J. Oral Maxillofac. Surg.* **2020**, *78*, 373.e371–373.e318. [CrossRef]
110. Chowdhury, S.K.R.; Saxena, V.; Rajkumar, K.; Shadamarshan, R.A. Evaluation of Total Alloplastic Temporomandibular Joint Replacement in TMJ Ankylosis. *J. Maxillofac. Oral Surg.* **2019**, *18*, 293–298. [CrossRef]
111. Bhargava, D.; Neelakandan, R.S.; Dalsingh, V.; Sharma, Y.; Pandey, A.; Pandey, A.; Beena, S.; Koneru, G. A three dimensional (3D) musculoskeletal finite element analysis of DARSN temporomandibular joint (TMJ) prosthesis for total unilateral alloplastic joint replacement. *J. Stomatol. Oral Maxillofac. Surg.* **2019**, *120*, 517–522. [CrossRef] [PubMed]
112. Mercuri, L.G. Costochondral Graft Versus Total Alloplastic Joint for Temporomandibular Joint Reconstruction. *Oral Maxillofac. Surg. Clin. N. Am.* **2018**, *30*, 335–342. [CrossRef]
113. Lotesto, A.; Miloro, M.; Mercuri, L.G.; Sukotjo, C. Status of alloplastic total temporomandibular joint replacement procedures performed by members of the American Society of Temporomandibular Joint Surgeons. *Int. J. Oral Maxillofac. Surg.* **2017**, *46*, 93–96. [CrossRef] [PubMed]
114. Ramos, A.; Mesnard, M. Christensen vs Biomet Microfixation alloplastic TMJ implant: Are there improvements? A numerical study. *J. Craniomaxillofac. Surg.* **2015**, *43*, 1398–1403. [CrossRef]
115. Neelakandan, R.S.; Raja, A.V.; Krishnan, A.M. Total Alloplastic Temporomandibular Joint Reconstruction for Management of TMJ Ankylosis. *J. Maxillofac. Oral Surg.* **2014**, *13*, 575–582. [CrossRef]
116. Burgess, M.; Bowler, M.; Jones, R.; Hase, M.; Murdoch, B. Improved outcomes after alloplastic TMJ replacement: Analysis of a multicenter study from Australia and New Zealand. *J. Oral Maxillofac. Surg.* **2014**, *72*, 1251–1257. [CrossRef] [PubMed]

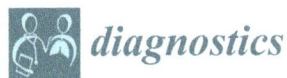

Review

Comprehensive Management of Rheumatic Diseases Affecting the Temporomandibular Joint

Lauren Covert [1], Heather Van Mater [1] and Benjamin L. Hechler [2,3,*]

1. Department of Pediatrics, Division of Rheumatology, Duke University Hospitals, Durham, NC 27710, USA; lauren.tam@duke.edu (L.C.); heather.vanmater@duke.edu (H.V.M.)
2. Department of Surgery, Division of Plastic, Maxillofacial, and Oral Surgery, Duke University Hospitals, Durham, NC 27710, USA
3. Department of Head and Neck Surgery and Communication Sciences, Duke University Hospitals, Durham, NC 27710, USA
* Correspondence: Benjamin.hechler@duke.edu

Abstract: The temporomandibular joint (TMJ) is a synovial joint and thus is vulnerable to the afflictions that may affect other joints in the fields of rheumatology and orthopedics. Too often temporomandibular complaints are seen strictly as dental or orofacial concerns. Similarly, patients with known rheumatic disease may not have their TMJs included in routine screening and monitoring protocols. The purpose of this review is to highlight the rheumatic conditions likely to affect the TMJ and outline medical and surgical management in these patients with a focus on the need for continued patient reassessment and monitoring.

Keywords: temporomandibular joint; temporomandibular disorder; rheumatic disease; juvenile idiopathic arthritis; rheumatoid arthritis; inflammatory arthritis

1. Introduction

The temporomandibular joint (TMJ) is a synovial joint of high functional significance. Although TMJ disorders (TMD) are often thought of as dental or orofacial phenomena, we must not forget that true intracapsular, diacapitular TMJ disease is an arthropathy. When significant intracapsular TMJ damage and dysfunction are present, occlusal imbalance or myofascial pain are never the cause, and an underlying arthropathy must be investigated. Similarly, patients with known rheumatic diseases should be investigated for TMJ involvement. Furthermore, it should be kept in mind that the young to middle-aged female population is the typical patient population presenting with autoimmune disorders and TMD [1]. It is thus crucial that rheumatologists, dentists, oral and maxillofacial surgeons (OMS), and head and neck surgeons are able to independently understand the TMJ's place in manifesting rheumatic diseases.

One-fifth to one-fourth of Americans report a doctor-diagnosed arthritic condition [2], with the Centers for Disease Control and Prevention (CDC) confirming that approximately 25% of US adults suffer from arthritis [3]. The World Health Organization (WHO) has quantified the worldwide morbidity of some of the most common arthritic conditions, with 25% of those with osteoarthritis (OA) unable to perform major daily activities of living, and 50% of those with rheumatoid arthritis (RA) unable to perform full-time job activities within 10 years of disease onset [4]. Although certain autoimmune rheumatic diseases are less common, their individual patient morbidity can be significantly more serious. The terminology used to refer to these musculoskeletal conditions is often inconsistent and confusing. Joint diseases should collectively be referred to as "arthropathies", although in the English language the term "arthritis" has been used extensively and in disparate contexts. Throughout this manuscript, "rheumatic diseases" is used to refer primarily to inflammatory autoimmune conditions, unless otherwise indicated (e.g., osteoarthritis).

Citation: Covert, L.; Mater, H.V.; Hechler, B.L. Comprehensive Management of Rheumatic Diseases Affecting the Temporomandibular Joint. *Diagnostics* **2021**, *11*, 409. https://doi.org/10.3390/diagnostics 11030409

Academic Editor: Luis Eduardo Almeida

Received: 13 February 2021
Accepted: 25 February 2021
Published: 27 February 2021

Publisher's Note: MDPI stays neutral with regard to jurisdictional claims in published maps and institutional affiliations.

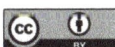

Copyright: © 2021 by the authors. Licensee MDPI, Basel, Switzerland. This article is an open access article distributed under the terms and conditions of the Creative Commons Attribution (CC BY) license (https:// creativecommons.org/licenses/by/ 4.0/).

Comprehensive management of the TMJ in rheumatic diseases is based upon the initial understanding of four important principles:

1.1. All TMD Should Be Considered as Potentially Secondary to an Underlying Systemic Condition

The first principle in understanding how to manage TMD in rheumatic diseases is simply the realization that TMD may be a manifestation of an underlying rheumatic condition. It can again not be overemphasized that true intracapsular, diacapitular TMJ disease is an arthropathy. Similar to how visualizing an oral lesion concerning for squamous cell carcinoma should prompt questions of weight loss or dysphagia, TMJ signs or symptoms should prompt questions of other joint involvement, constitutional symptoms, or synchronously or metachronously identified organ involvement.

1.2. TMD Presents Differently in Rheumatic Diseases Than in Non-Rheumatic TMD

Clinicians who frequently treat TMD in non-rheumatic patients are accustomed to a pattern of linear disease progression consistent with the Wilkes classification. Indeed, Wilkes commented on the "strong relation to the time course of the organic lesions present", with clinical, radiographic, and pathologic findings correlating well [5]. In rheumatic diseases—particularly autoimmune conditions requiring various medical interventions and those present in children and adolescents—the temporal progression of TMD may be unexpected, and a correlation between clinical and radiographic findings is not to be assumed.

1.3. Temporomandibular Joint Disease Is a Continuum

In science in general and medicine in particular, "cut offs" are often chosen by statistical optimization and therefore may not have strict clinical correlations. In reality, clinical continua are much more common. Accordingly, it is thus much more clinically relevant to follow parameters *within* an individual patient *across time* than to compare parameters *across* patients *at a single time point*. Patients who develop more severe systemic symptoms will be more likely to develop more severe TMJ symptoms.

1.4. Rheumatic Diseases Can also Manifest as Parotid Abnormalities

Although not the topic of this review, it should be realized that rheumatic conditions frequently affect not only the TMJ but the anatomically proximate parotid glands. Indeed, those with rheumatoid arthritis (RA) have been shown to have abnormal intra-parotid lymph nodes as compared to controls [6]. This gives further credence to principle one, that pre-auricular signs and symptoms should always be investigated in the context of known or potential rheumatic conditions. A corollary to this line of thought is that should a CT of the face be planned for evaluation of possible TMJ pathology, addition of IV contrast should be considered—assuming the patient's medical condition allows—in the event that TMJ, infratemporal fossa, or parotid soft tissue pathology is the true etiology (Figure 1).

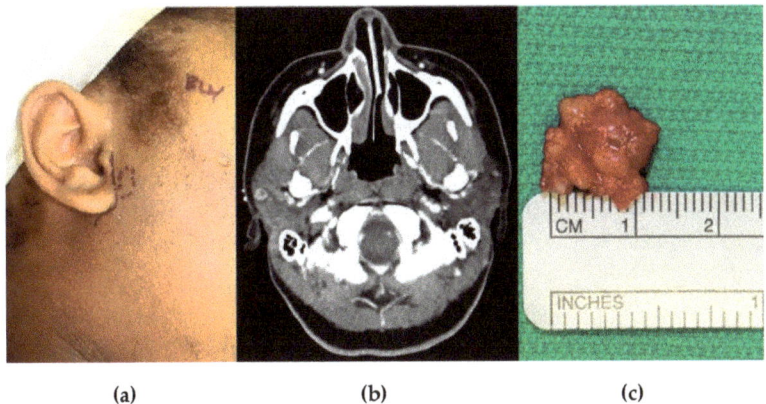

Figure 1. A 26-year-old female presented for evaluation with chief complaints of right TMJ popping and pre-auricular pain for one year. She reported a strong family history of both systemic lupus erythematosus and Sjogren Syndrome. C-reactive protein was elevated and anti-nuclear antibodies showed speckled and homogenous patterns in high titers. (**a**) Dotted line indicates location of pain per patient; (**b**) CT was intentionally obtained with contrast to evaluate for TMJ and soft tissue abnormalities. Note an intra-parotid lesion lying immediately lateral to the mandibular condyle; (**c**) Intra-parotid lesion removed and found to be a basal cell adenoma. The patient's symptoms resolved after treatment.

2. Rheumatic DISEASES Affecting the Temporomandibular Joint

As will be seen, many rheumatic diseases can affect the TMJ. Original reviews suggesting that those with rheumatoid arthritis (RA) will have bilateral, symmetric TMJ involvement while those with seronegative spondyloarthropathies (SNS) will have unilateral disease should be viewed with caution [7] (Figure 2). For example, a review of the currently reported TMJ ankylosis cases in ankylosing spondylitis (AS) patients in the English literature suggests that approximately half presented with bilateral ankylosis [8]. A corollary of this line of thought is the fact that no radiographic findings or clinical signs or symptoms are pathognomonic for a specific rheumatologic disease.

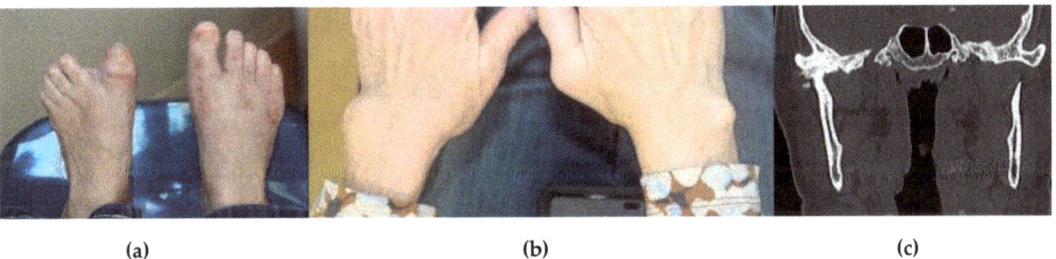

Figure 2. A 56-year-old female presented for evaluation with chief complaints of right TMJ pain and limited mandibular opening. Her history was most notable for long-standing RA refractory to multiple medications. (**a**) Bilateral toe involvement requiring Hoffman procedure; (**b**) Bilateral wrist involvement; (**c**) CT of the face showed early unilateral right TMJ ankylosis, lateral pannus formation, and heterotopic bone formation. The left TMJ was completely normal.

It should also be noted that the more infrequent a specific set of conditions is reported in the literature (e.g., significant TMJ disease in patients with a specific rheumatologic diagnosis), the more anecdotal the reports become. For example, a cursory review of the literature on TMJ disease in rheumatic diseases reveals many case reports of TMJ ankylosis; however, the astute reader must realize the entire reason such reports are worthy of case reports is their overall infrequency amongst a given population.

An abbreviated reference of diagnostic criteria for each condition which can manifest with TMJ dysfunction is presented in Table 1.

Table 1. Abbreviated summary of diagnostic criteria for various rheumatic diseases affecting the TMJ. Criteria provided have been commonly used for clinical and/or research purposes. Abbreviations: **ACR**—American College of Rheumatology; **ANA**—anti-nuclear antibodies; **ARA**—American Rheumatism Association (predecessor of the ACR); **ASAS**—Assessment of Spondyloarthritis International Society; **axSpA**—axial spondyloarthritis; **CASPAR**—Classification of Psoriatic Arthritis Study; **CCP**—cyclic citrullinated peptide; **CRP**—C-reactive protein; **ESR**—erythrocyte sedimentation rate; **EULAR**—European League Against Rheumatism; **FM**—fibromyalgia; **ILAR**—International League of Associations for Rheumatology; **JIA**—juvenile idiopathic arthritis; **PsA**—psoriatic arthritis; **RA**—rheumatoid arthritis; **RF**—rheumatoid factors; **SLE**—systemic lupus erythematosus; **SSc**—systemic sclerosis; **SSS**—symptom severity scale; **WPI**—widespread pain index.

Condition	Abbreviated Diagnostic Criteria	
JIA	**ILAR/EULAR (2001)** • Arthritis 6+ weeks • Age < 16 years at diagnosis • No other identifiable cause	
SSc	**ACR/EULAR (2013)** *Each item is weighted with total score ≥ 9 indicative of definite SSc* • Skin thickening of fingers • Fingertip lesions • Telangiectasias • Abnormal nailfold capillaries • Pulmonary arterial hypertension and/or interstitial lung disease • Raynaud phenomenon • Anti-centromere, -topoisomerase I, or -RNA polymerase III antibodies	
RA	**ARA (1987)** *4+ of the following* • Morning stiffness for 6+ weeks • Arthritis, 3+ joints, for 6+ weeks • Arthritis, hands, for 6+ weeks • Symmetric arthritis for 6+ weeks • Rheumatoid nodules • RF+ • Radiographic change	**ACR/EULAR (2010)** • Synovitis, 1+ joint • Absence of alternative diagnosis *AND* • Score of 6+ out of the following, which are weighted: • Number of involved joints • RF+ or anti-CCP+ • Elevated ESR or CRP • Symptoms 6+ weeks
SLE	**ACR (1997)** • 4+ of 11 criteria including mucocutaneous and major organ clinical criteria and immunologic laboratory criteria	**ACR/EULAR (2019)** • ANA+ or equivalent • At least one clinical criterion • Additional clinical or immunologic criteria are weighted and are additive towards a final score (≥10 = SLE)
axSpA	**ASAS (2009)** • 3+ months of back pain with onset prior to 45 years of age • IF sacroiliitis on imaging, 1+ SpA feature is required • IF no sacroiliitis on imaging, HLA-B27+ and 2+ SpA features are required	

Table 1. Cont.

Condition	Abbreviated Diagnostic Criteria	
PsA	**CASPAR (2006)** *3+ points from weighted items of the following* • Skin psoriasis • Nail lesions • Dactylitis • Negative RF • Juxta-articular bone formation	
FM	**ACR (1990)** • Widespread, chronic pain • 11+ of 18 tender points • No other identifiable cause	**ACR (2010)** • WPI ≥ 7 + SSS ≥ 5 <u>OR</u> WPI ≥ 3 + SSS ≥ 9 • Symptoms 3+ months • No other identifiable cause

2.1. Juvenile Idiopathic Arthritis

Juvenile idiopathic arthritis (JIA), formerly known as juvenile rheumatoid arthritis (JRA), is seen by many as the most concerning rheumatic condition associated with TMJ dysfunction given the risk of dentofacial deformity in the growing child. Consequently, it is the most studied rheumatic condition causing TMJ dysfunction. Its diagnosis per the International League of Associations for Rheumatology (ILAR) requires six weeks of arthritis in a patient under 16 years of age with the exclusion of other etiologic diagnoses [9]. Seven subcategories of the disease are recognized. It is reported that 17–87% of JIA patients will have TMJ involvement [10]. Of particular interest is that in JIA patients with acute TMJ arthritis up to 71% of cases may be asymptomatic and up to 63% may have normal findings on clinical exam [11]. Indeed, even when ultrasonic or MRI evaluation confirms joint effusion in these patients, the vast majority have been shown to be asymptomatic [12,13]. Because by definition the disease process begins in childhood or adolescence, the risk of dentofacial deformity is substantial.

2.2. Systemic Sclerosis/Scleroderma

Systemic sclerosis (SSc) is a heterogeneous group of disorders which like JIA can manifest in childhood (e.g., localized scleroderma) but is much more common in adults. For decades the mandible has been documented as a bone affected by the disease, both directly and indirectly [14,15]. Compared to the general population, even asymptomatic patients with SSc have decreased mandibular range of motion, although this can be confounded by soft tissue thickening resulting in micrognathia [16]. Although less common than other rheumatic diseases, SSc may be the rheumatic condition most associated with TMJ signs and symptoms, with multiple sources reporting >90% of SSc patients with TMJ signs and symptoms [17,18].

2.3. Rheumatoid Arthritis

Rheumatoid arthritis is characterized by polyarticular, erosive synovitis that is often relatively symmetrical and may present with significant extra-articular organ disease, a point made clear when it is recognized that those with RA have shorter lifespans than healthy controls [19]. It is reported that 5–86% of RA patients will have TMJ involvement, with 20–40% as a relatively consistent finding [20]. Similar to JIA, asymptomatic patients often have significant disease demonstrable on three-dimensional imaging. It has even been suggested that those with RA who are asymptomatic actually have a *higher* likelihood of TMJ degenerative disease detected on CT than symptomatic patients [21]. In contradistinction, symptoms may occur prior to overt TMJ signs, making disease monitoring via C-reactive protein (CRP), erythrocyte sedimentation rate (ESR), and number of involved systemic joints important [22,23]. The presence of anti-cyclic citrullinated protein antibodies has been shown to be significantly associated with development of TMD in RA patients [24]. Cervical spine involvement also appears to increase the likelihood of TMJ disease [25]. A consistent finding in RA patients with TMJ involvement is the predominant sign and symptom being TMJ sounds [17,26], with disease severity (defined by number of edematous joints) associated with TMJ sounds [19].

2.4. Systemic Lupus Erythematosus

Systemic lupus erythematosus (SLE) has for decades been seen as the quintessential autoimmune disorder. Compared to the other rheumatic diseases affecting the TMJ, patients with SLE are less likely to have TMJ signs or symptoms, and there is conflicting data as to whether their signs and symptoms are different from control populations [17,20,27]. A now classic study by Jonsonn compared 37 SLE patients to 37 dental patients (controls) and found significantly worse signs, symptoms, and radiographic condylar flattening in the SLE patients; however, the majority of the SLE cohort had long-standing disease, all but one had systemic arthritis and arthralgia, and radiographic TMJ changes were significantly more common in patients with renal involvement, suggesting that the high frequency of TMJ complaints may represent an overall more active SLE population. [28]. A more recent study did indeed correlate more severe TMJ dysfunction in SLE with increased number of immunosuppressive medications, presumably a surrogate for disease activity [29]. SLE is one of the few conditions where "avascular" or "aseptic" necrosis of the TMJs is mentioned [30–33]; however, most of these reports come from single groups without histologic analysis of condylar specimens with the only assumption being that because patients have been on glucocorticoids avascular necrosis is likely. Conversely, what is much more likely is inflammatory arthritic destruction.

2.5. Axial Spondyloarthritis (Ankylosing Spondylitis, Non-Radiographic Axial Spondyloarthritis)

Both ankylosing spondylitis (AS) and non-radiographic axial spondyloarthritis (nr-axSpA) are subcategories of the umbrella diagnosis of axial spondyloarthritis (axSpA). Both are considered SNS processes. As the name implies, axSpA primarily involves the axial skeleton, either with (AS) or without (nr-axSpA) plain radiographic evidence of disease. AS and nr-axSpA may be distinct disease phenotypes or simply the spectrum of a single underlying disease process, as over the course of five years 20% of nr-axSpA cases develop radiographic evidence of disease [34]. The majority of axSpA patients are HLA-B27 positive, although this test is not completely sensitive or specific for the disease [35]. The TMJ is reported to be involved in 3–22% of patients, with the literature mainly focusing on patients with AS [36]. A general pattern observed in the cases of TMJ ankyloses in axSpA patients is that (1) the rheumatologic diagnosis is often made many years prior to TMJ dysfunction and (2) essentially all patients developing TMJ ankylosis previously had developed cervical spine fusion [37].

2.6. Psoriatic Arthrits

Psoriatic arthritis (PsA) is also an SNS and is a disease process originally said to be found in 5–7% of patients with psoriasis [38] but now thought to occur in 15–25% given the increased awareness and diagnosis of the disease [39]. The clinical patterns of the arthritic component most specific to PsA, as originally described [40], include distal interphalangeal (DIP) arthritis and arthritis mutilans (destructive arthritis), although other patterns may be present with significant overlap to other conditions, most notably RA. Although the TMJ is an infrequently involved joint in PsA, it has indeed been described as the first joint involved in PsA [41]. Because of the relatively low number of reports of PsA affecting the TMJs, firm conclusions on prevalence are difficult to make [8], although a recent review has suggested approximately one-third of PsA patients have TMJ symptoms [42]. Review of reports to date, however, do suggest a tendency for those with PsA and subsequent TMD to have worse disease and a significant erosive component, possibly not surprising given the destructive arthritic pattern present in many with severe PsA [38,43].

2.7. Others

2.7.1. Osteoarthritis

Unlike the disorders described thus far, osteoarthritis (OA) is not a primary autoimmune inflammatory condition but a disease process marked by mechanical breakdown in the setting of abnormal forces or abnormal response to normal forces, with or without the presence of inflammation. Abnormal forces can be of increased magnitude (microtrauma) or increased frequency (microtrauma) [44], or normal forces can be applied to impaired articular cartilage or an abnormal disc-condyle complex [45]. Consequently, unilateral TMJ OA is often associated with asymmetric anatomy, asymmetric masticatory forces, or previous unilateral injury [46]. Unlike the axial or appendicular skeleton, obesity and occupation are not necessarily associated with OA of the TMJ. The diagnosis of TMJ osteoarthritis should, however, mirror the American College of Rheumatology (ACR) classification criteria for OA of the knee and hip: pain should be a primary symptom; joint stiffness, limited mobility, and crepitus will likely be present; radiographic evidence of erosion, subchondral cysts, subchondral sclerosis, and osteophytes are common; and elimination of autoimmune or infectious causes should be ensured [47,48].

2.7.2. Fibromyalgia

Although fibromyalgia (FM) is not a cause of intra-articular TMD, patients with FM often present with signs and symptoms concerning for inflammatory articular disease including pre-auricular pain, pain on mandibular function, limited mouth opening, and diurnal change in symptoms. At least one study has gone as far as to suggest that all patients with FM present with pain when the TMJs and retrodiskal tissues are palpated [49]. A recent systematic review revealed a strong association between FM and TMD; however, the overwhelming association was with regard to complaints of pain, particularly masticatory muscular pain [50]. In this way, the FM patient often has a higher symptom burden relative to any radiographic abnormality while the inflammatory arthritis patient is more likely to have a lower symptom burden relative to the degree of radiographic joint disease. It should be noted that TMJ arthritic disease can present in patients with FM, but FM is not the etiology.

2.7.3. Idiopathic Condylar Resorption

Although not a rheumatic inflammatory disease, idiopathic condylar resorption (ICR) must be mentioned as it presents nearly exclusively in adolescent and young women and thus demographically overlaps the patient population represented by systemic rheumatic conditions. Indeed, the original discussions on this phenomenon highlighted similarity to autoimmune resorption [51], although further investigations also emphasized what is now generally accepted as the role of hormones such as estrogen, prolactin, and endogenous steroids in this process [52]. Although ICR is usually symmetric, unlike rheumatic diseases it is not autoimmune and usually not inflammatory in nature, evidenced by the typical lack of synovitis and joint effusion on MRI even in the setting of active condylysis [53]. One frequently propagated misconception is that ICR is usually asymptomatic [54], when surveys actually suggest that the majority of ICR patients present with TMJ pain and myofascial pain [55]. ICR thus becomes a diagnosis of exclusion when symmetric condylysis is appreciated in a female patient whose rheumatologic work-up is otherwise negative.

3. Systemic Management of Rheumatic Diseases

While there are different types of inflammatory arthritides, as described above, systemic management across these distinct conditions share a similar approach and classes of medication including non-steroidal anti-inflammatory drugs (NSAIDs), corticosteroids, conventional and biologic disease-modifying antirheumatic drugs (DMARDs). Empirical practice with systemic treatment has beneficial effects on TMJ arthritis [56]. Goals of therapy for TMJ arthritis are similar to the treatment of arthritis in general—the cessation and prevention of joint damage, suppression of systemic disease, and eventual remission off medications [57]. Treatments for inflammatory arthritis are individualized based on severity of disease, number of joints involved, physical limitations and potential for joint damage [53].

Most of the literature regarding treatment of inflammatory TMJ arthritis with systemic medication is specific to JIA with a focus on an approach to normalize mandibular growth, reduce MRI-verified inflammation, and preserve osseous TMJ morphology. Current biologic medications have significantly decreased the extent of disability and need for major surgeries and joint replacement in JIA [57]. A retrospective study of 38 patients with JIA involving the TMJ, who were receiving systemic therapy, showed less severe osseous deformity and maintained normal mandibular ramus growth at 2 year follow up compared to baseline MRI. This contrasted to cohort studies with corticosteroid TMJ injections, in which TMJ deformity deteriorated and mandibular ramus growth was impaired [58].

Generally, however, there has been little evidence to guide management for TMJ arthritis. Most randomized controlled trials of DMARDs have not included TMJ involvement as an outcome, and there is minimal prospective data on medical therapy [59]. Consensus on treatment is lacking. In 2014, an 87-center multinational survey of pediatric rheumatologists worldwide showed that first-line treatment of TMJ arthritis varied with NSAIDs in 33%, non-biologic DMARDs in 36%, anti-TNF medication in 5%, and intra-articular steroid injection in 26% [60]. Furthermore, a cross-sectional survey of 52 academic OMS in the US revealed that the majority (81%) of JIA patients were being treated on average with 1–2 systemic medications, 13% on 3–4 medications and only 5% on no systemic medications [61]. It is worth noting that even with optimal medical management for peripheral arthritis in JIA, the TMJ is the most common joint that does not respond to initial therapy. Retrospective studies suggest that response to medical therapy of the TMJ may lag behind that of other joints for unclear reasons [62]. Consensus on treatment of TMJ arthritis in JIA is currently in development amongst pediatric rheumatologists within the US based on expert opinion.

3.1. NSAIDs

NSAIDs such as naproxen, ibuprofen, and indomethacin are commonly used as an initial therapy in inflammatory arthritis with or without TMJ involvement. NSAIDs inhibit cyclooxygenase (COX)-2 activity, reducing cytokine-induced destruction of the extracellular matrix of the TMJ [63]. While often part of a maintenance medication regimen, NSAIDs are only beneficial for reducing TMJ complaints in a minority of patients; more aggressive treatment with DMARDs is generally necessary [10]. In fact, NSAIDs are effective for TMJ arthritis for one-fourth to one-third of JIA patients but primarily in oligoarticular disease. They are often considered as adjunctive or bridge therapy to more definitive interventions for TMJ disease [57]. NSAIDs are usually well tolerated. Potential side effects include gastritis, gastrointestinal bleeding, headache, increased sun sensitivity, and hepatic and/or renal dysfunction [53].

3.2. Conventional DMARDs

Conventional DMARDs include sulfasalazine, leflunomide, and methotrexate. Methotrexate is the only medication with significant evidence in the treatment of TMJ arthritis [57] and is usually first line in practice for JIA with TMJ involvement. Weekly intramuscular injection of methotrexate has been shown to decrease cartilage degeneration in rabbits with antigen-induced arthritis but failed to eliminate arthritis completely [64]. Furthermore, in a cross-sectional study, Ince et al. demonstrated that methotrexate therapy may minimize TMJ destruction in polyarticular JIA. Methotrexate is a folic acid analog that inhibits dihydrofolate reductase, leading to inhibition of purine and thymine synthesis, a reduction in T and B cell activation, and antibody formation. The dosing range is 0.5 to 1 mg/kg weekly, or 15 mg/m^2, with a maximum dose of 25 mg weekly. It can be given by mouth or subcutaneously. Over sixty percent of patients with JIA benefit significantly, though given its slower onset of action, effects are usually not apparent until 4–6 months after initiation. Serious toxicity is uncommon, but side effects including nausea, anorexia, stomatitis, transient aminotransferase level elevation, and malaise 24 hours after administration are relatively common. Folic acid supplementation has been shown to decrease these common side effects [53].

3.3. Biologic DMARDs

Biologic DMARDs used in the treatment of TMJ inflammatory arthritis include tumor necrosis factor (TNF) inhibitors such as adalimumab, etanercept, and infliximab. These medications are usually administered systemically via subcutaneous injection (etanercept and adalimumab) or intravenous infusion (infliximab). Local therapy with intra-articular injection of infliximab has been attempted but has failed to show efficacy in improving acute or chronic synovitis, or in changing maximal incisional opening [59]. TNF inhibitors are generally given in combination with methotrexate for TMJ arthritis that is refractory to methotrexate alone. The decision on whether to initiate systemic TNF blockade when severe disease is identified or to wait until after failure of initial methotrexate is currently based on expert opinion [10]. TNF inhibition has been shown to reduce TMJ pain and improve oral function in the literature for adults, however there is not strong evidence for juvenile TMJ arthritis. Other biologic DMARDS may also be considered including tocilizumab and abatacept. Current consensus is that non-systemic JIA responds well to TNF inhibition and methotrexate while systemic JIA responds well to IL-1 and Il-6 blockade with medications such as canakinumab and tocilizumab, respectively [65]. Overall, biologic DMARDs are generally well tolerated and require minimal lab monitoring. The main adverse effect is increased risk of infection.

3.4. Timing of Systemic Therapy

While those with isolated TMJ arthritis may start with isolated steroid injection or irrigation, patients with polyarticular arthritis, or more systemic disease activity, benefit from antirheumatic medications. Systemic medications are generally optimized and continued until all aspects of disease including arthritis, uveitis, and systemic symptoms are well controlled. Once remission on medications is obtained, in pediatrics, treatment usually continues for at least 12–24 months before attempting to taper off, assuming the treatments are well tolerated. Recent recommendations in orthopedic literature include stopping patients' biologic medications one dose before any planned joint replacement and waiting 14 days or until wound healing is complete until restarting the medications. New recommendations include continuing conventional DMARDs such as methotrexate during the perioperative period [62].

3.5. Potential Side Effects of Other Systemic Therapy

It is worth mentioning that some rheumatic disease systemic therapies, particularly bisphosphonates and corticosteroids, can be associated with TMJ disease. Bisphosphonates are potent inhibitors of osteoclastic bone resorption and are known for their use in treating osteopenia and osteoporosis but are also used in the management of chronic nonbacterial osteomyelitis (CNO, also known in the OMS literature as diffuse sclerosing osteomyelitis (DSO) or primary chronic osteomyelitis (PCO)), a rheumatic condition of inflammatory bone destruction. Jaw osteonecrosis is a potential risk of bisphosphonate use and should be considered in patients treated with bisphosphonates who present with TMJ complaints. Corticosteroids are used more widely across many rheumatic conditions as part of both acute and maintenance therapy. The side effect profile of corticosteroids will not be discussed in depth here, but it is worth noting that the risk of osteoporosis, osteopenia, and avascular necrosis is much greater when a patient is on chronic corticosteroids.

3.6. Systemic Therapy for Non-Rheumatic Causes of TMJ Arthritis

Traditional treatment of TMJ osteoarthritis mainly includes NSAIDs. De Souza et al [66] demonstrated equivalent pain reduction with diclofenac sodium compared with occlusal splints as well as intra-articular injections of sodium hyaluronate or corticosteroid. Research more recently has investigated oral glucosamine as an adjunctive therapy for TMJ osteoarthritis treatment. In a double-blinded randomized controlled trial conducted by Yang et al [67], oral glucosamine hydrochloride added to hyaluronate sodium injection failed to have meaningful effect on pain at month 6 post-injection but did improve pain and function at month 12, suggesting possible efficacy after prolonged use.

Systemic treatment is not indicated for idiopathic condylar resorption (ICR), which was mentioned above as a diagnosis of exclusion and can be a mimicker of systemic rheumatic disease. While differentiating isolated TMJ JIA from ICR can be difficult, the distinction is crucial as systemic therapy is not warranted for ICR but a cornerstone of JIA management.

4. Assessment of the Temporomandibular Joint in Rheumatic Disease

As noted in the Introduction, a critically important distinction between TMJ disease presentation in rheumatic diseases and non-rheumatic TMD is the delay—or even complete absence—of clinical signs and symptoms relative to anatomic destruction in rheumatologic patients. Since providers who frequently treat non-rheumatic TMD patients often do not recommend imaging until significant signs or symptoms are present, a known rheumatic diagnosis should prompt the clinician to consider earlier application of imaging modalities in this patient population (Figure 3). This may alert the provider to situations where earlier initiation of non- or minimally-invasive treatments (conventional or biologic DMARD adjustment, arthrocentesis, intra-articular medicament application, etc.) may delay further joint destruction. The relapsing/remitting nature of some of these conditions, in concert with the use of DMARDs, NSAIDs, biologics, and the associated individual patient variations in response, complicate any expected association between signs, symptoms, and imaging findings which is usually more robust in the non-rheumatic patient.

4.1. Patient History

For the patient without a previous rheumatic diagnosis, new signs and/or symptoms of TMD should include a broad patient history including questions regarding constitutional symptoms, pain and dysfunction of other joints, back complaints, muscle weakness, and skin/nail lesions [8]. Questions specific to vasculitides, which may occur with rheumatic conditions, can also be helpful, particularly questions about new respiratory, ophthalmologic, mucosal, or renal abnormalities.

For all patients, with or without a previous rheumatic diagnosis, a more traditional history—one more pointed at orofacial musculoskeletal disease and osteoarthritis—still remains appropriate. Questions include those regarding headaches, earaches, recent or remote trauma, parafunctional habits, and bone and cartilage diseases. Patients should specifically be asked to quantify and qualify pain, clicking, crepitus, locking, dislocation, reduced opening, stiffness, change in diet, and sense of altered occlusion.

4.2. Clinical Examination

Although the TMJ clinical examination should always be comprehensive and is therefore not fundamentally different in patients with a known rheumatic disease, it does become helpful for the clinician to understand which metrics have been shown to be helpful in these patients.

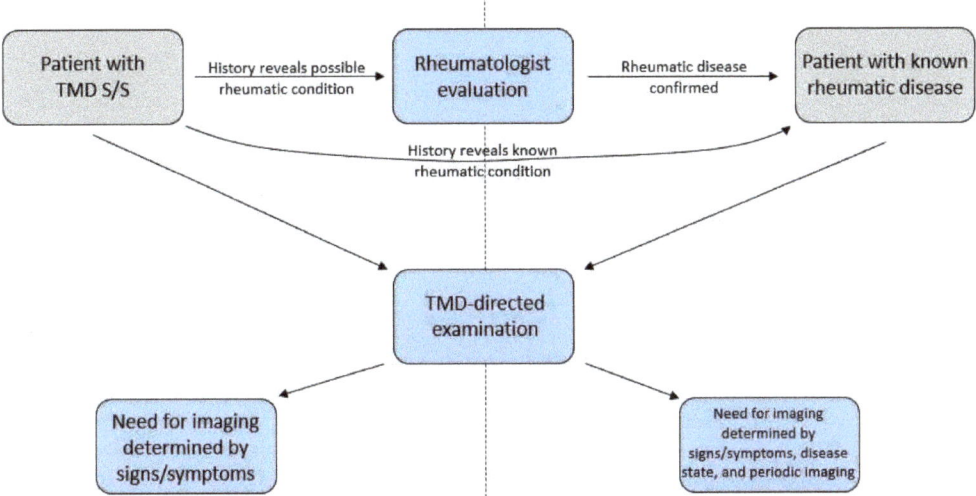

Figure 3. Basic framework for incorporating rheumatology referral and evaluation in patients presenting with signs and symptoms of a temporomandibular joint disorder. Patients found to have rheumatic diseases should undergo period TMJ imaging.

The Helkimo Clinical Dysfunction Index (Di) and Helkimo Anamnestic Index (Ai) are useful metrics for assessing and monitoring such patients [68]. While the Ai is technically subjective and thus truly part of the patient's history or subjective assessment, it is often recorded simultaneously during the clinical examination. Subjectively (Ai), the patient can be completely asymptomatic, mildly-moderately symptomatic (joint sounds, jaw fatigue, jaw stiffness), or severely symptomatic (trismus, locking, luxation, discoordination). Objectively (Di), mandibular range of motion, dysfunction with motion, and pain are measured, with significant weight being placed on end-stage pain and dysfunction (Table 2).

Table 2. Helkimo clinical dysfunction index (Di). The maximum score recorded from each domain is added to determine the total clinical dysfunction index score. Abbreviations: **MIO**—maximum incisal opening; mm—millimeter.

Domain	Criteria	Score
Mandibular Mobility	• MIO > 40 mm, excursions > 7 mm • MIO > 30 mm, excursions > 3 mm • MIO ≤ 30 mm, excursions ≤ 3 mm	0 1 5
TMJ Dysfunction	• No sounds/deviation on opening • Sounds and/or deviation > 2 mm • Locking and/or luxation	0 1 5
Muscle Pain	• No muscle pain • Pain on palpation at 1–3 sites • Pain on palpation at 4+ sites	0 1 5
TMJ Pain	• No tenderness to palpation • Lateral (superficial) TMJ pain • Posterior (deep) TMJ pain	0 1 5

Table 2. *Cont.*

Domain	Criteria	Score
Mandibular Movement Pain	• No pain • Pain with 1 movement • Pain with 2+ movements	0 1 5
	Di 0: 0 points—absence of dysfunction Di I: 1–4 points—mild dysfunction Di II: 5–9 points—moderate dysfunction Di III: 10–25 points—severe dysfunction	

The Helkimo indices have been most rigorously studied in the TMJ OA population. It should be noted, however, that OA patients often present for evaluation because of pain, and thus the translatability of these results to the autoimmune population—many who either do not have pain initially or at least have a weaker association between pain and clinical and radiographic signs—should be considered cautiously. Said another way, the Helkimo index alone may underestimate the degree of damage in inflammatory rheumatic disease. Strong associations between the Helkimo index and bony changes (condylar head or fossa) but not soft tissue changes (joint space size) have been reported when using CT [69,70].

Juvenile SLE patients have been found to have significantly worse Di scores than healthy controls, with the discrepancy due primarily to TMJ dysfunction and not pain. Even more specifically, it appears that decreased laterotrusive movements may be the first signs of dysfunction in this population [29]. This has been demonstrated in the RA population as well, where worse Di scores were found to be primarily due to decreased mandibular mobility and not necessarily worse pain [71]. On the contrary, others have found that both the Ai and Di were significantly worse in RA patients than control patients, and the Helkimo indices performed significantly better at discriminating RA versus control patients than other indices [1]. As noted previously, the relapsing/remitting nature of these conditions, in concert with the use of DMARDs and NSAIDs—which frequently are not reported or controlled for as confounders in studies—complicates the association between symptoms, particularly pain, and overall cumulative TMJ damage. Accordingly, duration of autoimmune disease alone does not necessarily correlate with worsening Helkimo indices [72]. Studies generally agree that the Helkimo index as a whole helps to discriminate patients with significant arthritic disease from those without significant TMJ involvement [73,74]. A qualitative summary of studies to date finds that decreased mandibular mobility and pain on mandibular function are the most commonly reported findings.

In addition to routine use of the Helkimo indices, international consensus guidelines have been established for orofacial examination in patients with juvenile idiopathic arthritis and can be extrapolated to the rheumatic TMD population in general [75,76]. These guidelines have resulted in a minimum recommended "short screening protocol" that includes assessment of TMJ pain in open and closed positions, mandibular deviation on opening, maximum incisal opening (MIO), frontal facial asymmetry, and facial profile. While the Helkimo indices focus more on grades of pain and dysfunction, the consensus guidelines are meant to screen for and monitor diacapitular disease activity and resulting dentofacial deformity. Monitoring in the rheumatic population will be further discussed below.

4.3. Imaging

4.3.1. Three-Dimensional Bone Imaging

Bony destruction is reliably associated with periods of more severe disease activity. Although erosions, cortical morphology, and subcortical changes can fluctuate over time, both two-dimensional and volumetric condylar changes appear to correlate with cumulative disease activity in the joint. In RA and JIA patients, CT and MRI reveal that condylar or ramal height, condylar volume, anteroposterior length, and mediolateral width are all associated with disease severity [77], although findings are not specific to inflammatory diseases and thus cannot be used to diagnose autoimmune TMJ disease [13]. The most unifying finding in active rheumatic TMJ disease—regardless of whether the condyle, ramus, or both are affected—is asymmetry [78].

It must not be forgotten that conventional radiographs remain a reasonable screening examination in asymptomatic patients without dysfunction per the Helkimo index, with the possible exception of JIA patients. Even in this population, however, it has been suggested that condylar asymmetry on screening panoramic is specific for joint damage [79], but a concern remains for low sensitivity and reproducibility with this modality compared with three-dimensional imaging [80]. In both osteoarthritic and RA patients it has been suggested that CT may not add much to the bony changes visible on plain radiographs [81].

4.3.2. Three-Dimensional Soft Tissue Imaging

MRI is the gold standard for soft tissue TMJ imaging including assessment of the articular disc, synovium, joint spaces, bone marrow, and surrounding musculature. This requires imaging protocols including fluid-sensitive (usually T2), pre-contrast T1 (usually fast spin echo, FSE), and post-contrast fat-saturated T1 sequences [82–84]. By far the most studied population is those with JIA, as this population is the most likely to lack signs and symptoms with significant disease activity. In a most extreme example, a study by Kellenberger et al. showed that 100% of control patients with joint effusions on MRI had pain while 0% of JIA patients with joint effusions had pain [85].

An enhancement ratio (ER) or enhancement value (EV), defined as the contrast enhancement of the superior joint space divided by that of a nearby muscle (often the longus capitis), has been described and validated in the JIA population [86,87]. Other semiquantitative MRI grading systems exist, with the OMERACT (Outcome Measures in Rheumatoid Arthritis and Clinical Trials) and EuroTMJoint (now TMJaw) research group having the most applicable systems [13]. These scoring systems evaluate inflammation (bone marrow edema, joint effusion, synovial thickening, joint enhancement) and damage (condylar flattening, erosions, and disc abnormality) and provide either a cumulative score that can be followed (OMERACT), similar to the Helkimo indices, or a progressive score (EuroTMJoint/TMJaw), similar to the Wilkes staging system.

4.3.3. Nuclear Medicine Imaging

Bone scintigraphy is a nuclear medicine examination based upon the premise that high bone turnover and/or osteoblastic activity—indicative of hyperplasia, active growth centers, or inflammatory turnover, among others—increases local uptake of radiopharmaceuticals which mimic pyrophosphate [88]. Accordingly, studies show that those with active rheumatic conditions have increased condylar uptake allowing reasonable discrimination from healthy controls and those with non-inflammatory TMJ OA, which seems to mirror discrimination by inflammatory laboratory markers (e.g., ESR, CRP) [89]. Similar findings using positron emission tomography (PET), where avidity is based upon increased glucose uptake in inflammatory environments, have been noted [90]. Nuclear medicine studies have no role in identifying TMJ OA [91].

4.3.4. Ultrasonography

In theory, ultrasonography (US) seems an ideal modality to evaluate the soft tissues of the TMJ, with the TMJ being relatively superficial and US being a continuous imaging modality conducive to dynamic imaging. Unfortunately, only a few studies have attempted to objectively compare US to the current gold standard for soft tissue imaging, MRI, in autoimmune TMJ disease [11,92,93]. Although some suggest that there is at least moderate correlation between US and MRI for the assessment of synovitis in childhood arthritis [93], a recent systematic review in the JIA population could not recommend US as a standard imaging modality in these patients [94].

5. Interventions for Temporomandibular Joint Dysfunction in Rheumatic Disease

Outcomes purportedly expected in the management of TMD in the rheumatic patient population should be reviewed with caution. A careful review of the available literature demonstrates that many authors reference studies involving non-rheumatic TMD patients. As the reader is already well aware, there are vast differences in presentation and outcomes in rheumatic and non-rheumatic TMD patients. Given the available evidence, an algorithm for management of rheumatic TMD patients is presented in Figure 4. Although this algorithm is based upon the TMJ Working Group's recommendations in the JIA patient [95], less emphasis is placed on the skeletal maturity of the patient and more emphasis is placed on the disease state and degree of patient dysfunction. The central role of the systemic rheumatologic management is also highlighted by this algorithm.

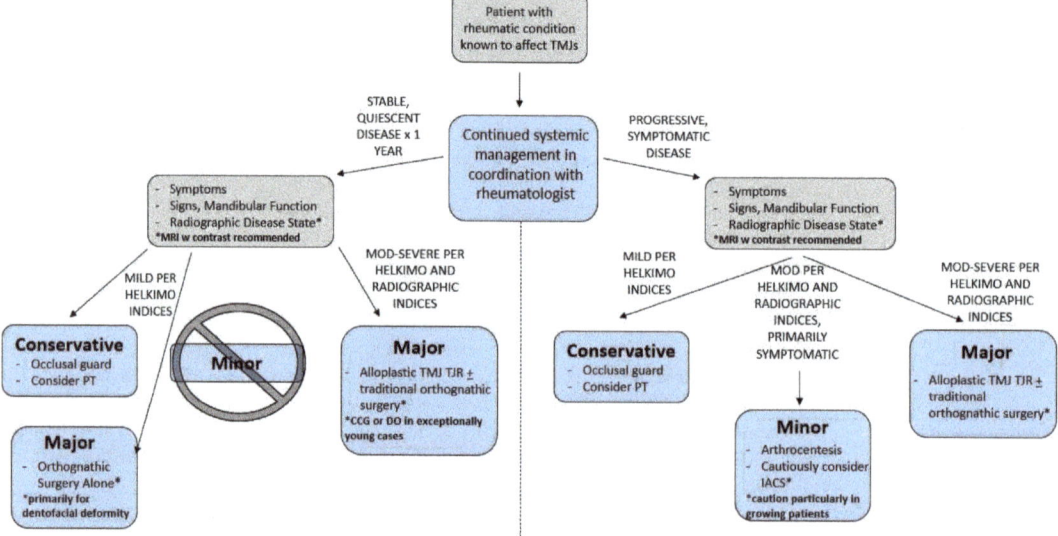

Figure 4. Recommended algorithm for treatment. Abbreviations: **CCG**—costochondral grafting; **DO**—distraction osteogenesis; **IACS**—intra-articular corticosteroids; mod—moderate; **PT**—physical therapy; **TJR**—total joint replacement.

5.1. Conservative Interventions

In non-rheumatic TMD patients, "conservative" interventions typically convey ideas of joint rest, diet alteration, occlusal guards, physical therapy, NSAIDs, and muscle relaxants. Although these certainly may also be beneficial for the rheumatic patient [96,97], the foundation of conservative management in these patients is systemic management of their inflammatory disease, as described above. That being said, self-directed physical therapy has shown effective in improving mandibular function, TMJ related pain, or both in patients with RA and AS [98,99]. In FM patients, tactile stimulation has been shown to improve sleep quality, quality of life, and TMD symptoms [100]. Low-level laser therapy for TMJ inflammatory arthritis has only been preliminarily investigated in animal models [101], and thus no conclusions regarding efficacy should be made.

Although many still propagate "occlusal equilibration" or "fixed prosthetics" for the treatment of TMD in general and TMJ OA or autoimmune diseases in particular [102,103], it should be made clear that no robust evidence supports these practices [104,105], and the senior author finds the continued use of these practices for this purpose highly misleading to patients. Although occlusal modification, including orthodontic treatment, can certainly improve facial appearance, masticatory function, and oral hygiene in these patients [106,107], it should not in any way be expected to improve rheumatic TMD.

5.2. Minor Procedures

Arthrocentesis and Intra-Articular Injection

It is well documented that arthrocentesis improves pain and dysfunction in patients with osteoarthritis, particularly Wilkes stages II, III, and IV [108,109]. Arthrocentesis with lysis and lavage alone likely improves pain and dysfunction in the rheumatic TMD population as well [110]; however, analysis is at times confounded by the fact that most rheumatic patients have traditionally also received intra-articular corticosteroid injection (IACS) at the conclusion of arthrocentesis [111]. A more recent study found that the IACS component does indeed improve the Helkimo index over arthrocentesis alone [112]. There is no question that TMJ IACS can at least temporarily improve symptoms in properly selected patients with active RA [111,113] or JIA [112], but concerns remain regarding long-term effects of IACS.

For example, multiple studies have specifically reported on the presence of heterotopic bone formation in JIA patients who have IACS, but a cause-and-effect relation has never been proven [83,114]. More recently, a retrospective review of JIA patients illustrated the complexity of the cause-and-effect relation, as the authors found that the total number of injections and time to first injection were associated with increased risk of heterotopic bone formation, yet they noted that children with more severe arthritis were likely to receive IACS [115]. Clearly, indiscriminate use of IACS should be avoided, and it should only be considered during active inflammation not responsive to medical management, preferably when confirmed by MRI [116]. Alternatively, consideration should be made for arthrocentesis with lysis and lavage *without* IACS, or with injection of hyaluronic acid [117].

More recently, intra-articular biologic injection (IAB) has been studied in the TMJ, with the first being a case report of IAB with infliximab in a patient with PsA unresponsive to both systemic infliximab and TMJ IACS [118]. Subsequent reports of IAB with infliximab in JIA patients show that although the injections appear safe, they do not affect jaw opening or improve inflammation or destruction as appreciated on MRI [119,120]. IAB with etanercept has been reported in rabbit [121] and rat [122] models of inflammatory TMJ arthritis and TMJ loading, respectively. The rabbit model showed that IAB with etanercept did not perform as well as systemic etanercept and performed no different than intra-articular saline injection. The rat model simply suggested that biochemical and biomechanical processes in the TMJ are likely driven in part by TNF-α. In conclusion, evidence to date does not support intra-articular biologic injection of the TMJs.

5.3. Major Procedures

5.3.1. Open Arthroplasty and Associated Procedures

Synovectomy and discectomy, or possibly discectomy alone, have been shown to improve mandibular function [123] and pain [124] in patients with rheumatic TMJ disease, including RA, AS, and PsA patients. The effectiveness of these procedures should be taken into context, however, as many of these studies were performed before the application of biologic DMARDs for autoimmune rheumatic diseases. Additionally, overly aggressive attempts at or simply multiplicity of open arthroplasties may complicate eventual joint replacement, if this is foreseen in the patient's future.

5.3.2. Orthognathic Surgery

Debate continues on the stability of orthognathic surgery results in patients with resorptive TMJ processes such as inflammatory rheumatic diseases and ICR. It should also be noted that this does not treat the underlying pathology but simply masks a subset of the orofacial manifestations. The optimistic hope is that if a patient's disease process is well controlled, the result will be stable. Unfortunately, this essentially can never be guaranteed, and therefore many "successes" end up being measured in the short term of months [125–128]. A patient with a process defined by condylar resorption electing to undergo orthognathic surgery alone must absolutely be informed that relapse is expected, TMJ pain and dysfunction are not expected to resolve, and only TMJ TJR will predictably result in long-term stability [129]. Thus, the patient best suited for orthognathic surgery alone is one with stably quiescent disease with relatively mild deformities.

Condylotomy—which has evolved to its current day form of essentially a vertical ramus osteotomy—has been documented as a treatment in active inflammatory TMD [103], but this represents a lack of understanding of the disease process and should not be performed.

5.3.3. Distraction Osteogenesis

Distraction osteogenesis (DO) of the mandibular rami has been reported in JIA patients. As would be expected for a treatment aimed primarily at altering the dentofacial abnormality without addressing the TMJ disease process itself, facial appearance and occlusal relationship were improved while long-term pain, mandibular mobility, and TMJ signs had either mixed results or continued progression [130,131]. It should also be noted that inclusion criteria in the only prospective study to date were unilateral TMJ involvement, inactive disease, and TMJs with "clinical and subjective good function" preoperatively [130]. Therefore, similar to the potential orthognathic patient, patients with a process defined by condylar resorption electing to undergo DO alone must absolutely be informed that relapse is expected, TMJ pain and dysfunction are not expected to resolve, and only TMJ TJR will predictably result in long-term stability.

5.3.4. Total Joint Replacement

Although historically costochondral grafting (CCG) has been performed in patients with rheumatic TMD [132–134], and although debate continues on the application of autogenous or alloplastic procedures for TMJ TJR in non-rheumatic end-stage joint disease, the senior author agrees with the idea that inflammatory TMJ destruction is best treated with alloplastic methods [135].

Guidelines have been put forth to guide physicians when prosthetic TMJ TJR may be appropriate, including in inflammatory joint disease [136]. Not surprisingly, the superiority of alloplastic TMJ TJR in non-rheumatic end-stage joint disease patients has been found to translate to the autoimmune population as well [137]. Outcomes of alloplastic TMJ TJR in RA, PsA, AS, SSc, and JIA patients have been reported, showing consistent improvement in associated pain and dysfunction [138–147]. The literature nearly unanimously suggests that patients with appropriate indications for TMJ TJR have seen improved, durable outcomes.

A legitimate concern in open surgery—particularly those involving alloplastic implantation—is the immunosuppressive therapies that many patients will be taking, particularly those patients with disease severe enough to require such surgery [116]. Studies of TMJ TJR often do not comment on perioperative medication management, although this is vitally important to success. Although developed with the American Association of Hip and Knee Surgeons (AAHKS), the ACR has published perioperative guidelines for management of antirheumatic medications in those undergoing arthroplasty [148]. As mentioned previously, conventional DMARDs should generally be continued through surgery while surgery should occur at the end of biologic DMARD dosing cycles, and the biologic should not be resumed until 14 or more days post-operatively (assuming no post-operative infectious or wound healing complications).

6. Monitoring of the Rheumatic Patient with Temporomandibular Joint Disease

There are minimal evidence-based or consensus guidelines for monitoring in rheumatic patients with TMD, with most available data pertaining to the JIA population. Consensus assessment methods were reached by the Temporomandibular Joint Juvenile Arthritis (TMJaw) Working Group for monitoring of TMJ arthritis and involvement in JIA patients in 2019 [95]. These include MRI with contrast, 3D scans (which may include CBCT or medical grade CT as appropriate), clinical examination, and patient-reported outcome measures. Consensus could not be reached to recommend the use of MRI without contrast, plain radiographs, or ultrasound in the monitoring of TMJ arthritis in these patients. The TMJaw group also proposed a clinical evaluation protocol for regular assessment of the TMJ joint in patients with JIA, which is applicable both for screening as well as following patients with a history of TMJ arthritis [75,76]. As discussed above, the components of the exam allow for a quick assessment of pain, range of motion, and dentofacial deformity and asymmetry, which when followed over time can assist in detecting subtle changes indicative of active or progressive disease. However, as previously stated, given the potential for active, erosive TMJ arthritis in asymptomatic or minimally symptomatic patients, there is also a need for imaging to both evaluate for initial disease, as well as to follow the course of TMJ arthritis during and after treatment. This is the case when following up after either TMJ arthrocentesis or initiation of systemic rheumatic medications. Given MRI with contrast is the gold standard for active synovitis, monitoring 6 months after a treatment is initiated or changed with an MRI is the most accurate for assessing whether there is ongoing disease activity that would warrant additional measures.

A survey of academic American OMS practice patterns in managing and monitoring JIA patients suggests that once inflammatory arthritic patients are deemed to be in remission, most are monitored at 6 to 12 month intervals [61]. However, this study also revealed that the average OMS often relies more on symptoms and plain radiography rather than MRI when following this patient population. This highlights the potential benefit of ongoing discussions between rheumatology and OMS to determine the best imaging modality for individual patients.

With regard to monitoring for disease activity and its effect on surgical treatment decisions, the TMJaw group recommends that a lack of progression over one year combined with contrasted MRI confirmation of quiescent disease serves as reasonable evidence to proceed with autologous reconstruction (e.g., costochondral grafting and/or orthognathic surgery). The unpredictability of the disease process, particularly in younger patients, should be considered however when deciding on surgical intervention. A suggested monitoring protocol is presented in Figure 5.

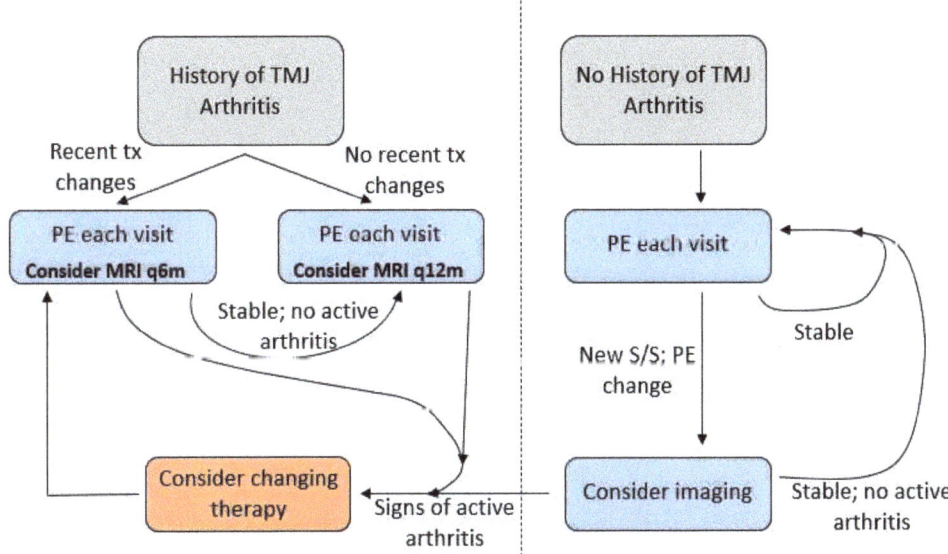

Figure 5. Recommended monitoring protocol. Abbreviations: q6m—every 6 months; q12m—every 12 months; PE—physical exam; S/S—signs and symptoms; tx—treatment.

Funding: This research received no external funding.

Institutional Review Board Statement: Not applicable.

Informed Consent Statement: Not applicable.

Conflicts of Interest: The authors declare no conflict of interest.

References

1. Da Cunha, S.C.; Nogueira, R.V.; Duarte, A.P.; Vasconcelos, B.C.; de Almeida, R.A. Analysis of helkimo and craniomandibular indexes for temporomandibular disorder diagnosis on rheumatoid arthritis patients. *Braz. J. Otorhinolaryngol.* **2007**, *73*, 19–26. [CrossRef]
2. Helmick, C.G.; Felson, D.T.; Lawrence, R.C.; Gabriel, S.; Hirsch, R.; Kwoh, C.K.; Liang, M.H.; Kremers, H.M.; Mayes, M.D.; Merkel, P.A.; et al. National Arthritis Data Workgroup. Estimates of the prevalence of arthritis and other rheumatic conditions in the United States: Part I. *Arthritis Rheum.* **2008**, *58*, 15–25. [CrossRef] [PubMed]
3. Centers for Disease Control and Prevention. Arthritis in America. 7 March 2017. Available online: https://www.cdc.gov/vitalsigns/arthritis/index.html (accessed on 10 October 2020).
4. World Health Organization. Chronic Rheumatic Conditions. Available online: https://www.who.int/chp/topics/rheumatic/en/ (accessed on 10 October 2020).
5. Wilkes, C.H. Internal derangements of the temporomandibular joint. Pathological variations. *Arch. Otolaryngol. Head Neck Surg.* **1989**, *115*, 469–477. [CrossRef]
6. Hirahara, N.; Kaneda, T.; Muraoka, H.; Fukuda, T.; Ito, K.; Kawashima, Y. Characteristic magnetic resonance imaging findings in rheumatoid arthritis of the temporomandibular joint: Focus on abnormal bone marrow sgnal of the mandibular condyle, pannus, and lymph node swelling in the parotid glands. *J. Oral Maxillofac. Surg.* **2017**, *75*, 735–741. [CrossRef]
7. Scutellari, P.N.; Orzincolo, C.; Ceruti, S. L'articolazione temporo-mandibolare nelle condizioni patologiche: Artrite reumatoide e spondiloartriti sieronegative. (The temporo-mandibular joint in pathologic conditions: Rheumatoid arthritis and seronegative spondyloarthritis). *Radiol. Med.* **1993**, *86*, 456–466.
8. Sidebottom, A.J.; Salha, R. Management of the temporomandibular joint in rheumatoid disorders. *Br. J. Oral Maxillofac. Surg.* **2013**, *51*, 191–198. [CrossRef]
9. Petty, R.E.; Southwood, T.R.; Manners, P.; Baum, J.; Glass, D.N.; Goldenberg, J.; He, X.; Maldonado-Cocco, J.; Orozco-Alcala, J.; Prieur, A.M.; et al. International League of Associations for Rheumatology. International League of Associations for Rheumatology classification of juvenile idiopathic arthritis: Second revision, Edmonton, 2001. *J. Rheumatol.* **2004**, *31*, 390–392.
10. Veldhuis, E.C.; Veldhuis, A.H.; Koudstaal, M.J. Treatment management of children with juvenile idiopathic arthritis with temporomandibular joint involvement: A systematic review. *Oral Surg. Oral Med. Oral Pathol. Oral Radiol.* **2014**, *117*, 581–589. [CrossRef]
11. Weiss, P.F.; Arabshahi, B.; Johnson, A.; Bilaniuk, L.T.; Zarnow, D.; Cahill, A.M.; Feudtner, C.; Cron, R.Q. High prevalence of temporomandibular joint arthritis at disease onset in children with juvenile idiopathic arthritis, as detected by magnetic resonance imaging but not by ultrasound. *Arthritis Rheum.* **2008**, *58*, 1189–1196. [CrossRef] [PubMed]
12. Melchiorre, D.; Falcini, F.; Kaloudi, O.; Bandinelli, F.; Nacci, F.; Matucci Cerinic, M. Sonographic evaluation of the temporo-mandibular joints in juvenile idiopathic arthritis. *J. Ultrasound* **2010**, *13*, 34–37. [CrossRef] [PubMed]
13. Kellenberger, C.J.; Junhasavasdikul, T.; Tolend, M.; Doria, A.S. Temporomandibular joint atlas for detection and grading of juvenile idiopathic arthritis involvement by magnetic resonance imaging. *Pediatr. Radiol.* **2018**, *48*, 411–426. [CrossRef]
14. Seifert, M.H.; Steigerwald, J.C.; Cliff, M.M. Bone resorption of the mandible in progressive systemic sclerosis. *Arthritis Rheum.* **1975**, *18*, 507–512. [CrossRef]
15. Osial, T.A., Jr.; Avakian, A.; Sassouni, V.; Agarwal, A.; Medsger, T.A., Jr.; Rodnan, G.P. Resorption of the mandibular condyles and coronoid processes in progressive systemic sclerosis (scleroderma). *Arthritis Rheum.* **1981**, *24*, 729–733. [CrossRef]
16. Ferreira, E.L.; Christmann, R.B.; Borba, E.F.; Borges, C.T.; Siqueira, J.T.; Bonfa, E. Mandibular function is severely impaired in systemic sclerosis patients. *J. Orofac. Pain* **2010**, *24*, 197–202.
17. Aliko, A.; Ciancaglini, R.; Alushi, A.; Tafaj, A.; Ruci, D. Temporomandibular joint involvement in rheumatoid arthritis, systemic lupus erythematosus and systemic sclerosis. *Int. J. Oral Maxillofac. Surg.* **2011**, *40*, 704–709. [CrossRef] [PubMed]
18. Crincoli, V.; Fatone, L.; Fanelli, M.; Rotolo, R.P.; Chialà, A.; Favia, G.; Lapadula, G. Orofacial Manifestations and Temporo-mandibular Disorders of Systemic Scleroderma: An Observational Study. *Int. J. Mol. Sci.* **2016**, *17*, 1189. [CrossRef]
19. Bessa-Nogueira, R.V.; Vasconcelos, B.C.; Duarte, A.P.; Góes, P.S.; Bezerra, T.P. Targeted assessment of the temporomandibular joint in patients with rheumatoid arthritis. *J. Oral Maxillofac. Surg.* **2008**, *66*, 1804–1811. [CrossRef] [PubMed]
20. Aceves-Avila, F.J.; Chávez-López, M.; Chavira-González, J.R.; Ramos-Remus, C. Temporomandibular joint dysfunction in various rheumatic diseases. *Reumatismo* **2013**, *65*, 126–130. [CrossRef] [PubMed]
21. Cordeiro, P.C.; Guimaraes, J.P.; de Souza, V.A.; Dias, I.M.; Silva, J.N.; Devito, K.L.; Bonato, L.L. Temporomandibular joint involvement in rheumatoid arthritis patients: Association between clinical and tomographic data. *Acta Odontol. Latinoam.* **2016**, *29*, 123–129. [PubMed]

22. Celiker, R.; Gökçe-Kutsal, Y.; Eryilmaz, M. Temporomandibular joint involvement in rheumatoid arthritis. Relationship with disease activity. *Scand. J. Rheumatol.* **1995**, *24*, 22–25. [CrossRef]
23. Yoshida, A.; Higuchi, Y.; Kondo, M.; Tabata, O.; Ohishi, M. Range of motion of the temporomandibular joint in rheumatoid arthritis: Relationship to the severity of disease. *Cranio* **1998**, *16*, 162–167. [CrossRef] [PubMed]
24. Mortazavi, N.; Babaei, M.; Babaee, H.; Kazemi, H.H.; Mortazavi, R.; Mostafazadeh, A. Evaluation of the prevalence of temporomandibular joint involvement in rheumatoid arthritis using research diagnostic criteria for temporomandibular disorders. *J. Dent.* **2018**, *15*, 332–338. [CrossRef]
25. Redlund-Johnell, I. Severe rheumatoid arthritis of the temporomandibular joints and its coincidence with severe rheumatoid arthritis of the cervical spine. *Scand. J. Rheumatol.* **1987**, *16*, 347–353. [CrossRef]
26. Ozcan, I.; Ozcan, K.M.; Keskin, D.; Bahar, S.; Boyacigil, S.; Dere, H. Temporomandibular joint involvement in rheumatoid arthritis: Correlation of clinical, laboratory and magnetic resonance imaging findings. *B ENT* **2008**, *4*, 19–24. [PubMed]
27. Crincoli, V.; Piancino, M.G.; Iannone, F.; Errede, M.; Di Comite, M. Temporomandibular disorders and oral features in systemic lupus erythematosus patients: An observational study of symptoms and signs. *Int. J. Med. Sci.* **2020**, *17*, 153–160. [CrossRef]
28. Jonsson, R.; Lindvall, A.M.; Nyberg, G. Temporomandibular joint involvement in systemic lupus erythematosus. *Arthritis Rheum.* **1983**, *26*, 1506–1510. [CrossRef] [PubMed]
29. Fernandes, E.G.; Savioli, C.; Siqueira, J.T.; Silva, C.A. Oral health and the masticatory system in juvenile systemic lupus erythematosus. *Lupus* **2007**, *16*, 713–719. [CrossRef]
30. Grinin, V.M.; Maksimovskiĭ, I.M.; Nasonova, V.A. Asepticheskiĭ nekroz visochno-nizhnecheliustnogo sustava pri sistemnoĭ krasnoĭ volchanke [Aseptic necrosis of the temporomandibular joint in systemic lupus erythematosus]. *Stomatologiia* **1999**, *78*, 23–27. [PubMed]
31. Grinin, V.M. Kontseptsiia patogeneza okkliuzionnykh narusheniĭ pri zabolevaniiakh visochno-nizhnecheliustnogo sustava [The concept of the pathogenesis of occlusive disorders in diseases of the temporomandibular joint]. *Stomatologiia* **1995**, *74*, 29–32.
32. Grinin, V.M.; Nasonova, V.A.; Maksimovskiĭ, I.M.; Ternovoĭ, S.K.; Sinitsyn, V.E.; Smirnov, A.V. Differentsial'naia diagnostika avaskuliarnogo nekroza visochno-nizhnecheliustnogo sustava pri sistemnoĭ krasnoĭ volchanke [The differential diagnosis of avascular necrosis of the temporomandibular joint in systemic lupus erythematosus]. *Stomatologiia* **2000**, *79*, 23–25. [PubMed]
33. Szántó, D.; Bohátka, L.; Csokonay, L.; Schiefner, G.; Boross, G.; Jáger, M.; Barzó, P. A capitulum mandibulae avascularis necrosisa systemás lupus erythematosusban [Avascular necrosis of the mandibular condyle in systemic lupus erythematosus]. *Orv. Hetil.* **1986**, *127*, 3187–3190.
34. Costantino, F.; Zeboulon, N.; Said-Nahal, R.; Breban, M. Radiographic sacroiliitis develops predictably over time in a cohort of familial spondyloarthritis followed longitudinally. *Rheumatology* **2017**, *56*, 811–817. [CrossRef] [PubMed]
35. Mathieu, A.; Paladini, F.; Vacca, A.; Cauli, A.; Fiorillo, M.T.; Sorrentino, R. The interplay between the geographic distribution of HLA-B27 alleles and their role in infectious and autoimmune diseases: A unifying hypothesis. *Autoimmun. Rev.* **2009**, *8*, 420–425. [CrossRef] [PubMed]
36. Davidson, C.; Wojtulewski, J.A.; Bacon, P.A.; Winstock, D. Temporo-mandibular joint disease in ankylosing spondylitis. *Ann. Rheum. Dis.* **1975**, *34*, 87–91. [CrossRef] [PubMed]
37. Li, J.M.; Zhang, X.W.; Zhang, Y.; Li, Y.H.; An, J.G.; Xiao, E.; Yan, Y.B. Ankylosing spondylitis associated with bilateral ankylosis of the temporomandibular joint. *Oral Surg. Oral Med. Oral Pathol. Oral Radiol.* **2013**, *116*, e478–e484. [CrossRef] [PubMed]
38. Koorbusch, G.F.; Zeitler, D.L.; Fotos, P.G.; Doss, J.B. Psoriatic arthritis of the temporomandibular joints with ankylosis. Literature review and case reports. *Oral Surg. Oral Med. Oral Pathol.* **1991**, *71*, 267–274. [CrossRef]
39. Alinaghi, F.; Calov, M.; Kristensen, L.E.; Gladman, D.D.; Coates, L.C.; Jullien, D.; Gottlieb, A.B.; Gisondi, P.; Wu, J.J.; Thyssen, J.P.; et al. Prevalence of psoriatic arthritis in patients with psoriasis: A systematic review and meta-analysis of observational and clinical studies. *J. Am. Acad. Dermatol.* **2019**, *80*, 251–265. [CrossRef]
40. Wright, V.; Moll, J.M. Psoriatic arthritis. *Bull. Rheum. Dis.* **1971**, *21*, 627–632. [CrossRef]
41. Farronato, G.; Garagiola, U.; Carletti, V.; Cressoni, P.; Bellintani, C. Psoriatic arthritis: Temporomandibular joint involvement as the first articular phenomenon. *Quintessence Int.* **2010**, *41*, 395–398.
42. Dervis, E.; Dervis, E. The prevalence of temporomandibular disorders in patients with psoriasis with or without psoriatic arthritis. *J. Oral Rehabil.* **2005**, *32*, 786–793. [CrossRef]
43. Badel, T.; Savić Pavičin, I.; Krapac, L.; Zadravec, D., Rosić, D. Psoriatic arthritis and temporomandibular joint involvement—Literature review with a reported case. *Acta Dermatovenerol. Croat.* **2014**, *22*, 114–121.
44. Okeson, J. *Management of Temporomandibular Disorders and Occlusion*, Mosby: New York, NY, USA, 2019.
45. Tanaka, E.; Detamore, M.S.; Mercuri, L.G. Degenerative disorders of the temporomandibular joint: Etiology, diagnosis, and treatment. *J. Dent. Res.* **2008**, *87*, 296–307. [CrossRef] [PubMed]
46. Matsumoto, R.; Ioi, H.; Goto, T.K.; Hara, A.; Nakata, S.; Nakasima, A.; Counts, A.L. Relationship between the unilateral TMJ osteoarthritis/osteoarthrosis, mandibular asymmetry and the EMG activity of the masticatory muscles: A retrospective study. *J. Oral Rehabil.* **2010**, *37*, 85–92. [CrossRef] [PubMed]
47. Altman, R.; Asch, E.; Bloch, D.; Bole, G.; Borenstein, D.; Brandt, K.; Christy, W.; Cooke, T.D.; Greenwald, R.; Hochberg, M. Development of criteria for the classification and reporting of osteoarthritis. Classification of osteoarthritis of the knee. Diagnostic and Therapeutic Criteria Committee of the American Rheumatism Association. *Arthritis Rheum.* **1986**, *29*, 1039–1049. [CrossRef] [PubMed]

48. Altman, R.; Alarcón, G.; Appelrouth, D.; Bloch, D.; Borenstein, D.; Brandt, K.; Brown, C.; Cooke, T.D.; Daniel, W.; Feldman, D. The American College of Rheumatology criteria for the classification and reporting of osteoarthritis of the hip. *Arthritis Rheum.* **1991**, *34*, 505–514. [CrossRef] [PubMed]
49. Balasubramaniam, R.; Laudenbach, J.M.; Stoopler, E.T. Fibromyalgia: An update for oral health care providers. *Oral Surg. Oral Med. Oral Pathol. Oral Radiol. Endodontol.* **2007**, *104*, 589–602. [CrossRef] [PubMed]
50. Ayouni, I.; Chebbi, R.; Hela, Z.; Dhidah, M. Comorbidity between fibromyalgia and temporomandibular disorders: A systematic review. *Oral Surg. Oral Med. Oral Pathol. Oral Radiol.* **2019**, *128*, 33–42. [CrossRef]
51. Arnett, G.W.; Milam, S.B.; Gottesman, L. Progressive mandibular retrusion—Idiopathic condylar resorption: Part I. *Am. J. Orthod. Dentofac. Orthop.* **1996**, *110*, 8–15. [CrossRef]
52. Abubaker, A.O.; Raslan, W.F.; Sotereanos, G.C. Estrogen and progesterone receptors in temporomandibular joint discs of symptomatic and asymptomatic persons: A preliminary study. *J. Oral Maxillofac. Surg.* **1993**, *51*, 1096–1100. [CrossRef]
53. Abramowicz, S.; Kim, S.; Prahalad, S.; Chouinard, A.F.; Kaban, L.B. Juvenile arthritis: Current concepts in terminology, etiopathogenesis, diagnosis, and management. *Int. J. Oral Maxillofac. Surg.* **2016**, *45*, 801–812. [CrossRef]
54. Huang, Y.L.; Pogrel, M.A.; Kaban, L.B. Diagnosis and management of condylar resorption. *J. Oral Maxillofac. Surg.* **1997**, *55*, 114–119. [CrossRef]
55. Alsabban, L.; Amarista, F.J.; Mercuri, L.G.; Perez, D. Idiopathic condylar resorption: A survey and review of the literature. *J. Oral Maxillofac. Surg.* **2018**, *76*, 2316.e1–2316.e13. [CrossRef]
56. Stoustrup, P.; Twilt, M.; Herlin, T. Systemic treatment for temporomandibular joint arthritis in juvenile idiopathic arthritis. *J. Rheumatol.* **2020**, *47*, 793–795. [CrossRef]
57. Carrasco, R. Juvenile idiopathic arthritis overview and involvement of the temporomandibular joint. *Oral Maxillofac. Surg. Clin. N. Am.* **2015**, *27*, 1–10. [CrossRef]
58. Bollhalder, A.; Patcas, R.; Eichenberger, M.; Muller, L.; Schroeder-Kohler, S.; Saurenmann, R.K.; Kellenberger, C.J. Magnetic resonance imaging followup of temporomandibular Joint inflammation, deformation, and mandibular growth in juvenile idiopathic arthritis patients receiving systemic treatment. *J. Rheumatol.* **2020**, *47*, 909–916. [CrossRef]
59. Stoll, M.L.; Kau, C.H.; Waite, P.D.; Cron, R.Q. Temporomandibular joint arthritis in juvenile idiopathic arthritis, now what? *Pediatr. Rheumatol.* **2018**, *16*, 32. [CrossRef] [PubMed]
60. Foeldvari, I.; Tzaribachev, N.; Cron, R.Q. Results of a multinational survey regarding the diagnosis and treatment of temporomandibular joint involvement in juvenile idiopathic arthritis. *Pediatr. Rheumatol.* **2014**, *12*, 6. [CrossRef]
61. Kinard, B.E.; Abramowicz, S. Juvenile idiopathic arthritis practice patterns among oral and maxillofacial surgeons. *J. Oral Maxillofac. Surg.* **2017**, *75*, 2333.e1–2333.e8. [CrossRef] [PubMed]
62. Granquist, E.F. Treatment of the temporomandibular Joint in a child with juvenile idiopathic arthritis. *Oral Maxillofac. Surg. Clin. N. Am.* **2018**, *30*, 97–107. [CrossRef] [PubMed]
63. Wang, X.D.; Zhang, J.N.; Gan, Y.H.; Zhou, Y.H. Current understanding of pathogenesis and treatment of TMJ osteoarthritis. *J. Dent. Res.* **2015**, *94*, 666–673. [CrossRef] [PubMed]
64. Rafayelyan, S.; Meyer, P.; Radlanski, R.J.; Minden, K.; Jost-Brinkmann, P.G.; Präger, T.M. Effect of methotrexate upon antigen-induced arthritis of the rabbit temporomandibular joint. *J. Oral Pathol. Med.* **2015**, *44*, 614–621. [CrossRef] [PubMed]
65. Nilbo, P.; Pruunsild, C.; Voog-Oras, U.; Nikopensius, T.; Jagomagi, T.; Saag, M. Contemporary management of TMJ involvement in JIA patients and its orofacial consequences. *EPMA J.* **2016**, *7*, 12.
66. De Souza, R.F.; Lovato da Silva, C.H.; Nasser, M.; Fedorowicz, Z.; Al-Muharrqai, M.A. Interventions for managing temporomandibular joint osteoarthritis. *Cochrane Database Syst. Rev.* **2012**, *2012*. [CrossRef]
67. Yang, W.; Lie, W.; Miao, C.; Sun, H.; Li, L.; Li, C. Oral glucosamine hydrochloride combined with hyaluronate sodium intraarticular injection for temporomandibular joint osteoarthritis: A double blind randomized controlled trial. *J. Oral Maxillofac. Surg.* **2018**, *76*, 2066–2073. [CrossRef] [PubMed]
68. Helkimo, M. Studies on function and dysfunction of the masticatory system. II. Index for anamnestic and clinical dysfunction and occlusal state. *Sven Tandlak. Tidskr.* **1974**, *67*, 101–121.
69. Su, N.; Liu, Y.; Yang, X.; Luo, Z.; Shi, Z. Correlation between bony changes measured with cone beam computed tomography and clinical dysfunction index in patients with temporomandibular joint osteoarthritis. *J. Craniomaxillofac. Surg.* **2014**, *42*, 1402–1407. [CrossRef]
70. Hiltunen, K.; Vehkalahti, M.M.; Peltola, J.S.; Ainamo, A. A 5-year follow-up of occlusal status and radiographic findings in mandibular condyles of the elderly. *Int. J. Prosthodont.* **2002**, *15*, 539–543. [PubMed]
71. Gleissner, C.; Kaesser, U.; Dehne, F.; Bolten, W.W.; Willershausen, B. Temporomandibular joint function in patients with longstanding rheumatoid arthritis—I. Role of periodontal status and prosthetic care—A clinical study. *Eur. J. Med. Res.* **2003**, *8*, 98–108.
72. Witulski, S.; Vogl, T.J.; Rehart, S.; Ottl, P. Evaluation of the TMJ by means of clinical TMD examination and MRI diagnostics in patients with rheumatoid arthritis. *Biomed. Res. Int.* **2014**, *328560*. [CrossRef] [PubMed]
73. Capurso, U.; De Michelis, B.; Giaretta Agosti, G.; Lepore, L. Compromissione funzionale dell'apparato masticatorio nell'artrite reumatoide giovanile [Compromised function of the masticatory apparatus in juvenile rheumatoid arthritis]. *Minerva Ortognatod.* **1989**, *7*, 47–52.

74. Capurso, U.; Scutellari, P.N.; Orzincolo, C.; Calura, G. La compromissione dell'articolazione temporo-mandibolare nell'artrite reumatoide [Involvement of the temporomandibular joint in rheumatoid arthritis]. *Radiol. Med.* **1989**, *78*, 299–304.
75. Stoustrup, P.; Herlin, T.; Spiegel, L.; Rahimi, H.; Koos, B.; Pedersen, T.K.; Twilt, M. Temporomandibular joint juvenile arthritis working group. standardizing the clinical orofacial examination in juvenile idiopathic arthritis: An interdisciplinary, consensus-based, short screening protocol. *J. Rheumatol.* **2020**, *47*, 1397–1404. [CrossRef]
76. Stoustrup, P.; Twilt, M.; Spiegel, L.; Kristensen, K.D.; Koos, B.; Pedersen, T.K.; Küseler, A.; Cron, R.Q.; Abramowicz, S.; Verna, C.; et al. EuroTM joint Research Network. Clinical orofacial examination in juvenile idiopathic arthritis: International consensus-based recommendations for monitoring patients in clinical practice and research studies. *J. Rheumatol.* **2017**, *44*, 326–333. [CrossRef]
77. Youssef Mohamed, M.M.; Dahaba, M.M.; Farid, M.M.; Ali Elsayed, A.M. Radiographic changes in TMJ in relation to serology and disease activity in RA patients. *Dentomaxillofac. Radiol.* **2020**, *49*, 20190186. [CrossRef] [PubMed]
78. Koos, B.; Gassling, V.; Bott, S.; Tzaribachev, N.; Godt, A. Pathological changes in the TMJ and the length of the ramus in patients with confirmed juvenile idiopathic arthritis. *J. Craniomaxillofac. Surg.* **2014**, *42*, 1802–1807. [CrossRef]
79. Piancino, M.G.; Cannavale, R.; Dalmasso, P.; Tonni, I.; Filipello, F.; Perillo, L.; Cattalini, M.; Meini, A. Condylar asymmetry in patients with juvenile idiopathic arthritis: Could it be a sign of a possible temporomandibular joints involvement? *Semin. Arthritis Rheum.* **2015**, *45*, 208–213. [CrossRef]
80. Poveda-Roda, R.; Bagan, J.; Carbonell, E.; Margaix, M. Diagnostic validity (sensitivity and specificity) of panoramic X-rays in osteoarthrosis of the temporomandibular joint. *Cranio* **2015**, *33*, 189–194. [CrossRef] [PubMed]
81. Modgil, R.; Arora, K.S.; Sharma, A.; Negi, L.S.; Mohapatra, S.; Pareek, S. TMJ arthritis imaging: Conventional radiograph vs. CT scan—Is CT actually needed? *Curr. Rheumatol. Rev.* **2019**, *15*, 135–140. [CrossRef] [PubMed]
82. Kellenberger, C.J.; Abramowicz, S.; Arvidsson, L.Z.; Kirkhus, E.; Tzaribachev, N.; Larheim, T.A. Recommendations for a standard magnetic resonance imaging protocol of temporomandibular joints in juvenile idiopathic arthritis. *J. Oral Maxillofac. Surg.* **2018**, *76*, 2463–2465. [CrossRef]
83. Lochbühler, N.; Saurenmann, R.K.; Müller, L.; Kellenberger, C.J. Magnetic resonance imaging assessment of temporomandibular Joint Involvement and mandibular growth following corticosteroid injection in juvenile idiopathic arthritis. *J. Rheumatol.* **2015**, *42*, 1514–1522. [CrossRef]
84. Miller, E.; Inarejos Clemente, E.J.; Tzaribachev, N.; Guleria, S.; Tolend, M.; Meyers, A.B.; von Kalle, T.; Stimec, J.; Koos, B.; Appenzeller, S.; et al. Imaging of temporomandibular joint abnormalities in juvenile idiopathic arthritis with a focus on developing a magnetic resonance imaging protocol. *Pediatr. Radiol.* **2018**, *48*, 792–800. [CrossRef] [PubMed]
85. Kellenberger, C.J.; Bucheli, J.; Schroeder-Kohler, S.; Saurenmann, R.K.; Colombo, V.; Ettlin, D.A. Temporomandibular joint magnetic resonance imaging findings in adolescents with anterior disk displacement compared to those with juvenile idiopathic arthritis. *J. Oral Rehabil.* **2019**, *46*, 14–22. [CrossRef]
86. Resnick, C.M.; Vakilian, P.M.; Breen, M.; Zurakowski, D.; Caruso, P.; Henderson, L.; Nigrovic, P.A.; Kaban, L.B.; Peacock, Z.S. Quantifying temporomandibular joint synovitis in children with juvenile idiopathic arthritis. *Arthritis Care Res.* **2016**, *68*, 1795–1802. [CrossRef]
87. Buch, K.; Peacock, Z.S.; Resnick, C.M.; Rothermel, H.; Kaban, L.B.; Caruso, P. Regional differences in temporomandibular joint inflammation in patients with juvenile idiopathic arthritis: A dynamic post-contrast magnetic resonance imaging study. *Int. J. Oral Maxillofac. Surg.* **2020**, *49*, 1210–1216. [CrossRef]
88. Epstein, J.B.; Rea, A.; Chahal, O. The use of bone scintigraphy in temporomandibular joint disorders. *Oral Dis.* **2002**, *8*, 47–53. [CrossRef]
89. Shim, J.S.; Kim, C.; Ryu, J.J.; Choi, S.J. Correlation between TM joint disease and rheumatic diseases detected on bone scintigraphy and clinical factors. *Sci. Rep.* **2020**, *10*, 4547. [CrossRef]
90. Mupparapu, M.; Oak, S.; Chang, Y.C.; Alavi, A. Conventional and functional imaging in the evaluation of temporomandibular joint rheumatoid arthritis: A systematic review. *Quintessence Int.* **2019**, *50*, 742–753. [PubMed]
91. Kang, J.H.; An, Y.S.; Park, S.H.; Song, S.I. Influences of age and sex on the validity of bone scintigraphy for the diagnosis of temporomandibular joint osteoarthritis. *Int. J. Oral Maxillofac. Surg.* **2018**, *47*, 1445–1452. [CrossRef]
92. Müller, L.; Kellenberger, C.J.; Cannizzaro, E.; Ettlin, D.; Schraner, T.; Bolt, I.B.; Peltomäki, T.; Saurenmann, R.K. Early diagnosis of temporomandibular joint involvement in juvenile idiopathic arthritis: A pilot study comparing clinical examination and ultrasound to magnetic resonance imaging. *Rheumatology* **2009**, *48*, 680–685. [CrossRef]
93. Kirkhus, E.; Gunderson, R.B.; Smith, H.J.; Flatø, B.; Hetlevik, S.O.; Larheim, T.A.; Arvidsson, L.Z. Temporomandibular joint involvement in childhood arthritis: Comparison of ultrasonography-assessed capsular width and MRI-assessed synovitis. *Dentomaxillofac. Radiol.* **2016**, *45*, 20160195. [CrossRef] [PubMed]
94. Hechler, B.L.; Phero, J.A.; Van Mater, H.; Matthews, N.S. Ultrasound versus magnetic resonance imaging of the temporomandibular joint in juvenile idiopathic arthritis: A systematic review. *Int. J. Oral Maxillofac. Surg.* **2018**, *47*, 83–89. [CrossRef]
95. Resnick, C.M.; Frid, P.; Norholt, S.E.; Stoustrup, P.; Peacock, Z.S.; Kaban, L.B.; Pedersen, T.K.; Abramowicz, S.; Temporomandibular Joint Juvenile Arthritis (TMJaw) working group. An algorithm for management of dentofacial deformity resulting from juvenile idiopathic arthritis: Results of a multinational consensus conference. *J. Oral Maxillofac. Surg.* **2019**, *77*, 1152.e1–1152.e33. [CrossRef] [PubMed]

96. Isola, G.; Ramaglia, L.; Cordasco, G.; Lucchese, A.; Fiorillo, L.; Matarese, G. The effect of a functional appliance in the management of temporomandibular joint disorders in patients with juvenile idiopathic arthritis. *Minerva Stomatol.* **2017**, *66*, 1–8. [PubMed]
97. Stoustrup, P.; Küseler, A.; Kristensen, K.D.; Herlin, T.; Pedersen, T.K. Orthopaedic splint treatment can reduce mandibular asymmetry caused by unilateral temporomandibular involvement in juvenile idiopathic arthritis. *Eur. J. Orthod.* **2013**, *35*, 191–198. [CrossRef] [PubMed]
98. Tegelberg, A.; Kopp, S. Short-term effect of physical training on temporomandibular joint disorder in individuals with rheumatoid arthritis and ankylosing spondylitis. *Acta Odontol. Scand.* **1988**, *46*, 49–56. [CrossRef]
99. Tegelberg, A.; Kopp, S. A 3-year follow-up of temporomandibular disorders in rheumatoid arthritis and ankylosing spondylitis. *Acta Odontol. Scand.* **1996**, *54*, 14–18. [CrossRef]
100. Adiels, A.M.; Helkimo, M.; Magnusson, T. Tactile stimulation as a complementary treatment of temporomandibular disorders in patients with fibromyalgia syndrome. A pilot study. *Swed. Dent. J.* **2005**, *29*, 17–25. [PubMed]
101. Khozeimeh, F.; Moghareabed, A.; Allameh, M.; Baradaran, S. Comparative evaluation of low-level laser and systemic steroid therapy in adjuvant-enhanced arthritis of rat temporomandibular joint: A histological study. *Dent. Res. J.* **2015**, *12*, 215–223.
102. Shoohanizad, E.; Garajei, A.; Enamzadeh, R.; Yari, A. Nonsurgical management of temporomandibular joint autoimmune disorders. *AIMS Public Health* **2019**, *6*, 554–567. [CrossRef]
103. Puricelli, E.; Corsetti, A.; Tavares, J.G.; Luchi, G.H. Clinical-surgical treatment of temporomandibular joint disorder in a psoriatic arthritis patient. *Head Face Med.* **2013**, *9*, 11. [CrossRef]
104. List, T.; Axelsson, S. Management of TMD: Evidence from systematic reviews and meta-analyses. *J. Oral Rehabil.* **2010**, *37*, 430–451. [CrossRef] [PubMed]
105. Koh, H.; Robinson, P.G. Occlusal adjustment for treating and preventing temporomandibular joint disorders. *Cochrane Database Syst. Rev.* **2003**, *31*. [CrossRef]
106. Kuroda, S.; Kuroda, Y.; Tomita, Y.; Tanaka, E. Long-term stability of conservative orthodontic treatment in a patient with rheumatoid arthritis and severe condylar resorption. *Am. J. Orthod. Dentofac. Orthop.* **2012**, *141*, 352–362. [CrossRef]
107. Ferri, J.; Potier, J.; Maes, J.M.; Rakotomalala, H.; Lauwers, L.; Cotelle, M.; Nicot, R. Temporomandibular joint arthritis: Clinical, orthodontic, orthopaedic and surgical approaches. *Int. Orthod.* **2018**, *16*, 545–561. [CrossRef] [PubMed]
108. Leibur, E.; Jagur, O.; Voog-Oras, Ü. Temporomandibular joint arthrocentesis for the treatment of osteoarthritis. *Stomatologija* **2015**, *17*, 113–117. [PubMed]
109. Nitzan, D.W.; Price, A. The use of arthrocentesis for the treatment of osteoarthritic temporomandibular joints. *J. Oral Maxillofac. Surg.* **2001**, *59*, 1154–1159. [CrossRef] [PubMed]
110. Gynther, G.W.; Holmlund, A.B. Efficacy of arthroscopic lysis and lavage in patients with temporomandibular joint symptoms associated with generalized osteoarthritis or rheumatoid arthritis. *J. Oral Maxillofac. Surg.* **1998**, *56*, 147–151. [CrossRef]
111. Trieger, N.; Hoffman, C.H.; Rodriguez, E. The effect of arthrocentesis of the temporomandibular joint in patients with rheumatoid arthritis. *J. Oral Maxillofac. Surg.* **1999**, *57*, 537–540. [CrossRef]
112. Antonarakis, G.S.; Courvoisier, D.S.; Hanquinet, S.; Dhouib, A.; Carlomagno, R.; Hofer, M.; Scolozzi, P. Benefit of temporomandibular joint lavage with intra-articular steroids versus lavage alone in the management of temporomandibular joint involvement in juvenile idiopathic arthritis. *J. Oral Maxillofac. Surg.* **2018**, *76*, 1200–1206. [CrossRef]
113. Vallon, D.; Akerman, S.; Nilner, M.; Petersson, A. Long-term follow-up of intra-articular injections into the temporomandibular joint in patients with rheumatoid arthritis. *Swed. Dent. J.* **2002**, *26*, 149–158.
114. Ringold, S.; Thapa, M.; Shaw, E.A.; Wallace, C.A. Heterotopic ossification of the temporomandibular joint in juvenile idiopathic arthritis. *J. Rheumatol.* **2011**, *38*, 1423–1428. [CrossRef]
115. Stoll, M.L.; Amin, D.; Powell, K.K.; Poholek, C.H.; Strait, R.H.; Aban, I.; Beukelman, T.; Young, D.W.; Cron, R.Q.; Waite, P.D. Risk Factors for Intraarticular Heterotopic Bone Formation in the Temporomandibular Joint in Juvenile Idiopathic Arthritis. *J. Rheumatol.* **2018**, *45*, 1301–1307. [CrossRef]
116. O'Connor, R.C.; Fawthrop, F.; Salha, R.; Sidebottom, A.J. Management of the temporomandibular joint in inflammatory arthritis: Involvement of surgical procedures. *Eur. J. Rheumatol.* **2017**, *4*, 151–156. [CrossRef] [PubMed]
117. Kopp, S.; Akerman, S.; Nilner, M. Short-term effects of intra-articular sodium hyaluronate, glucocorticoid, and saline injections on rheumatoid arthritis of the temporomandibular joint. *J. Craniomandib. Disord.* **1991**, *5*, 231–238. [PubMed]
118. Alstergren, P.; Larsson, P.T.; Kopp, S. Successful treatment with multiple intra-articular injections of infliximab in a patient with psoriatic arthritis. *Scand. J. Rheumatol.* **2008**, *37*, 155–157. [CrossRef] [PubMed]
119. Stoll, M.L.; Morlandt, A.B.; Teerawattanapong, S.; Young, D.; Waite, P.D.; Cron, R.Q. Safety and efficacy of intra-articular infliximab therapy for treatment-resistant temporomandibular joint arthritis in children: A retrospective study. *Rheumatology* **2013**, *52*, 554–559. [CrossRef] [PubMed]
120. Stoll, M.L.; Vaid, Y.N.; Guleria, S.; Beukelman, T.; Waite, P.D.; Cron, R.Q. Magnetic resonance imaging findings following intraarticular infliximab therapy for refractory temporomandibular joint arthritis among children with juvenile idiopathic arthritis. *J. Rheumatol.* **2015**, *42*, 2155–2159. [CrossRef] [PubMed]
121. Kristensen, K.D.; Stoustrup, P.; Küseler, A.; Pedersen, T.K.; Nyengaard, J.R.; Hauge, E.; Herlin, T. Intra-articular vs. systemic administration of etanercept in antigen-induced arthritis in the temporomandibular point. Part I: Histological effects. *Pediatr. Rheumatol. Online J.* **2009**, *7*, 5. [CrossRef] [PubMed]

122. Sperry, M.M.; Yu, Y.H.; Kartha, S.; Ghimire, P.; Welch, R.L.; Winkelstein, B.A.; Granquist, E.J. Intra-articular etanercept attenuates pain and hypoxia from TMJ loading in the rat. *J. Orthop. Res.* **2020**, *38*, 1316–1326. [CrossRef]
123. Bjørnland, T.; Larheim, T.A. Synovectomy and diskectomy of the temporomandibular joint in patients with chronic arthritic disease compared with diskectomies in patients with internal derangement. A 3-year follow-up study. *Eur. J. Oral Sci.* **1995**, *103*, 2–7. [CrossRef]
124. Bjornland, T.; Larheim, T.A.; Haanaes, H.R. Surgical treatment of temporomandibular joints in patients with chronic arthritic disease: Preoperative findings and one-year follow-up. *Cranio* **1992**, *10*, 205–210. [CrossRef]
125. Leshem, D.; Tompson, B.; Britto, J.A.; Forrest, C.R.; Phillips, J.H. Orthognathic surgery in juvenile rheumatoid arthritis patients. *Plast. Reconstr. Surg.* **2006**, *117*, 1941–1946. [CrossRef]
126. Pagnoni, M.; Amodeo, G.; Fadda, M.T.; Brauner, E.; Guarino, G.; Virciglio, P.; Iannetti, G. Juvenile idiopathic/rheumatoid arthritis and orthognathic surgery without mandibular osteotomies in the remittent phase. *J. Craniofac. Surg.* **2013**, *24*, 1940–1945. [CrossRef] [PubMed]
127. Oye, F.; Bjørnland, T.; Støre, G. Mandibular osteotomies in patients with juvenile rheumatoid arthritic disease. *Scand. J. Rheumatol.* **2003**, *32*, 168–173. [CrossRef] [PubMed]
128. Thaller, S.R.; Cavina, C.; Kawamoto, H.K. Treatment of orthognathic problems related to scleroderma. *Ann. Plast. Surg.* **1990**, *24*, 528–533. [CrossRef] [PubMed]
129. Mercuri, L.G.; Handelman, C.S. Idiopathic condylar resorption: What should we do? *Oral Maxillofac. Surg. Clin. N. Am.* **2020**, *32*, 105–116. [CrossRef]
130. Nørholt, S.E.; Pedersen, T.K.; Herlin, T. Functional changes following distraction osteogenesis treatment of asymmetric mandibular growth deviation in unilateral juvenile idiopathic arthritis: A prospective study with long-term follow-up. *Int. J. Oral Maxillofac. Surg.* **2013**, *42*, 329–336. [CrossRef] [PubMed]
131. Mackool, R.L.; Shetye, P.; Grayson, B.; McCarthy, J.G. Distraction osteogenesis in a patient with juvenile arthritis. *J. Craniofac. Surg.* **2006**, *17*, 387–390. [CrossRef] [PubMed]
132. Ferguson, J.W.; Luyk, N.H.; Parr, N.C. A potential role for costo-chondral grafting in adults with mandibular condylar destruction secondary to rheumatoid arthritis—A case report. *J. Craniomaxillofac. Surg.* **1993**, *21*, 15–18. [CrossRef]
133. MacIntosh, R.B.; Shivapuja, P.K.; Naqvi, R. Scleroderma and the temporomandibular joint: Reconstruction in 2 variants. *J. Oral Maxillofac. Surg.* **2015**, *73*, 1199–1210. [CrossRef]
134. Felix, V.B.; Cabral, D.R.; de Almeida, A.B.; Soares, E.D.; de Moraes Fernandes, K.J. Ankylosis of the temporomandibular joint and reconstruction with a costochondral graft in a patient with juvenile idiopathic arthritis. *J. Craniofac. Surg.* **2017**, *28*, 203–206. [CrossRef]
135. Keyser, B.R.; Banda, A.K.; Mercuri, L.G.; Warburton, G.; Sullivan, S.M. Alloplastic total temporomandibular joint replacement in skeletally immature patients: A pilot survey. *Int. J. Oral Maxillofac. Surg.* **2020**, *49*, 1202–1209. [CrossRef]
136. Sidebottom, A.J. UK TMJ replacement surgeons; British Association of Oral and Maxillofacial Surgeons. Guidelines for the replacement of temporomandibular joints in the United Kingdom. *Br. J. Oral Maxillofac. Surg.* **2008**, *46*, 146–147. [CrossRef] [PubMed]
137. Mehra, P.; Henry, C.H.; Giglou, K.R. Temporomandibular joint reconstruction in patients with autoimmune/connective tissue disease. *J. Oral Maxillofac. Surg.* **2018**, *76*, 1660–1664. [CrossRef] [PubMed]
138. Mehra, P.; Wolford, L.M.; Baran, S.; Cassano, D.S. Single-stage comprehensive surgical treatment of the rheumatoid arthritis temporomandibular joint patient. *J. Oral Maxillofac. Surg.* **2009**, *67*, 1859–1872. [CrossRef] [PubMed]
139. Hechler, B.L.; Matthews, N.S. Role of alloplastic reconstruction of the temporomandibular joint in the juvenile idiopathic arthritis population. *Br. J. Oral Maxillofac. Surg.* **2021**, *59*, 21–27. [CrossRef] [PubMed]
140. Brown, Z.; Rushing, D.C.; Perez, D.E. Alloplastic temporomandibular joint reconstruction for patients with juvenile idiopathic arthritis. *J. Oral Maxillofac. Surg.* **2020**, *78*, 1492–1498. [CrossRef] [PubMed]
141. Mishima, K.; Yamada, T.; Sugahara, T. Evaluation of respiratory status and mandibular movement after total temporomandibular joint replacement in patients with rheumatoid arthritis. *Int. J. Oral Maxillofac. Surg.* **2003**, *32*, 275–279. [CrossRef] [PubMed]
142. Saeed, N.R.; McLeod, N.M.; Hensher, R. Temporomandibular joint replacement in rheumatoid-induced disease. *Br. J. Oral Maxillofac. Surg.* **2001**, *39*, 71–75. [CrossRef]
143. O'Connor, R.C.; Saleem, S.; Sidebottom, A.J. Prospective outcome analysis of total replacement of the temporomandibular joint with the TMJ Concepts system in patients with inflammatory arthritic diseases. *Br. J. Oral Maxillofac. Surg.* **2016**, *54*, 604–609. [CrossRef]
144. Felstead, A.M.; Revington, P.J. Surgical management of temporomandibular joint ankylosis in ankylosing spondylitis. *Int. J. Rheumatol.* **2011**, 854167. [CrossRef] [PubMed]
145. Manemi, R.V.; Fasanmade, A.; Revington, P.J. Bilateral ankylosis of the jaw treated with total alloplastic replacement using the TMJ concepts system in a patient with ankylosing spondylitis. *Br. J. Oral Maxillofac. Surg.* **2009**, *47*, 159–161. [CrossRef] [PubMed]

146. Balon, P.; Vesnaver, A.; Kansky, A.; Kočar, M.; Prodnik, L. Treatment of end stage temporomandibular joint disorder using a temporomandibular joint total prosthesis: The Slovenian experience. *J. Craniomaxillofac. Surg.* **2019**, *47*, 60–65. [CrossRef]
147. Lypka, M.; Shah, K.; Jones, J. Prosthetic temporomandibular joint reconstruction in a cohort of adolescent females with juvenile idiopathic arthritis. *Pediatr. Rheumatol. Online J.* **2020**, *18*, 68. [CrossRef]
148. Goodman, S.M.; Springer, B.; Guyatt, G.; Abdel, M.P.; Dasa, V.; George, M.; Gewurz-Singer, O.; Giles, J.T.; Johnson, B.; Lee, S.; et al. 2017 American College of Rheumatology/American Association of Hip and Knee Surgeons guideline for the perioperative management of antirheumatic medication in patients with rheumatic diseases undergoing elective total hip or total knee arthroplasty. *J. Arthroplast.* **2017**, *32*, 2628–2638. [CrossRef] [PubMed]

MDPI
St. Alban-Anlage 66
4052 Basel
Switzerland
Tel. +41 61 683 77 34
Fax +41 61 302 89 18
www.mdpi.com

Diagnostics Editorial Office
E-mail: diagnostics@mdpi.com
www.mdpi.com/journal/diagnostics

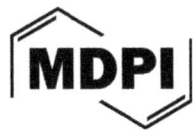

www.ingramcontent.com/pod-product-compliance
Lightning Source LLC
LaVergne TN
LVHW070358100526
838202LV00014B/1340